The
Renal Biopsy

VIRGINIA A. LIVOLSI, MD
Series Editor

Published

Forthcoming

MPP

8

GARY STRIKER, MD
Director, Division of Kidney,
Urologic, and Hematologic Diseases
National Institutes of Health
Bethesda, Maryland

LILIANE J. STRIKER, MD
Chief, Renal Cell Biology Section
National Institutes of Health
Bethesda, Maryland

VIVETTE D'AGATI, MD
Professor of Pathology
Director, Renal Pathology Laboratory
Columbia University
College of Physicians and Surgeons
New York, New York

The Renal Biopsy

MAJOR PROBLEMS IN PATHOLOGY

third edition

W.B. SAUNDERS COMPANY
A Division of Harcourt Brace & Company
PHILADELPHIA LONDON TORONTO MONTREAL SYDNEY TOKYO

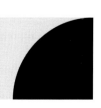

W.B. SAUNDERS COMPANY
A Division of Harcourt Brace & Company

The Curtis Center
Independence Square West
Philadelphia, Pennsylvania 19106

Library of Congress Cataloging-in-Publication Data

The renal biopsy / Gary Striker, Liliane J. Striker, Vivette D'Agati. — 3rd ed.

p.   cm. — (Major problems in pathology; v. 8)

Liliane Striker's name appears first on the second edition.
Includes bibliographical references and index.

ISBN 0–7216–6412–1

1. Kidneys—Needle biopsy.   2. Kidneys—Diseases—Diagnosis.
   I. Striker, Liliane J.   II. D'Agati, Vivette.   III. Title.   IV. Series.
   [DNLM: 1. Kidney Diseases—diagnosis.   2. Biopsy—methods.
   3. Kidney—pathology.   W1 MA492X v. 8 1997 / WJ 302 S917u 1997]

RC904.S75 1997   616.6′ 10758—dc20

DNLM/DLC   96–28905

THE RENAL BIOPSY, Third Edition   ISBN 0–7216–6412–1

Printed in the United States of America.

Last digit is the print number: 9   8   7   6   5   4   3   2   1

Preface

The approach used in this text is intended to be very practical, that is, to provide a guide to the interpretation of renal biopsies. The assumption is made that the reader is primarily interested in this text to aid in the interpretation of renal biopsies, rather than seeking a reference text on renal diseases. A number of splendid clinical and pathologic anatomy texts are available that meet the latter needs, and only those aspects of renal disease that are pertinent to renal biopsy interpretation are included herein. Similarly, the references found at the end of each section are representative rather than inclusive. We have deliberately chosen to restrict the number of references; instead we have provided a list of more comprehensive reference texts of renal diseases below.

Although we have elected to use the diagrams and many illustrations from the previous editions, the focus, format, and text have been completely redirected.

The patient population from which we have drawn our experience reflects that of Western Europe (Hôpital Tenon, Dr. Liliane Morel-Maroger Striker), the Atlantic Seaboard (Columbia University, Dr. Vivette D'Agati), and the Pacific Northwest (University of Washington, Dr. Gary Striker). The age range of the patients is similarly broad, extending from infants to the elderly. Finally, the breadth of our experience encompasses nearly 20,000 renal biopsies over a period of almost 30 years. There is no particular geographic focus, but few tropical diseases are covered in this text.

The wise consultation and advice of many clinicians and pathologists in guiding and shaping our approaches to renal biopsy interpretation are gratefully acknowledged. It is possible to mention but a few: Drs. G. Richet and J. P. Mery (Paris), Drs. C. L. Pirani and G. Appel (New York), and Dr. W. C. Couser (Washington).

REFERENCE TEXTS

Royer P, Habib R, Mathieu H, Broyer M: Pediatric Nephrology. Philadelphia, W.B. Saunders Co., 1974.

Churg J, Sobin LH, et al. (eds): Renal Disease: Classification and Atlas of Glomerular Diseases. Tokyo, Igaku-shoin, 1980.

Spargo BH, Seymour AE, Ordóñez NG: Renal Biopsy Pathology with Diagnostic and Therapeutic Implications. New York, John Wiley and Sons, 1980.

Cameron JS, Glassock RJ (eds): The Nephrotic Syndrome. New York, M. Dekker, 1988.

Cameron JS, Davison AS, Grunfeld JP, Kerr D, Ritz E (eds): Oxford Textbook of Clinical Nephrology. Oxford, Oxford University Press, 1992.

Heptinstall RH: Pathology of the Kidney. Boston, Little, Brown & Co., 1992.

Grishman E, Churg J, Needle MA, Venkataseshan VS (eds): The Kidney in Collagen-Vascular Diseases. New York, Raven Press, 1993.

Tisher CC, Brenner BM (eds): Renal Pathology with Clinical and Functional Correlations. Philadelphia, JB Lippincott, 1994.

Massry SG, Glassock RJ (eds): Textbook of Nephrology. Baltimore, Williams & Wilkins, 1995.

Jacobson HR, Striker GE, Klahr S (eds): The Principles and Practice of Nephrology. St. Louis, Mosby–Year Book, 1995.

Silva F, D'Agati VD, Nadasdy T (eds): Renal Biopsy Interpretation. Churchill Livingstone, New York, 1996.

Droz D, Lantz B (eds): La Biopsie Renale. Paris, Editions INSERM, 1996.

Contents

1

ROLE OF THE RENAL BIOPSY IN THE EVALUATION OF RENAL DISEASE

A renal biopsy provides one of the few objective measurements of the type, nature, site, extent, and state of evolution of renal diseases. As pointed out by Conrad Pirani, a renal biopsy cannot substitute for a comprehensive clinical and laboratory investigation; rather, these approaches are complementary. Further, it is rarely a good practice that the same person be responsible for both the clinical and pathologic aspects of the patient workup. As in the clinical workup, it is critical that a single pathologist be responsible for the interpretation and integration of the renal biopsy findings, i.e., the light, immunofluorescence, electron microscopic, and morphometric data.

Our current ability to interpret and understand the changes revealed at biopsy continues to evolve, based on both basic research and clinical studies. Indeed, many techniques that have previously been restricted to the research laboratory can now be applied to the renal biopsy by the inventive, insightful pathologist. The purpose of this chapter is to provide a practical approach to renal biopsy using currently available methods and to explore the questions that can now be addressed by means of renal biopsy.

The single purpose of the diagnosis must be kept in mind—that is, to provide sufficient accurate information on which to base an approach to both a treatment plan and prognosis. Thus, it is no longer justified to examine a renal biopsy specimen by other than the most modern and sophisticated methods available to modern pathologists. These include, at the very minimum, detailed light and immunofluorescence microscopic studies using various stains or probes for immune reactants and other native or foreign proteins indicated by the particular clinical and laboratory picture. Electron microscopic evaluation of a sufficient sample of the various compartments is required in certain categories of disease and provides information of interest in most renal biopsies. Finally, the value of glomerular morphometry has become clearer in the detection and delineation of glomerular diseases. Only after this type of study can one render an opinion that does justice to the patient, to the clinician, and to the tissue obtained at considerable expense and a certain amount of risk.

Accurate interpretation requires detailed knowledge of the structure and function of a normal kidney, from infancy to adulthood. In addition, it is necessary to have an appreciation of the general responses of tissues to injury and those that are particular to the individual regions of the kidney. Finally, each compartment must be assessed separately and in the most quantitative manner available for the observations at hand.

The basic features that can be assessed are shown in Figures 1–1 to 1–34.

Text continued on page 35

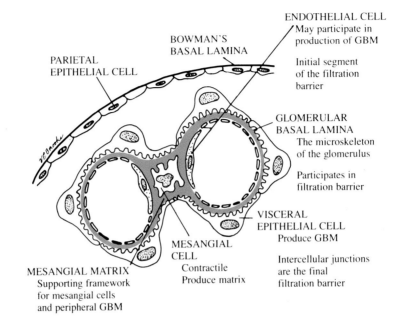

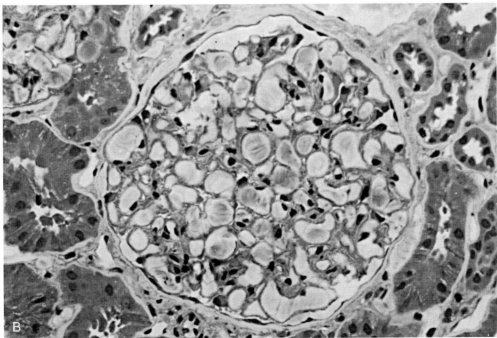

Figure 1–1. Normal glomerulus. *A*, Diagram. *B*, Hematoxylin and eosin stain (H&E), ×300.

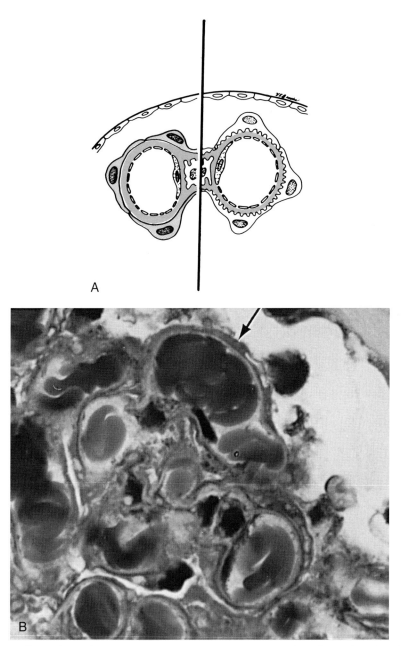

A

B

Figure 1–2. Epithelial cellular change, podocyte spreading. *A,* Diagram of a glomerular visceral epithelial cell, cytoplasmic spreading. *B,* **Minimal change disease.** High-power light micrograph of a methacrylate-embedded specimen. Podocyte swelling and spreading can be seen over most of the peripheral glomerular basement membranes *(arrow).* (H&E, ×1000.)

Illustration continued on following page

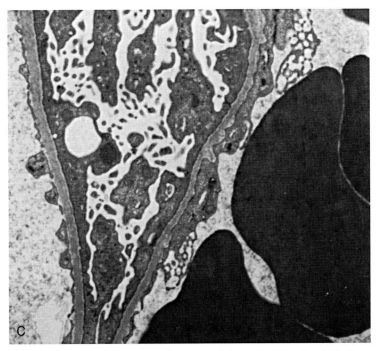

Figure 1–2 *Continued C,* Two adjacent loops show effacement of the epithelial cells, which form a nearly continuous sheet of cytoplasm. The basement membrane and the endothelial cell cytoplasm are not affected. (Electron micrograph, ×5000.)

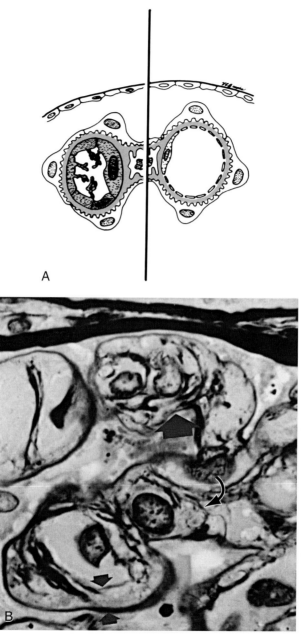

Figure 1–3. Endothelial cell change, swelling. *A*, Diagram of endothelial cell injury, manifested by swelling, surface irregularities, and hypercellularity. *B*, **Toxemia of pregnancy.** At higher power, the widened subendothelial spaces are clearly visible *(small arrows)*. The luminal aspect of the endothelial cell cytoplasm *(curved arrow)* is widely separated from the glomerular basement membrane by deposits *(large arrow)*. (Periodic acid–silver methenamine [PASM], ×1200.)

Illustration continued on following page

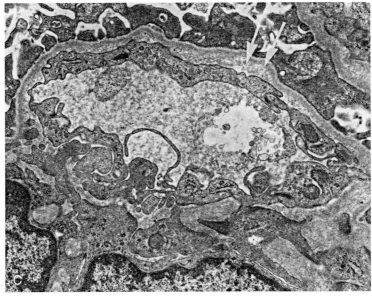

Figure 1–3 *Continued C,* At higher power, the widened subendothelial spaces are clearly visible. The luminal aspect of the endothelial cell cytoplasm *(double arrows)* is widely separated from the glomerular basement membrane by deposits *(light arrows).* (Electron micrograph, ×2000.)

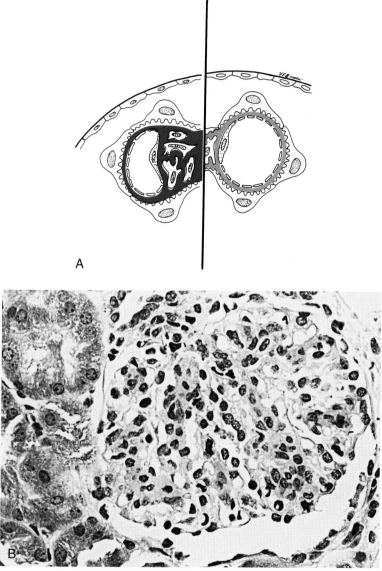

Figure 1–4. Hypercellularity, mesangial. *A,* Diagram of mesangial cell hypercellularity. Note that although this diagram depicts hypercellularity limited to the mesangium, it is often impossible to differentiate mesangial cells from endothelial cells. *B,* There is a marked, global increase in the number of mesangial cells. The mesangial matrix, tuft lumina, and basement membranes are not affected. (H&E, ×500.)

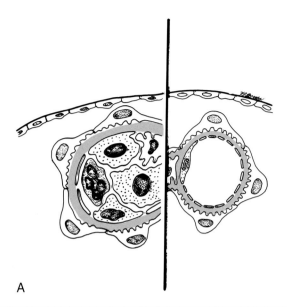

A

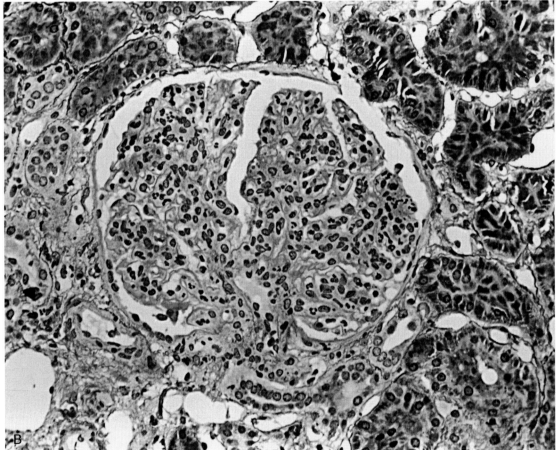

B

Figure 1–5. Hypercellularity, inflammation. *A,* Diagram of inflammatory cell infiltration by neutrophils and macrophages, accompanied by proliferation of resident glomerular cells. *B,* **Acute poststreptococcal glomerulonephritis.** The vascular spaces are occluded by intracapillary proliferation and infiltrating polymorphonuclear leukocytes. (H&E, ×500.)

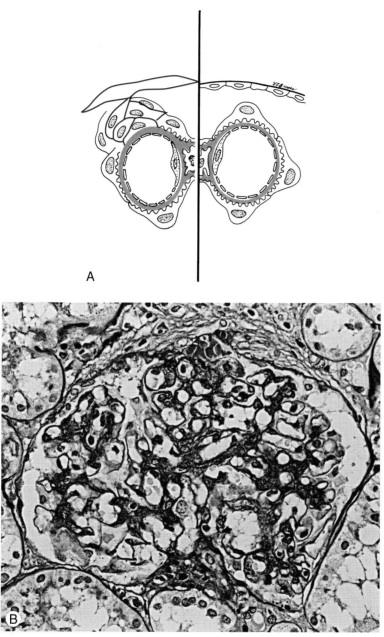

Figure 1–6. Hypercellularity, epithelial, synechia. *A,* Diagram of segmental epithelial cell proliferation, resulting in the formation of a synechia. *B,* **Focal segmental glomerulosclerosis in a patient with IgA nephropathy.** There is an area of hyalinosis with an adjacent synechia. Bowman's capsular basement membrane is multilaminated in the area of the synechia. The adjacent loops appear unremarkable. (PAS, ×630.)

Illustration continued on following page

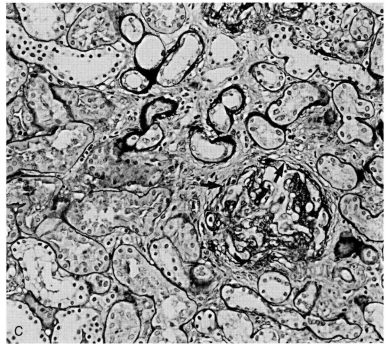

Figure 1–6 *Continued C*, **Hypercellularity, epithelial, synechia (organized). IgA nephropathy, severe chronic lesion.** There is severe mesangial sclerosis with partial disorganization of the tuft architecture and a large organized synechia *(arrows)*. (PAS, ×200.)

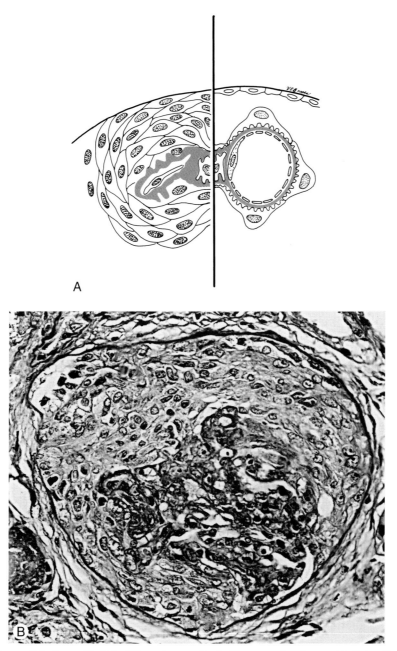

A

B

Figure 1–7. Hypercellularity, epithelial, diffuse (crescent). *A,* Diagram of diffuse epithelial cell proliferation. *B,* **Crescentic glomerulonephritis.** There is diffuse proliferation of glomerular epithelial cells, which completely occupy the urinary space. The underlying glomerular tuft is compressed and collapsed. (PASM, ×400.)

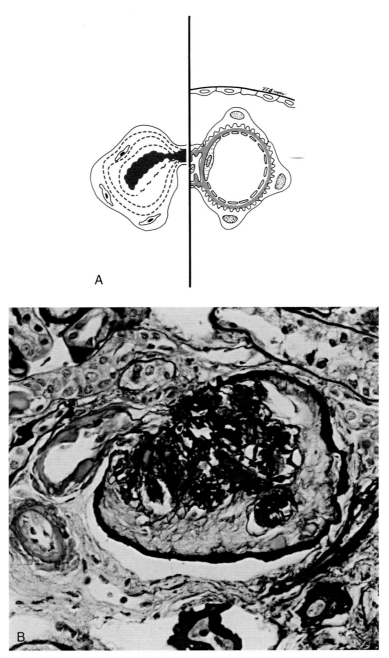

A

Figure 1–8. Sclerosis, obsolescence. *A,* Diagram of a fibrotic, shrunken (i.e., obsolescent) glomerulus. *B,* Organization of the crescent results in complete fibrosis (i.e., obsolescent glomerulus). Fragments of Bowman's capsule can still be recognized but the capsule has been interrupted over most of its perimeter. (PASM, ×150.)

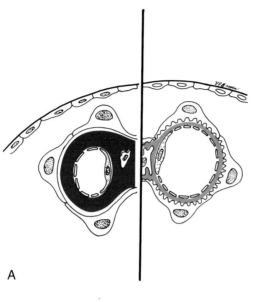

A

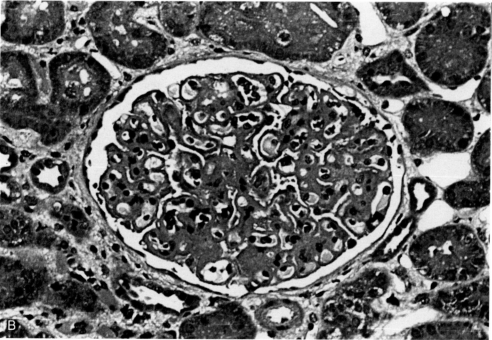

Figure 1–9. Glomerular basement membrane, thickening. *A,* Diagram of diffuse thickening of the glomerular basement membrane and an increase in the amount of the mesangial matrix. *B,* **Membranous nephropathy, Stage 2.** The major histologic change is diffuse thickening of the basement membranes, which gives the impression that the membranes are ''stiff.'' Silver staining is necessary to reveal the spikes and deposits. (H&E, ×300.)

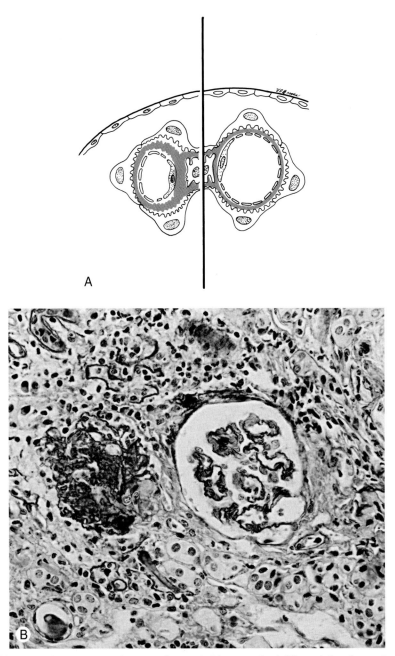

Figure 1–10. **Glomerular basement membrane, collapse.** *A,* Diagram of wrinkling of the glomerular basement membrane. This change is most marked near the mesangial region and results in narrowing of the lumen. *B,* **Benign nephrosclerosis.** Wrinkling, retraction, and collapse of the loops with loss of lumen. Interstitial fibrosis and focal tubular atrophy are present. (PASM, ×180.)

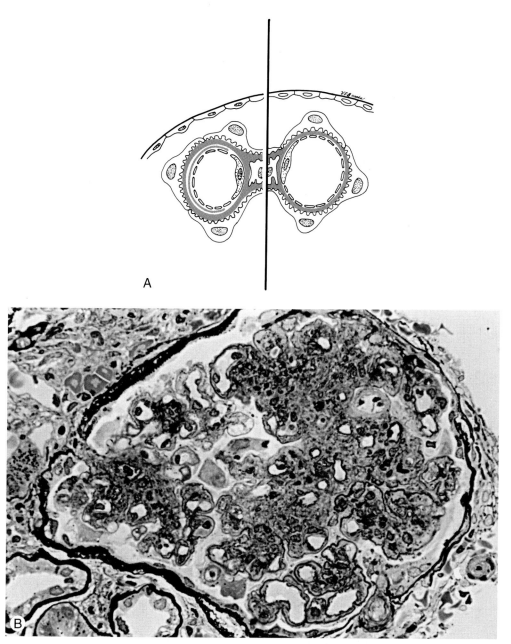

Figure 1–11. Glomerular basement membrane, duplication. *A,* Diagram of the formation of a second layer of basement membrane in the subendothelial space. *B,* **Membranoproliferative glomerulonephritis Type I.** The architecture of the glomerulus is distorted by the large masses of mesangial matrix, giving it a lobular appearance. There are widespread "double-contoured" basement membranes, the so-called "tram tracks." (PASM, ×400.)

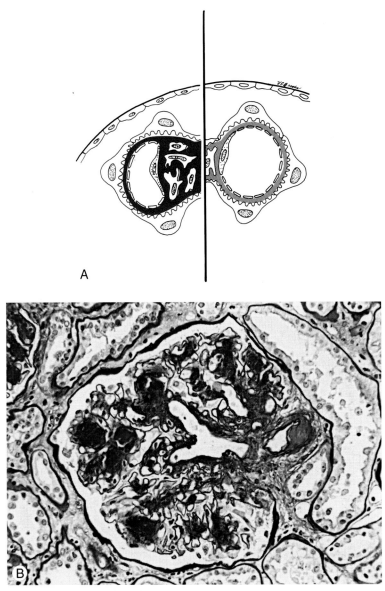

Figure 1–12. Mesangial matrix, sclerosis. *A,* Diagram of mesangial sclerosis. Note that the sclerosis is frequently preceded by mesangial hypercellularity. *B,* **Diabetic nephropathy.** There is diffuse mesangial hypercellularity and mesangial sclerosis. The basement membranes of the glomerulus, Bowman's capsule, and the tubules are thickened. A large arteriolar hyalin deposit is noted at the hilum. (PAS, ×300.)

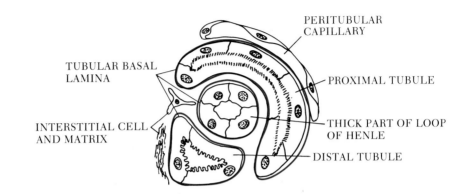

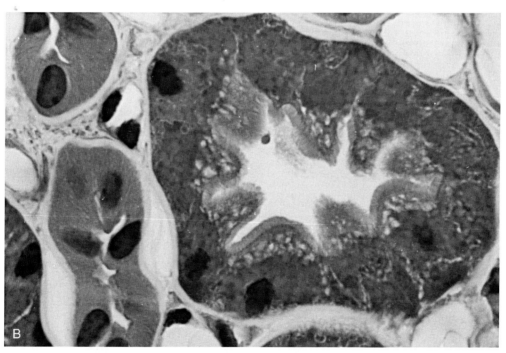

Figure 1–13. Normal tubules and interstitium. *A,* Diagram of the tubulointerstitial compartment. *B,* The morphology of the tubules and interstitium is well preserved in this methacrylate-embedded specimen. (H&E, ×1200.)

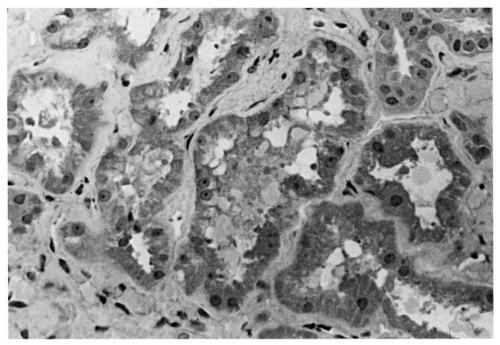

Figure 1–14. Tubules, cell injury. Acute tubular necrosis. The proximal tubular epithelium shows changes varying from vacuolation to frank necrosis. (H&E, ×300.)

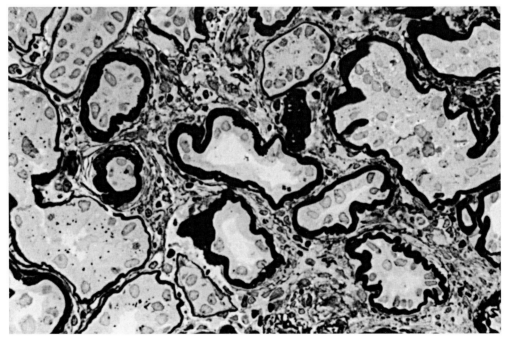

Figure 1–15. Tubules, basement membrane thickening. Diabetic nephropathy. The tubular basement membranes are thickened, especially in the areas of interstitial fibrosis. The interstitium contains an increased amount of connective tissue and scattered inflammatory cells. (Jones methenamine silver, ×300.)

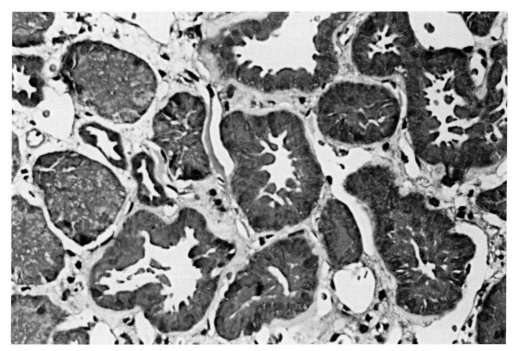

Figure 1–16. Interstitium, edema. Acute tubular necrosis, early. The interstitial spaces are filled with fluid, separating capillaries from the tubules. (Masson's trichrome, ×300.)

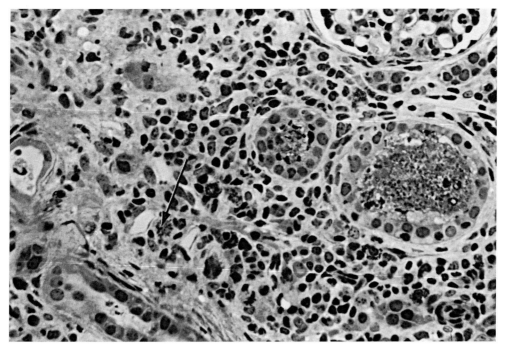

Figure 1–17. Interstitium, inflammation. Acute interstitial nephritis, nonsteroidal anti-inflammatory drugs. The intense interstitial infiltrate and edema are associated with interrupted (breaks) tubular basement membranes *(arrow)*. There is also tubulitis. (PAS, ×400.)

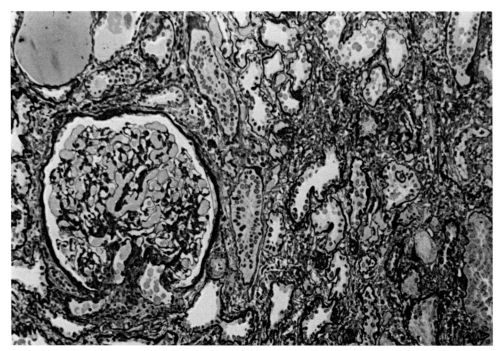

Figure 1–18. Interstitium, fibrosis. Chronic interstitial nephritis, analgesic abuse. The tubules show irregular atrophy, low-lying epithelium, and thickened basement membranes. The interstitium is increased in amount, in an irregular fashion. The glomerulus is relatively normal. (PASM, ×250.)

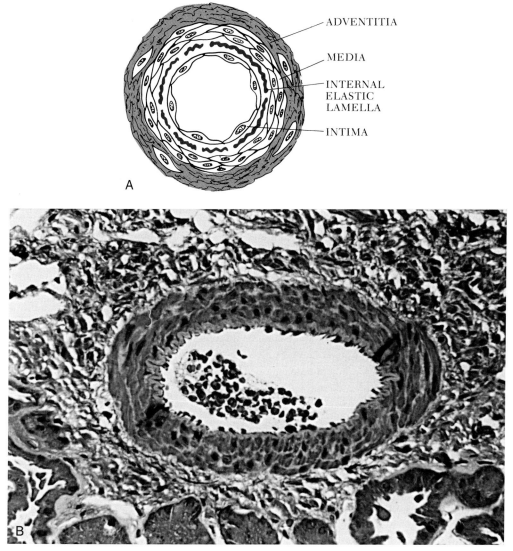

Figure 1–19. Artery, normal. *A,* Diagram of a normal artery. *B,* Normal artery in a methacrylate-embedded specimen. (H&E, ×300.)

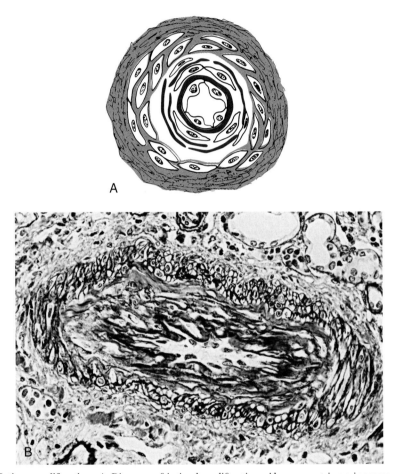

Figure 1–20. Intima, proliferation. *A*, Diagram of intimal proliferation. Also present is an increase in the amount of extracellular matrix. *B*, **Arteriosclerosis.** The multiple lamellae (duplication) in the subintima are visible in this silver-stained preparation. The endothelium is prominent. (PASM, ×300.)

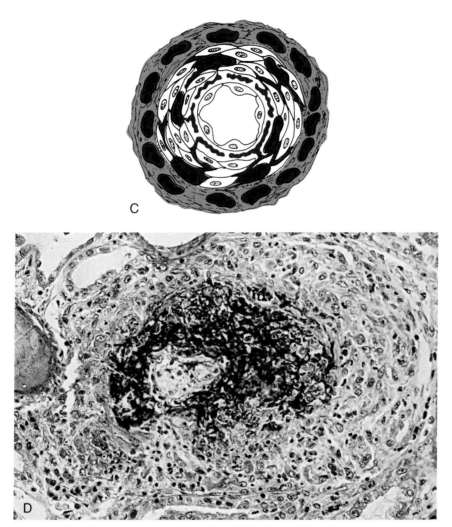

Figure 1–20 *Continued C,* **Intima, inflammatory cell infiltrate.** Diagram of infiltration of the vascular wall with inflammatory cells. *D,* **Polyarteritis nodosa.** The wall of this small artery is destroyed by a dense, circumferential inflammatory cell infiltrate with fibrinoid necrosis of the intima. (Phosphotungstic acid hematoxylin, ×250.)

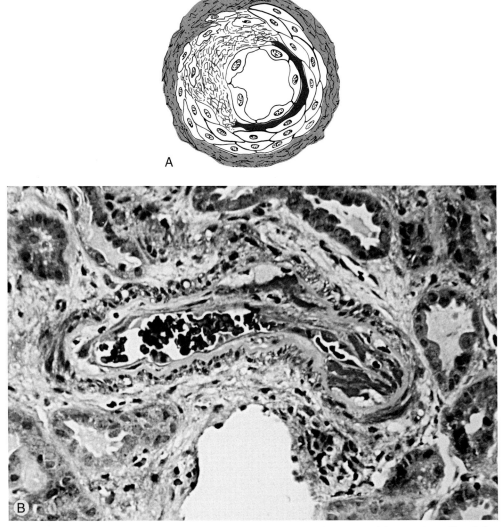

Figure 1–21. Intima, fibrin deposits. Polyarteritis nodosa. *A,* Diagram of disruption of the vascular wall and deposition of fibrin in the damaged area. *B,* Deposits of fibrin/fibrinogen lie in the areas of necrosis seen by light microscopy. (Masson's trichrome, ×250.)

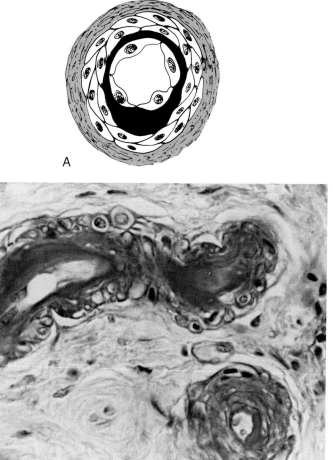

A

B

Figure 1–22. Intima, hyalin deposits. *A*, Diagram of a large hyalin deposit in the subintima. *B*, **Diabetic nephropathy.** The wall of one arteriole contains massive hyalin deposits. (PAS, ×400.)

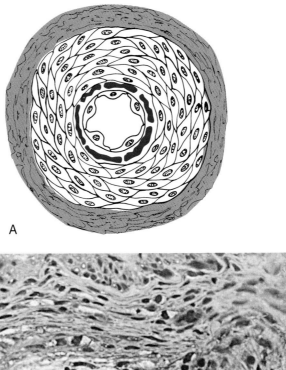

A

B

Figure 1–23. Media, hypercellularity. *A,* Diagram of marked medial hypercellularity. *B,* The medial layer of this artery is widened and contains an increased number of smooth muscle cell nuclei. (Masson's trichrome, ×150.)

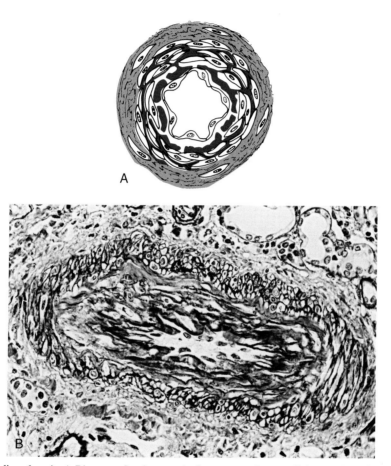

Figure 1–24. Media, sclerosis. *A*, Diagram of an increase in the amount of extracellular matrix in the media of an artery. *B*, **Arteriosclerosis.** The multiple lamellae (duplication) in the subintima are visible in this silver-stained preparation. Note the thickened basement membrane surrounding each smooth muscle cell in the media. Compare to Figure 1–20. The endothelium is prominent. (PASM, ×300.)

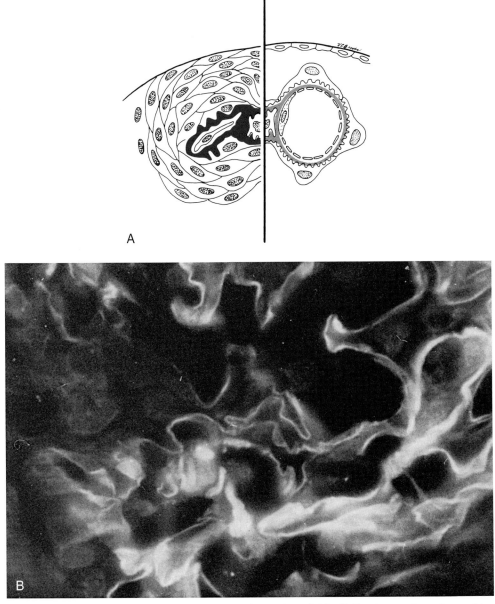

Figure 1–25. Deposits, linear. *A,* Diagram of crescentic glomerulonephritis. *B,* **Goodpasture's syndrome.** Linear IgG deposits outline the glomerular basement membranes. (Immunofluorescence micrograph, ×400.)

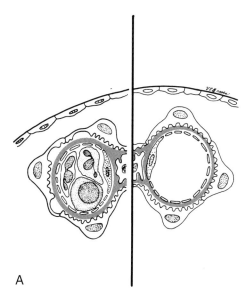

A

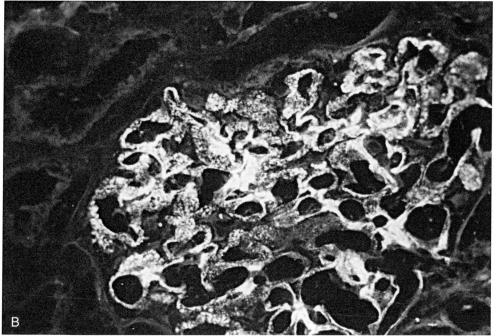

B

Figure 1–26. Deposits, subepithelial, granular. *A,* Diagram of irregular, subepithelial deposits in postinfectious glomeru-lonephritis. *B,* **Lupus nephritis, Class V.** Large numbers of subepithelial deposits of IgG are seen, also deposits in the mesangial and subendothelial regions. (Immunofluorescence micrograph, ×400.)

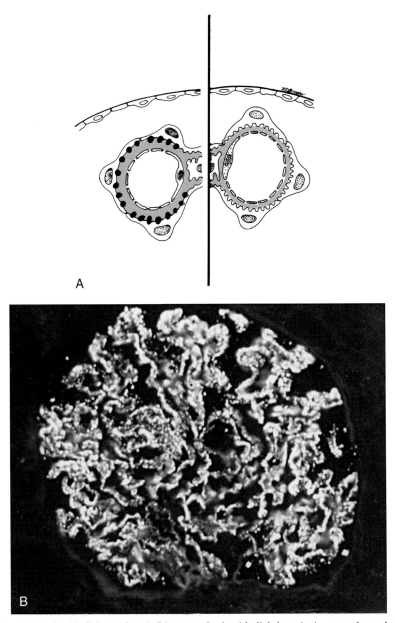

A

B

Figure 1–27. **Deposits, subepithelial, regular.** *A,* Diagram of subepithelial deposits in a regular, subepithelial distribution. This pattern is characteristic of membranous glomerulonephritis. *B,* **Membranous nephropathy, Stage 2 or Stage 3.** Granular deposits of IgG covering the epithelial aspect of the basement membrane. (Immunofluorescence micrograph, ×250.)

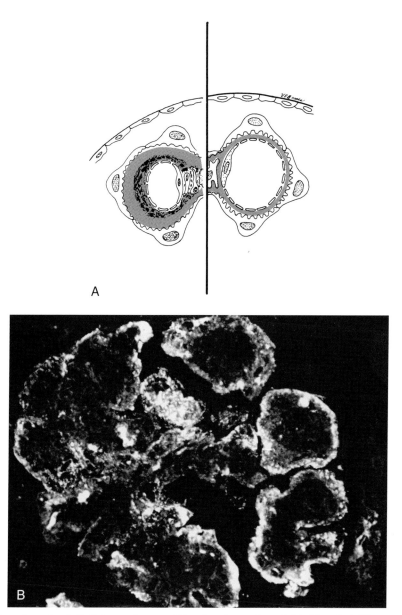

Figure 1–28. Deposits, subendothelial, membranoproliferative glomerulonephritis, Type I. *A,* Diagram of large, subendothelial deposits with thickened basement membranes. *B,* Nearly continuous, bulky C3 deposits outline the glomerular basement membranes. The mesangial regions are not affected. (Immunofluorescence micrograph, ×400.)

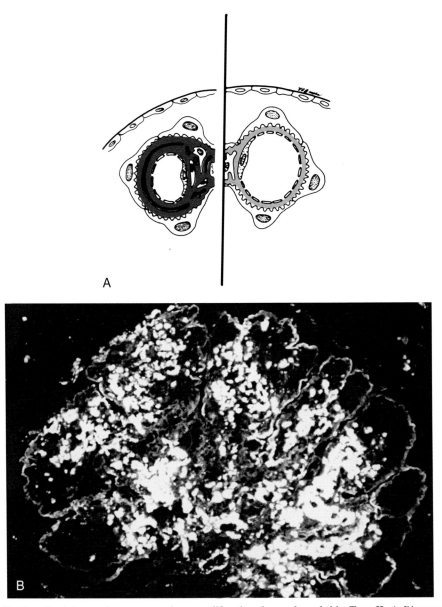

Figure 1–29. Deposits, intramembranous, membranoproliferative glomerulonephritis, Type II. *A,* Diagram of deposits within a very thickened glomerular basement membrane. *B,* **Dense deposit disease.** The mesangium contains brightly staining punctate C3 deposits, and the glomerular basement membranes are faintly stained. (Immunofluorescence micrograph, ×400.)

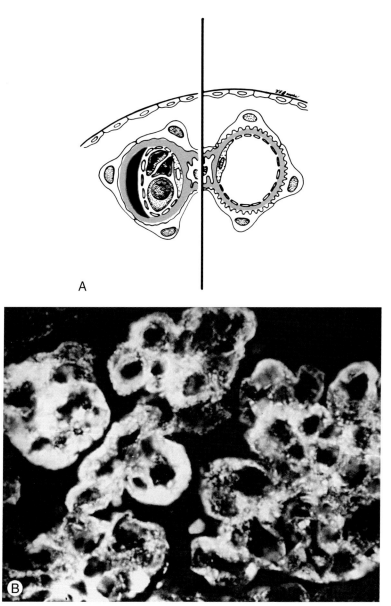

A

B

Figure 1–30. Deposits, subendothelial (systemic lupus erythematosus). *A,* Diagram of diffuse, large subendothelial deposits. *B,* **Lupus nephritis, Class IV.** The regions of the wire loops contain large deposits of IgG. There are also granular mesangial deposits. (Immunofluorescence micrograph, ×500.)

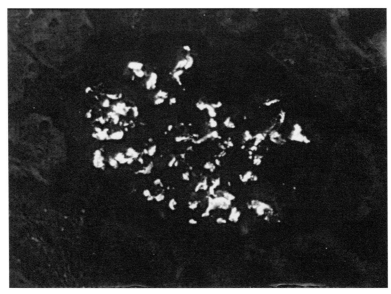

Figure 1–31. Deposits, mesangial, IgA nephropathy. There are heavy, irregular deposits in each mesangial region. All glomeruli are affected. (Immunofluorescence micrograph, anti-IgA, ×250.)

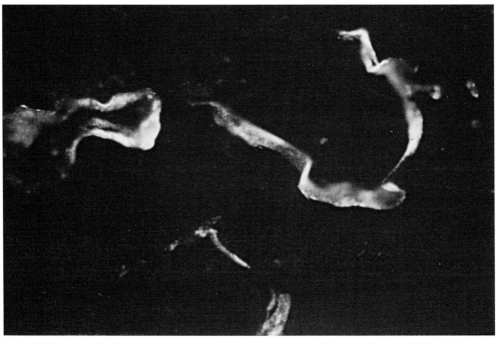

Figure 1–32. Deposits, tubular basement membranes, linear. Acute interstitial nephritis, methicillin. Linear deposits of IgG are present along the tubular basement membranes. (Immunofluorescence micrograph, ×400.)

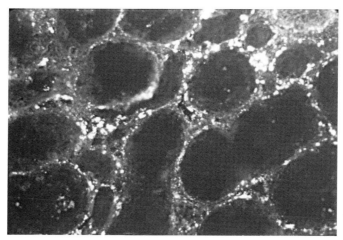

Figure 1–33. Deposits, tubular basement membranes, granular. Chronic interstitial nephritis. Sjögren disease. There are granular IgG deposits along the tubular basement membranes. (Immunofluorescence micrograph, ×400.)

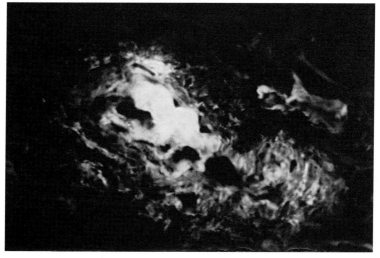

Figure 1–34. Deposits, artery. The vascular wall contains large aggregates of deposits without clear margins. (Immunofluorescence micrograph, antifibrin/fibrinogen antigens, ×250.)

GLOSSARY OF DESCRIPTIVE TERMS

Terms Relating to Distribution/ Structure

Apoptosis. Programmed cell death, characterized by a series of steps beginning with nuclear condensation and fragmentation and ending in engulfment of the cell by neighboring sister cells or inflammatory cells.

Diffuse. Involving all or almost all glomeruli.

Focal. Involving less than 50% of glomeruli.

Hyalinosis. Acellular material that stains red with eosin and periodic acid–Schiff (PAS) but is unstained by periodic acid–silver methenamine (PASM). Contents include serum proteins, other glycoproteins, and lipids.

Mesangiolysis. Disruption of mesangium, with loss of both the anatomic boundaries and stainable matrix. May be present in intravascular thrombosis.

Necrosis. Loss of structure, with disruption of local cells and extracellular matrix, often associated with fibrin deposition.

Obsolescence. Total loss of normal glomerular architecture due to replacement by sclerosis (scarring).

Sclerosis. Increase in one or several of the extracellular matrix components, as well as the appearance of new connective tissue elements. The sclerotic areas often stain positively with PAS, Masson's trichrome, and PASM. The absence of staining by one of these reagents may be useful in determining the nature of the extracellular matrix.

Segmental. Involving portions of individual glomeruli.

Terms Relating to Proliferation

Adhesions or synechiae. Localized crescents or bridges of connective tissue between the glomerular vascular loops and Bowman's capsule.

Crescent. Cellular proliferation and/or infiltration composed of glomerular epithelial cells, macrophages, and interstitial cells. If Bowman's capsule has been disrupted, crescents rapidly become sclerotic, resulting in glomerular obsolescence.

Endocapillary. Within vascular (capillary) loops.

Mesangial. Within the mesangium.

Terms Relating to Deposits

Intramembranous. Within the basement membrane.

Linear glomerular basement membrane. Outlining the peripheral glomerular basement membranes of all glomeruli, but not the mesangium.

Mesangial. Within the mesangium.

Subendothelial. Between the glomerular basement membrane and the endothelium.

Subepithelial or epimembranous. Located between the glomerular basement membrane and the podocytes.

Use of these terms and guidelines will allow categorization of a lesion and documentation of its nature and extent. Glomerular diseases are observed more commonly in renal biopsy specimens than are lesions in the tubulointerstitial or vascular regions. This distribution reflects the biopsy policies of the nephrology community, which are biased toward the use of a renal biopsy in patients with proteinuria, a reliable sign of glomerular disease. In addition, laboratory tests to detect early lesions in other renal compartments that lead to progressive kidney failure are very limited.

INITIAL APPROACH TO THE RENAL BIOPSY

The interpretation should be approached systematically, logically, and practically. The first consideration is the nature of the questions that can and should be addressed:

1. What is the nature of the injury—that is, is it inflammatory, proliferative, sclerotic, deposition of foreign material, or a mixture?
2. What is the site of the lesion? (Nephron segment)
   a. Glomeruli
   b. Tubules
   c. Interstitium
   d. Blood vessels
3. What is its distribution—that is, focal or diffuse?
4. What is the severity—that is, mild, moderate, or severe?
5. Is there evidence/possibility of repair?

After completing this analysis, the next step is to put these observations in context with the disease process and the patient, in consultation with the clinician. A summation, diagnosis, and interpretation can then be constructed.

SELECTED READINGS

1. Churg J, Sobin LH: Renal Disease. Classification and Atlas of Glomerular Disease. Tokyo, Igaku-Shoin Ltd, 1982.
2. Corwin HL, Schwartz MM, Lewis EJ: The importance of sample size in the interpretation of the renal biopsy. Am J Nephrol 8:85, 1988.
3. Kashgarian M, Hayslett JP, Spargo BH: Teaching monograph. Am J Pathol 89:187, 1977.
4. Marcussen N, Olsen S, Larsen S, et al: Reproducibility of the WHO classification of glomerulonephritis. Clin Nephrol 44:220, 1995.
5. Morel-Maroger L: The value of renal biopsy. Am J Kidney Dis 1:244, 1982.
6. Morel-Maroger L, Leathem A, Richet G: Glomerular abnormalities in nonsystemic diseases. Relationship between findings by light microscopy and immunofluorescence in 433 renal biopsy specimens. Am J Med 53:170, 1972.
7. Neilson EG: Pathogenesis and therapy of interstitial nephritis. Kidney Int 39:518, 1991.
8. Nolasco F, Cameron J, Hartley B, et al: Intraglomerular T cells and monocytes in nephritis: Study with monoclonal antibodies. Kidney Int 31:1160, 1987.
9. Pirani CL, Salinas-Madrigal L, Koss M: Evaluation of percutaneous renal biopsy. In Sommer SC (ed): Kidney Pathology Decennial. New York, Appleton-Century-Crofts, 1975, pp 109–163.
10. Schwartz MM, Bidani AK, Lewis EJ: Glomerular epithelial cell structure and function in chronic proteinuria induced by homologous protein load. Lab Invest 55:673, 1986.

2

RELATIONSHIP BETWEEN STRUCTURE AND FUNCTION

Glomerular Filtration Rate

We and others have found that the measurement of the glomerular filtration rate does not provide a good indication of the underlying renal disease. In our studies, sequential patients from a renal consultation clinic were evaluated without regard to the underlying type or stage of renal disease. We found that there is no correlation between glomerular changes and the glomerular filtration rate, as determined by the clearance of inulin (Fig. 2–1). The best correlation was between the glomerular filtration rate and interstitial disease (Fig. 2–2). At that time we suggested that interstitial fibrosis reflected nephron dropout and/or tubular damage. Recent findings confirm this speculation but also show that one of the most important determinants of glomerular filtration rate is the filtration surface area. The filtration surface area can be accurately determined only by renal biopsy, using morphometric techniques. The measurements must be made by electron microscopy. It now appears that as long as the filtration surface area can be increased, the glomerular filtration rate remains at or near normal levels in the presence of increasing glomerular damage. These data help explain the lack of correlation between renal structure and function obtained in the past.

Proteinuria (Albumin Excretion Rate)

One of the earliest signs of progressive, non-inflammatory glomerular lesions is protein-uria. This is particularly useful in the examination of diabetic patients, in whom it is useful to measure the albumin excretion rate (AER) in the milligram range, since it has been clearly established that those with an AER greater than 100 mg per 24 hours are very likely to develop progressive glomerular disease. However, it is also clear that the absence of an elevated AER does not exclude the presence of fixed diabetic glomerular lesions.

REPRODUCIBILITY OF INTERPRETATION BETWEEN PATHOLOGISTS

The utility of any analytic method depends upon its reproducibility within the same environment, and its acceptance and use by other experts. This has been assessed by a group of European renal pathologists, using the World Health Organization classification. The analysis was restricted to light microscopy. They found that there is good agreement for minimal change, membranous glomerulonephritis, focal glomerulonephritis, and crescentic glomerulonephritis. It is interesting that the diagnoses in which there was the least agreement are membranoproliferative glomerulonephritis and diffuse mesangial proliferative glomerulonephritis. Agreement on the diagnosis of membranoproliferative glomerulonephritis might have been improved by the use of immunofluorescence and electron microscopy. The relative lack of diagnostic agreement on

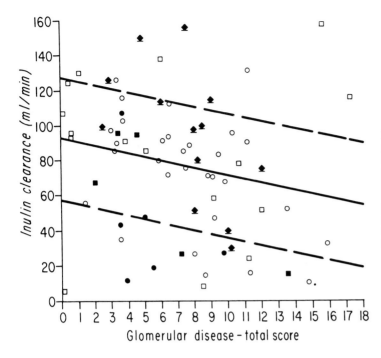

Figure 2–1. Relationship between inulin clearance and glomerular disease. Regression line *(solid line)* is y = 92 − 0.02x and SEE (standard error of the estimate) *(dashed line)* is 39. The poor correlation is apparent. Symbols refer to cases belonging to conventional diagnostic groups: ◆, acute glomerulonephritis; ○, chronic glomerulonephritis; ●, interstitial nephritis; ■, nephrosclerosis; □, miscellaneous.

the diagnosis of diffuse mesangial proliferative glomerulonephritis suggests that the determination of the number of mesangial cells is quite subjective and likely requires morpho-

metric analysis to determine cell number, as well as other techniques to determine cell turnover if proliferation is to be precisely evaluated.

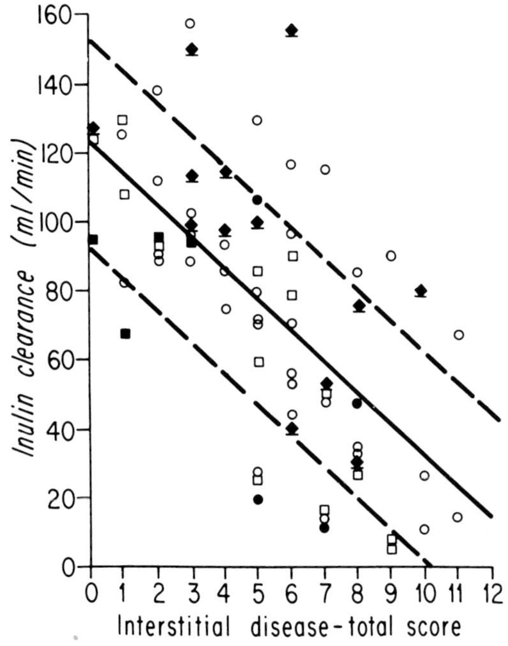

These data show that the interpretation of the histologic aspects of renal biopsy specimens, at least those of glomerular disease, is reproducible among geographically dispersed laboratories, which lends practicality and credibility to its use as a diagnostic tool.

CONCLUSION

The renal biopsy not only reveals the type and the extent of renal injury, but also it allows detection and quantification long before injury can be measured by other methods. Use of the renal biopsy as a research and clinical tool remains an underutilized resource. The advent of immunofluorescence and electron microscopy added to its usefulness almost three decades ago, and these are now routine measures. We and others have begun to apply modern molecular and cellular biologic techniques to the direct assessment of renal biopsy specimens. Unfortunately, these are not sufficiently tested nor economical enough to be used routinely.

Figure 2–2. Relationship between inulin clearance and interstitial disease. The regression line *(solid line)* is y = 122 − 8.8x and SEE *(dashed line)* is 31. The symbols are the same as in Figure 2–1.

SELECTED READINGS

1. Bohle A, MacKensen-Haen S, Gise HV: Significance of tubulointerstitial changes in the renal cortex for the excretory function and concentration ability of the kidney: A morphometric contribution. Am J Nephrol 7:421, 1987.
2. Risdon RA, Sloper JC, De Wardener HE: Relationship between renal function and histologic changes found in renal biopsy specimens from patients with persistent glomerulonephritis. Lancet 2:363, 1968.
3. Schainuck LI, Striker GE, Cutler RE, et al: Structural-functional correlations in renal disease. II. The correlations. Hum Pathol 1:631, 1970.
4. Striker GE, Schainuck LI, Cutler RE, et al: Structural-functional correlations in renal disease. I. A method for assaying and classifying histopathologic changes in renal disease. Hum Pathol 1:615, 1970.

HANDLING AND PREPARATION OF SPECIMENS

3

The ability to recognize and correctly interpret a renal biopsy specimen requires proper handling of the tissue at all stages of its preparation. Immunofluorescence microscopy is essentially always necessary as an adjunct to light microscopy. Electron microscopy is required in many instances, but this technique may be available only in selected centers. Other special methods may also be required.

The nephrologist (and the pathologist) referring specimens must confer with the receiving pathologist regarding the locally preferred methods of transport. In addition, an adequate clinical and laboratory workup is always required for interpretation of the biopsy findings.

The pathologist may be given two kinds of renal biopsy specimens: wedge samples and needle samples. Wedge biopsy specimens always include the cortex as well as a greater sample of renal tissue than needle biopsy specimens, but they are the exception in the usual pathology practice. In most instances, renal tissue is obtained with a needle, and the amount of tissue available is fairly limited.

HANDLING THE GROSS SPECIMEN

Ideally, the pathologist or a histology technician should attend the biopsy procedure to ensure that the tissue is handled properly. If this is not the case, several guidelines will help in obtaining the tissue in the most appropriate state for processing. It is critical to handle the tissue delicately to avoid crushing or tearing the specimen. The cores must be cut with a sharp blade on dental wax, using a slicing rather than a crushing motion. Wide-mouth pipettes or wooden sticks may be used to place the tissue fragments into appropriate containers. Forceps should never be used.

Two separate cores of tissue should be obtained whenever possible. If a small dissecting microscope is available, the first core should be examined for the presence of glomeruli and directly immersed in a bottle of the fixative chosen for light microscopy. Glomeruli are recognizable with a hand lens as tiny reddish structures of less than 1-mm diameter. The second core may be partitioned for immunofluorescence and electron microscopy.

If only one core of tissue is available, it should be bisected longitudinally. One half can then be processed for light microscopy. The second half is transected vertically, half being used for immunofluorescence microscopy and half for electron microscopy. The tissue for electron microscopy can be immediately fixed in the fixative of choice.

The tissue for immunofluorescence microscopy may be stored in a Petri dish and covered with a sterile gauze moistened with sterile TRIS (tris[hydroxymethyl]aminomethane) buffer or phosphate-buffered saline (PBS). The tissue should not be carried on ice because it may become partially frozen. Freezing should be accomplished by snap-freezing the tissue in liquid nitrogen or on dry ice. The tissue must not be cut in a cryostat or placed in a freezer before proper snap-freezing. If the tissue cannot be frozen within 2 hours, special transport media allow adequate, if not ideal, preservation of samples for longer periods (up to 36 hours).

In the case of wedge biopsies, ten 1 × 1 × 1 mm pieces of tissue should be placed in fixative for electron microscopy. One slice measuring 3 × 3 × 2 mm should be set aside for immunofluorescence microscopy, and the remainder should be placed in a fixative appropriate for light microscopy.

PREPARATION FOR SECTIONING

Light Microscopy

Fixation

Several fixatives have been proposed for light microscopy. The critical points are to choose a fixative that allows the preparation of thin (3-μm) sections and to use multiple stains. The most frequently used fixatives include Duboscq-Brazil or alcoholic Bouin's solution, 10% neutral-buffered formalin, Zenker-formol, Carnoy's solution, or paraformaldehyde. Paraformaldehyde has the advantage of being a reasonable fixative for both light and electron microscopy. Carnoy's solution allows immunofluorescence microscopy, since many antigens are preserved in this fixative.

A needle biopsy specimen requires a minimum fixation of 1 hour, whereas wedge biopsy specimens require several hours. The tissue is then processed overnight. The exact sequence of washes may vary and is best determined in the individual laboratory.

Embedding Medium

Paraffin

Paraffin is the most commonly used embedding medium. Paraffins with a high melting point allow the technician reproducibly to obtain thin sections for light microscopy. For immunofluorescence microscopy, one should use a low-melting point paraffin.

Glycol Methacrylate

Glycol methacrylate is used by several laboratories for light microscopy. The exact procedure depends on the manufacturing source.

The blocks are quite hard, allowing one to obtain sections of 1- to 2-μm thickness routinely, using a JB-4 microtome and a glass knife. The chief advantages of this method are that shrinkage of the tissue is less than in paraffin-embedded specimens and resolution is better because of the thinness of the section. The three main disadvantages are the hygroscopic tendency of the plastic (which results in variation in ease of sectioning because of variations in the ambient humidity), difficulty in storage of the blocks in a condition suitable for future resectioning, and an increased staining time. Most of the standard stains have been altered for use in this medium, and the results are quite satisfactory.

If sections less than 2 μm are obtained, the stains may be too pale for viewing easily, and satisfactory photographs may be difficult to obtain.

Cutting

We prefer to place three to four sections on each glass slide. Multiple sections should be cut, and the glass slides should be numbered, which is a useful precaution in the event of focal lesions.

Staining

A battery of stains is used. From paraffin blocks we obtain 12 slides cut at 3 to 4 μm and one at 8 μm. Slide numbers 1, 3, 6, and 12 are stained with hematoxylin and eosin (H&E). Slide 5 is stained with phosphotungstic acid–hematoxylin (PTAH) for fibrin. Slide 7 is stained with periodic acid–Schiff (PAS), which accentuates basement membranes, mesangial matrix, and the brush border of proximal tubular epithelial cells. Various pathologic alterations are also emphasized with this stain, including hyalinosis, cryoglobulin precipitates, and Tamm-Horsfall protein. Slide 8 is stained with a combination of methenamine silver and PAS with an H&E counterstain. This combination helps in the evaluation of lesions involving basement membranes. It is especially useful for photomicrography. Slide 9 is stained with Masson's trichrome, which accentuates fibrosis. It is often possible to detect subepithelial deposits with this stain. The slide containing the thickest sections, number 13, is used for Congo red staining in those specimens in which there is a suspicion of amyloid deposits. A thick section is required to provide sufficient dye binding for visualization by po-larizing microscopy.

The intervening unstained slides can be used for other stains such as those for reticulin or elastin.

Immunofluorescence Microscopy

After it has been properly snap-frozen, the tissue may be stored at $-70°$ C. (However, storage for periods exceeding 4 to 6 weeks results in desiccation, rendering the tissue un-interpretable.) The tissue is then cut in a cryo-stat at a temperature between -25 and $-20°$ C. The sections may not exceed 6 μm and ideally should be 3 to 4 μm in thickness. The slides are fixed for 5 to 10 minutes in acetone, dried at room temperature, washed in buf-fered saline, and covered for 30 minutes with a drop of fluorescein-labeled antiserum in a moist chamber that is light shielded. After sev-eral washes with buffer, the slides are mounted using buffered glycerol. It is possible to delay fading by adding phenylenediamine to the mounting medium.

Paraffin-embedded sections may also be suit-able for immunofluorescence microscopy, when snap-freezing is not an available option. In this case the most suitable method of fixa-tion is methyl-Carnoy's solution, at least 1 hour at 4° C. Embedding in low-melting-point paraf-fin is an absolute requirement to preserve anti-genicity. Following sectioning, the sections must be lightly trypsinized, using 1% tissue culture–grade trypsin for 5 to 10 minutes at 37° C. This method is suitable for immune reactants and many extracellular matrix com-ponents. It is also useful for proliferation cell nuclear antigen (PCNA) and bromodeoxyuri-dine (BrdU) staining to assess mitogenesis. For some antigens, treating the sections with so-dium dodecyl sulfate (SDS) may be the best method to visualize denatured antigens.

The sections are then examined using a fluorescence microscope equipped with appro-priate excitation and barrier filters. The sec-tions should be photographed, because the fluorescence fades on exposure to both ultravi-olet and incident light. They also fade within a few weeks in storage, even without exposure.

Immunoperoxidase

This technique is not as useful for the identi-fication of proteins in extracellular deposits as it is in the identification of cell surface mark-ers. Nonetheless, some use it on fixed and embedded specimens when frozen tissue is not available for immunofluorescence microscopy or when glomeruli are not present in the mate-rial obtained for frozen sectioning. Many in-vestigators have discussed the vagaries of the technique, including the requirement that the section must be glued to the slides and that the tissue sections require trypsin digestion before exposure to the antibodies. Digestion is used in an attempt to expose antigenic sites. The advantages of this method compared with immunofluorescence microscopy are that fro-zen tissue is not necessary and that slides are available as a permanent record. The disadvan-tage is that the technique still gives inconsis-tent results in many laboratories because of the presence of a high background.

Electron Microscopy

Fixation and Embedding

Many fixatives do not readily penetrate renal tissue. Thus, it is important that the fragments be no larger than $1 \times 1 \times 1$ mm. The most widely used fixative is 3% phosphate-buffered glutaraldehyde. This solution is diluted from a stock solution of 25% glutaraldehyde. The diluted solution has a shelf life of no more than 2 months, even when refrigerated. At room temperature, 3% glutaraldehyde deterio-rates within a few hours. Carson's fixative (4% formaldehyde and 1% glutaraldehyde) is an alternate fixative that is available commer-cially. Fixatives containing glutaraldehyde are not appropriate for light microscopy unless the free aldehyde groups are blocked. Other-wise, the staining patterns are altered and the tissue becomes brittle and difficult to cut in a paraffin-embedded block.

After fixation for a minimum of 2 hours, the tissue is rinsed in buffer, postfixed in 1% osmium tetroxide, dehydrated, and embed-ded.

If no glomeruli are present in the material prepared for electron microscopy, the tissue remaining in the light microscopy block can be used. The area of the light microscopy block containing glomeruli is identified and cut from the block. The fragment is rinsed several times in xylene to remove the paraffin. The tissue can then be processed for electron microscopy. The preservation of morphology is less than optimal, but it is often satisfactory for the recognition of significant alterations.

Sectioning and Staining

Thick sections (1 μm) are cut with glass knives and stained with toluidine blue to choose appropriate areas for thin sectioning. In the presence of a diffuse, uniform renal lesion, any region of the cortex that contains all the representative elements may be suitable. When the lesions are focal or irregular in severity, several representative areas should be chosen. Thin sections (60 to 90 μm) are then cut and stained with uranyl acetate and lead citrate.

Examination

Evaluation of the thin section should include an assessment of all compartments. The section should first be examined at low power. It is helpful to develop a systematic method of assessing the elements of each compartment. For instance, an examination of the glomerulus might include the peripheral vascular wall, all three glomerular cell types (endothelial, epithelial, and mesangial), and the extracellular matrix (glomerular basement membranes and mesangial matrix). An increase in mesangial cell number and matrix is best evaluated with the light microscope because of the small sample size and propensity for sampling errors by electron microscopy. However, the presence and location of immune deposits or amyloid may be best detected and documented by electron microscopy. The several tubular segments should be examined for alterations of either the epithelial cells or tubular basement membranes. The blood vessels, often overlooked, should be carefully evaluated for both cellular and extracellular matrix changes,

including the presence of hyalin or other changes related to hypertension. The distribution of interstitial changes is best documented using the light microscope.

Other Specialized Techniques

One new technique is in situ hybridization. This technique still belongs in the category of a research tool and requires specialized laboratories. Thus, applications to clinical problems remain for the future. It has been extensively used for detection of growth factors or of viral material.

Needle aspiration of the kidney is being used in evaluating renal transplants for the presence of rejection in some centers (see Chapter 11). This technique does not have a place in the evaluation of most renal diseases, because the specimen consists of isolated cells.

Another new method is the use of the polymerase chain reaction, following reverse transcription, to assess mRNA levels in different regions of the kidney. We have used this technique to examine the levels of collagens, glycoproteins, and growth factors and their receptors in glomeruli that had been isolated by microdissection.

SELECTED READINGS

1. Agodoa LY, Striker GE, Chi E: Glycomethacrylate embedding of renal biopsy specimens for light microscopy. Am J Clin Pathol 64:655, 1975.
2. Koehler JK: Advanced Techniques in Biological Electron Microscopy. Berlin, Springer-Verlag, 1973.
3. Striker LJ, Peten EP, Yang CW, Striker GE: Molecular approach to human kidney biopsies. *In* Schlondorff D, Bonventre JV (eds): Molecular Nephrology; Kidney Function in Health and Disease. New York, Marcel Dekker, 1995, pp 771–781.

Chapter

4

PRIMARY GLOMERULAR DISEASE OF UNKNOWN ETIOLOGY

MINIMAL LESION

The terms *minimal change nephrotic syndrome, minimal change disease, minimal change,* and *lipoid nephrosis* encompass a clinicopathologic entity that consists of the nephrotic syndrome in association with a specific configurational change that is limited to the visceral epithelial cells of the glomerulus. For the sake of brevity and consistency, we will refer to this syndrome as minimal change. This syndrome is defined by the presence of normal-appearing glomeruli by light and immunofluorescence microscopy, with an electron microscopic lesion consisting only of effacement of the pedicels. The result is that the urinary side of the glomerular basement membrane is covered by a homogeneous layer of epithelial cell cytoplasm rather than the complex interdigitation of pedicels from adjacent cells.

Note that *irregular* effacement of pedicels is a common feature of multiple glomerular lesions associated with proteinuria. Recently it has been suggested that there is a subset of patients with the idiopathic nephrotic syndrome who have enlarged glomeruli and are at increased risk for the development of focal sclerosing lesions and progression to renal failure. Thus, it may be useful to measure glomeruli in patients with the idiopathic nephrotic syndrome who are resistant to steroid therapy or relapse frequently.

Pathogenesis

The pathogenesis of minimal change is unknown, but one of the current beliefs is that

one mediator of the disease is a low-molecular-weight substance derived from T-lymphocytes. The effect of this substance could be to alter the podocytes so that the charge and size-selective characteristics of the glomerular vascular wall are altered. The net result of this change is the development of proteinuria. This hypothesis is strengthened by the rapid response of the proteinuria and pedicel effacement to steroid therapy, the presence of this clinical and morphologic entity in patients with certain malignancies of T-lymphocytes, and recent experimental evidence.

Patient Presentation

Minimal change is the most common underlying disease in nephrotic children. It is most frequently seen after 2 years of age, with a peak incidence at age 3 years. It is much more common in boys than in girls. Curiously, adults of both sexes are affected equally often.

The syndrome is characterized by multiple exacerbations and remissions, sometimes over a period of years, with long intervals between incidents. The precipitating events are not known, but minimal change has been associated with allergic reactions. The onset is heralded by the development of progressive edema and selective proteinuria (i.e., albuminuria). Hypertension and hematuria are rare and when present should lead to the suspicion of another type of renal disease.

Few children now undergo a biopsy unless

44

they do not respond to steroids, thus, few pathologists have the opportunity to see this disease by renal biopsy. The sole exceptions are those few patients with this syndrome who do not show a prompt response to steroid therapy and in whom the nephrotic syndrome is severe enough to prompt the question of treatment with more aggressive therapeutic agents.

Although the overwhelming majority of children with the nephrotic syndrome have this renal picture, it is much less frequent in adults, in whom it accounts for approximately 20% of patients presenting with the idiopathic nephrotic syndrome. Therefore, adults are much more likely to undergo renal biopsy before a trial of steroid therapy is undertaken.

Histology

Light Microscopy

Because the diagnosis of minimal change depends on the absence of obvious glomerular lesions or hypertrophy by light microscopy, it is imperative that multiple sections of each biopsy sample are prepared and examined thoroughly and measured morphometrically (Figs. 4–1 and 4–2). The glomeruli of children are smaller than those of adults and may appear to be hypercellular to pathologists who do not often examine pediatric renal tissue. If there is any question about cellularity or extracellular matrix changes by light micros-

copy, normal tissue from a child of similar age should be used for comparison.

The peripheral vascular loops may occasionally appear to be dilated but are otherwise normal. The podocyte cytoplasm appears swollen or vacuolated. The pedicel abnormalities (i.e., effacement) may be apparent in sections of methacrylate-embedded tissue (Fig. 4–3).

No cellular proliferation or mesangial matrix change is seen.

There is some controversy in the current literature about whether minimal change, mesangial proliferative glomerulonephritis, and focal or segmental glomerulonephritis are all part of a continuum. It has been said that a transition between these different diseases is possible. However, we are of the strong opinion that minimal change belongs in a separate category based on its morphologic appearance and clinical behavior. In our combined experience, we are not aware of any patient who has progressed from minimal change to any sclerosing or proliferative disease. However, it should be carefully stated that this conclusion is based on the study of biopsy specimens in which multiple sections have been examined by light, immunofluorescence, and electron microscopy and includes only those cases in which an adequate sample of renal tissue has been available for study. In the absence of this type of detailed search, focal lesions may be missed. The recent data on enlarged glomeruli being reliable markers for the presence of focal glomerulosclerosis require the routine measurement of glomerular size. If glomerular size is increased, a detailed search for the presence of focal lesions should be undertaken.

Only very minor changes are ordinarily present in the extraglomerular regions. They consist mainly of slight interstitial widening, apparently due to edema, and the presence of hyalin droplets in the cytoplasm of the proximal tubules. In biopsies of older patients, lesions in the tubulointerstitial or vascular compartments may be present as a consequence of arteriosclerosis.

Immunofluorescence Microscopy

The characteristic feature of this disease is the complete absence of immune reactants, fibrin, and other foreign materials. Some have suggested that a small amount of IgM and C3 may be found, but most agree that the hallmark of minimal change is the lack of depos-

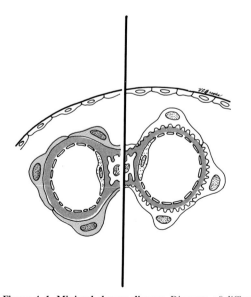

Figure 4–1. Minimal change disease. Diagram of diffuse podocyte effacement.

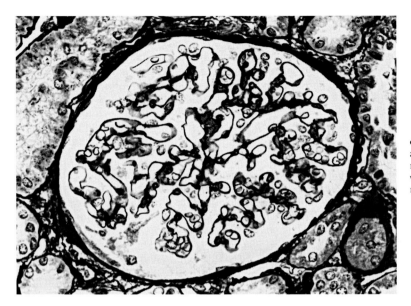

Figure 4–2. Minimal change disease. The basement membrane and mesangial regions are unremarkable. The vascular spaces are widely patent. (Jones methenamine silver, ×500.)

its, i.e., a negative immunofluorescence pattern.

Electron Microscopy

The electron microscopic changes are essentially restricted to the glomerular visceral epi-

thelial cells, thus some have dubbed minimal change the "epithelial cell disease." The characteristic podocyte abnormality is the complete effacement of the pedicels, resulting in a smooth and homogeneous layer of epithelial cell cytoplasm that lacks interdigitations (Fig. 4–4). In the past, this change in the architec-

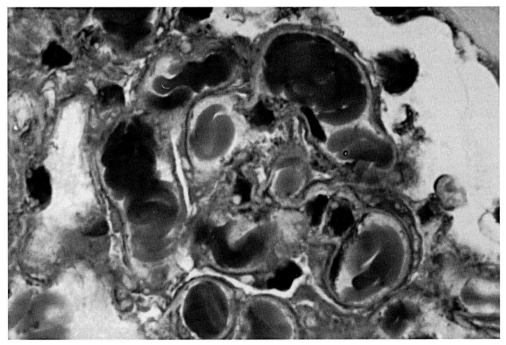

Figure 4–3. Minimal change disease. High-power light micrograph of a methacrylate-embedded specimen. Podocyte swelling and spreading can be seen over most of the peripheral glomerular basement membranes. (Hematoxylin and eosin, ×1000.)

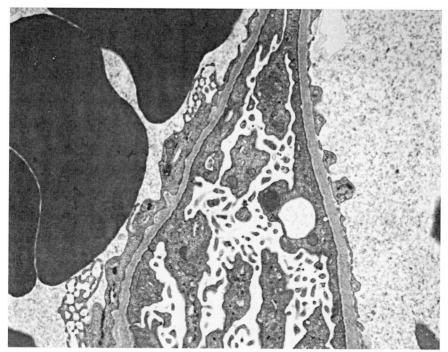

Figure 4–4. Minimal change disease. Two adjacent loops show effacement of the epithelial cells, which form a nearly continuous sheet of cytoplasm. The basement membrane and the endothelial cell cytoplasm are not affected. (Electron micrograph, ×5000.)

ture of the visceral epithelial cells was called fusion. However, scanning electron microscopy reveals the loss of the normal finger-like interdigitations (pedicels) between adjacent visceral epithelial cells, rather than fusion of the outer envelopes of adjacent cells. The epithelial cell processes, adjacent to and covering the peripheral basement membrane, are thickened but otherwise appear normal. The cytoplasm in the body of the epithelial cells may contain many large, clear vacuoles as well and an apparent increase in the number of other cell organelles. The urinary surface of the epithelial cells may also contain an increased number of microvilli; this change has been called microvillous transformation.

One clue to the presence of a focal lesion is that the pedicel spreading is less diffuse and regular. This stands in sharp contrast to that in minimal change, in which pedicel spreading is almost monotonous in its regularity and diffuseness.

The lamina rara externa, the lamina densa, and the lamina rara interna all appear normal.

The endothelial cell cytoplasm may also appear somewhat more prominent than normal, but quantitative studies of pore size have not been performed.

The mesangial cells and matrix appear normal.

No deposits are seen.

Prognosis

The outcome in children has been extensively studied, and a few long-term studies in adults have been reported. The outcome in most children is complete remission of the nephrotic syndrome after steroid therapy. Although there may be multiple exacerbations of the disease, each seems to be sensitive to steroid therapy. The podocyte changes rapidly revert to a normal appearance after steroid therapy, coincident with the disappearance of proteinuria. More than 70% of children have only one or a small number of episodes of the nephrotic syndrome. In our experience, when there has been a course other than that just described, careful reassessment of the original biopsy material has revealed either enlarged glomeruli or a lesion previously overlooked. In these cases, control of the nephrotic syndrome often requires the continuous administration of steroids (so-called steroid dependence) or addition of a cytotoxic agent.

Although the disorder is much less common in adults, several studies suggest that the prognosis in adults appears to be similar to that in children.

It remains to be firmly established whether or not a relationship exists among the various forms of nephrotic syndrome. Thus, IgM disease, mesangial proliferative glomerulonephritis, and like categories with demonstrable morphologic abnormalities should be considered as separate entities. The fact that they all are idiopathic, all are associated with the nephrotic syndrome, and may have at least a temporary response to steroid administration does not provide sufficient justification to place them into a category entitled minimal change, in our opinion.

SELECTED READINGS

1. Black DAK, Rose G, Brewer DB: Controlled trial of prednisone in adult patients with the nephrotic syndrome. Br Med J 3:421, 1970.
2. Churg J, Habib R, White RHR: Pathology of the nephrotic syndrome in children. Lancet 1:1299, 1970.
3. Fogo A, Hawkins EP, Berry PL, et al: Glomerular hypertrophy in minimal change disease predicts subsequent progression to focal glomerular sclerosis. Kidney Int 38:115, 1990.
4. Lee HS, Lim SC: The significance of glomerular hypertrophy in focal segmental glomerulosclerosis. Clin Nephrol 44:349, 1995.
5. Trompeter RS, Hicks J, Lloyd BW, et al: Long-term outcome for children with minimal-change nephrotic syndrome. Lancet 1:368, 1985.

FOCAL AND SEGMENTAL GLOMERULOSCLEROSIS AND COLLAPSING GLOMERULOPATHY

Focal and segmental glomerulosclerosis has many synonyms, including *focal sclerosis*, *focal hyalinosis*, and *focal glomerulosclerosis*. It is defined by the presence of localized areas of sclerosis within the glomerular tufts. Another condition recently described, known as collapsing glomerulopathy, will be described in this section, although it is not clear whether it is a variant of focal and segmental glomerulosclerosis or a separate entity.

Focal and segmental glomerulosclerosis is one of the common histologic lesions in the idiopathic nephrotic syndrome in adults; it is much less common in children. For this reason and also because many of the patients with this disease respond to steroid treatment, this entity was initially considered to be part of the group of diseases or syndromes collectively referred to as *lipoid nephrosis*. This term should now be considered to have only historic significance, because most investigators now believe that minimal change nephrotic syndrome, focal sclerosis, and IgM mesangial nephropathy are separate disorders. Others consider them to be a group of diseases with a common pathogenesis and a continuous spectrum of lesions. It is not our purpose to resolve this controversy, but the presence of areas of sclerosis, hyalinosis, or synechiae in a patient with an idiopathic nephrotic syndrome portends a different clinical course than in a patient with no lesions in the renal biopsy specimen. Namely, patients with histologic lesions are more likely to respond poorly to (or remain dependent on) steroids and have an increased risk of recurrence, as well as a propensity to progress to end-stage renal disease. In the presence of the nephrotic syndrome, some patients progress to end-stage renal disease in a period of 5 to 10 years. In addition, the risk of recurrence of the lesions in renal transplants is quite high.

Patients who have these histologic lesions but who do not have the nephrotic syndrome have a low risk of developing end-stage renal disease. Some focal and segmental sclerotic lesions, usually in the absence of hyalin material, may result from pre-existing acute lesions (e.g., infectious glomerulonephritis). Thus these scarred lesions may represent a benign outcome of an acute, severe glomerulonephritis and must be clearly distinguished from the progressive conditions just described. In these cases of "resolved glomerulonephritis," the patients seldom have significant proteinuria. In fact, if the nephrotic syndrome is present, this sequence of events and the diagnosis of postinfectious glomerulonephritis must be questioned.

Segmental and focal sclerosis may be seen in other diseases, such as acquired immunodeficiency syndrome and heroin nephropathy (see Chapter 5). It may also be observed in patients with nephron ablation, unilateral agenesis, or segmental hypoplasia. In fact, occasional areas of segmental hyalinosis may complicate most chronic glomerular diseases.

Pathogenesis

There is increasing evidence that proteinuria in these disorders is secondary to a loss in the permselectivity of the glomerular filtration barrier. There is some controversy about the nature of the physiopathology—that is, whether the change is a loss in the size selectivity, the charge, or some combination. The most current evidence suggests that a loss in size selectivity is the most significant change. A loss in charge selectivity also occurs; it can be recognized by the loss of the glomerular polyanion layer by light microscopic stains. The loss of glomerular polyanion could be either the cause or the result of the visceral epithelial cell lesions.

In experimental models, glomerulosclerosis seems to progress relentlessly, even though the initial stimulus is no longer present. This also seems to be the case in humans. Recent studies indicate that many factors may influence the presence and rate of progression, including dietary protein and lipids, elevated intravascular pressure, regulators of vascular tone, growth factors, and arachidonic acid metabolites. We have shown that glomerulosclerosis is associated with changes in the turnover of specific basement membrane constituents, and the exact pattern varies with disease type.

Primary focal glomerulosclerosis is the primary lesion found in 7 to 10% of children and adults presenting with the nephrotic syndrome. In children, there is a male predominance, whereas there is no difference between the sexes in adults. We found focal glomerulosclerosis in 57 nephrotic adults out of a total of 250 patients who presented with the nephrotic syndrome at Tenon Hospital, Paris, between 1965 and 1974.

Immunologic causes of this disease have also been proposed. The strongest case for this hypothesis comes from the observation that proteinuria develops shortly after renal function appears in some allograft recipients whose primary disease was focal sclerosis. Other observations that suggest a role for immunologic factors are reports that certain events, including atopy, bee stings, and upper respiratory tract infections, may precede the onset of proteinuria.

There may be a familial propensity to develop the nephrotic syndrome. Although the genetic basis of these disorders has not been clearly established, patients with minimal change or focal and segmental glomerulosclerosis are more likely to have an affected family member than can be explained on the basis of chance alone. In support of a genetic basis is the recent observation that this syndrome is much more common in those with African ancestry than in others.

Patient Presentation

As in minimal change disease the nephrotic syndrome associated with focal and segmental glomerulosclerosis is characterized by the rapid development of edema; however, in focal sclerosis the proteinuria is nonselective. Patients with focal sclerosis tend to have microscopic hematuria more commonly than those with minimal lesion. Hypoalbuminemia and hypercholesterolemia are prominent. Complement levels are normal.

Histology

Light Microscopy

The lesion of focal glomerulosclerosis is not specific and should always be interpreted along with the clinical and laboratory data. Table 4–1 lists the various clinicopathologic syndromes associated with focal sclerosing lesions, and this lengthy list is not complete.

Many glomeruli appear normal, contrasting with those in which segmental glomerulosclerosis is found. It is not uncommon, however, in the so-called unaffected areas to observe a small increase in the number of mesangial nuclei, sometimes associated with a mild in-

Table 4–1. Conditions That May Be Associated with Focal / Segmental Glomerulosclerosis*

Clinical Conditions	Hyalinosis
Idiopathic nephrotic syndrome	+
Asymptomatic proteinuria	+
Obesity	−
Unilateral renal agenesis	+
Obstructive or reflux nephropathy	+
Heroin-associated nephropathy	+
HIV-associated nephropathy	+
Postinfectious glomerulonephritis (resolving glomerulonephritis)	−
Systemic lupus erythematosus (treated)	−
Vasculitis (treated)	−
Glycogenosis	+
Sickle cell disease	−
Alport's syndrome	−
Familial deficiency of lecithin-cholesterol acyltransferase	+

*Excluding congenital disorders appearing before age 1 year.

crease in the amount of extracellular matrix. The affected glomeruli contain limited areas of sclerosis, which may be associated with disappearance of the local vascular spaces. The sclerotic areas are adjacent to, and part of, synechiae (Fig. 4–5). The sclerotic areas often contain large, eosinophilic deposits referred to as hyalin. The deposits are periodic acid–Schiff (PAS) or trichrome positive and are not stained with silver stains. They may resemble fibrin in hematoxylin and eosin (H&E) preparations. In the vicinity of the hyalin lesions, foam cells or vacuoles containing lipid may be encountered. It is now well accepted that the foam cells represent macrophages.

In nonobsolescent glomeruli, the affected mesangial spaces contain large accumulations of extracellular matrix. The mesangial spaces may later become obliterated by the confluence of segmental lesions, resulting in masses of eosinophilic material occupying the area of several lobules. In this latter case, the hyalinized masses may be connected to Bowman's capsule via a connective tissue bridge that occludes a part of the urinary space (Fig. 4–6). Occasionally, synechiae are outlined by visceral epithelial cells, and the adjacent Bowman's capsule cells are prominent, giving the false impression that this is a localized crescent. Bowman's capsule is usually multilaminated in the immediate vicinity of the

bridge (synechia) between the glomerular vascular loops and the capsule. The rest of the capsule may be normal. This finding is so characteristic that the presence of localized multilaminations in a section suggests that a synechia exists in the glomerulus, even though it may not be seen in the section under examination (Fig. 4–7).

In the affected glomeruli, there appears to be a clear-cut line of demarcation between the affected and nonaffected segments. Whether the rest of the "normal" glomerulus contains normal cells and extracellular matrix awaits the development of more sensitive methods of analysis. The segmental lesions may affect the vascular pole, but they are otherwise randomly distributed throughout the glomerular tufts. It is our impression that synechiae are often located in the vicinity of the urinary pole. This has been referred to as the "tip" lesion and has been described as a separate lesion, a conclusion that has not been fully documented (Fig. 4–8). The podocytes and occasionally the mesangial cells in this area contain lipid vacuoles. The tip lesion may be the only abnormality in some cases, and patients with this lesion appear to follow a course similar to that of others with focal and segmental glomerulosclerosis.

Finally, the proportion of affected glomeruli and the extension of the lesions within the

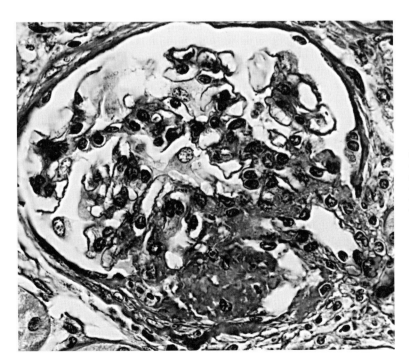

Figure 4–5. Focal segmental glomerulosclerosis. There is an area of hyalinosis with an adjacent synechia. Bowman's capsular basement membrane is multilaminated in the area of the synechia. The adjacent loops appear unremarkable. (Periodic acid–Schiff, ×630.)

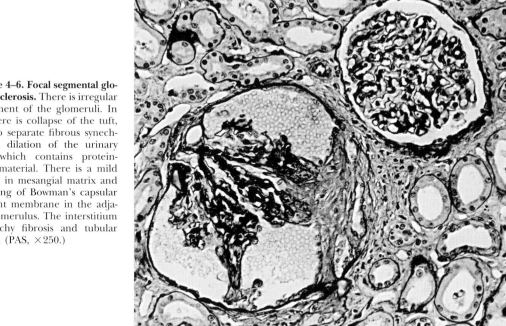

Figure 4–6. Focal segmental glomerulosclerosis. There is irregular involvement of the glomeruli. In one, there is collapse of the tuft, with two separate fibrous synechiae and dilation of the urinary space, which contains proteinaceous material. There is a mild increase in mesangial matrix and thickening of Bowman's capsular basement membrane in the adjacent glomerulus. The interstitium has patchy fibrosis and tubular atrophy. (PAS, ×250.)

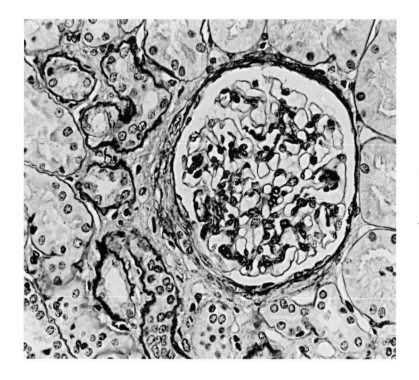

Figure 4–7. Focal segmental glomerulosclerosis. Early lesion showing segmental thickening of Bowman's capsule basement membrane and an increase in the adjacent mesangial matrix. (PAS, ×250.)

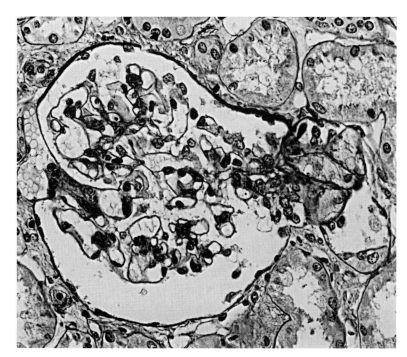

Figure 4–8. Focal segmental glomerulosclerosis, tip lesion. The urinary pole is the site of several foam cells that lie within the loops in a synechia. (PAS, ×400.)

individual glomeruli require an adequate sample. Based on autopsy cases, Rich (see reference 6) found that the lesion preferentially affects the juxtamedullary glomeruli. This pattern has not been established as a necessary condition to make the histologic diagnosis, but it is often difficult to state precisely the anatomic localization of glomeruli in biopsy specimens. The glomeruli appear hypertrophic. Some pathologists using morphometric techniques have postulated that there is a subgroup of patients, with minimal changes and large glomeruli, who will develop overt focal sclerosis. As the lesion progresses, it has been thought that the sclerotic lesions enlarge and obliterate progressively larger areas of the tuft. In areas adjacent to the sclerotic zones, the mesangial areas may be seen to be thickened.

The presence of one or a few isolated obsolescent glomeruli in a biopsy specimen has led some to append the diagnosis of "global sclerosis." Whether this represents a subset of focal glomerular sclerosis is open to question. When patients have advanced renal failure, most glomeruli may appear obsolescent. In these patients, there is clear evidence of the underlying focal sclerosing process in the remaining glomeruli. The areas of hyalinosis tend to persist even when the basic architecture of the tufts has been extensively modified by scarring.

The interstitium shows irregular areas of fibrosis, which may contain mononuclear inflammatory cells. One commonly finds small aggregates of foam cells in association with these interstitial lesions. Foam cells, once thought to be a marker of hereditary nephritis, seem rather to reflect the presence of proteinuria.

The tubules show focal atrophy with localized thickening of their basement membranes. These changes coincide with the interstitial lesions (see Fig. 4–7). In some instances, these foci of atrophy provide the only clue to the presence of focal glomerulosclerosis. Thus, the presence of tubulointerstitial changes around a glomerulus should lead one to examine multiple additional sections in a search for a focal and segmental glomerular lesion.

Protein, granular, and red blood cell casts in the tubules are common, but if proteinaceous casts are extremely large and prominent, causing massive dilation of tubules, one should think of human immunodeficiency virus (HIV) infection or heroin nephropathy. As in other glomerular lesions, the state of the interstitial change is the compartment most closely correlated with the glomerular filtration rate.

The blood vessel lesions parallel the glomerular changes. The arterioles and the juxtaglomerular vasculature often show hyalinosis or so-called fibrinoid material resembling that in the glomeruli. Duplication and thickening of the elastic laminae of the middle-sized arteries is common, as is smooth cell hyperplasia. These changes often herald hypertension.

Immunofluorescence Microscopy

The glomeruli do not contain significant amounts of immunoglobulin, complement components, or fibrin except for the areas of sclerosis. In the sclerotic areas, one finds large aggregates of IgM that are often seen in combination with C3 (Fig. 4–9). C1q is also common in these areas. Bowman's capsule and tubular basement membranes may also contain irregular aggregates of C3. The membrane attack complex antigens of the complement proteins are invariably present in the areas of sclerosis, and some report that these areas also contain IgG. The arterioles often contain IgM and C3 (a common finding in many arteriolar diseases).

Some patients also have minute, comma-like IgM deposits in the mesangial areas. It is difficult to delineate the difference between these minimal deposits and the larger deposits present in the so-called IgM mesangial nephropathy. Small, granular deposits of C3 may codistribute with the IgM, but they are also very discrete.

Electron Microscopy

In the nonsclerotic areas, there may be some degree of epithelial change characterized by irregular flattening and widening of the pedicels. The cytoplasm of the podocytes contains an increased number of organelles of various types and frequently has large empty vacuoles, leading some to say that there are "pseudocysts" in the cells. The peripheral areas of sclerosis are characterized by an increase in the amount of extracellular material that seems to envelop and encase the peripheral basement membrane. One is often able to recognize the original glomerular basement membrane as a wrinkled, dark structure within the sclerotic zone. In the area of a synechia, this matrix meets and fuses with the thickened Bowman's capsule (Fig. 4–10). Thus, the new mass of extracellular material forms the bridge between the glomerular tuft and the capsule, rather than the original basement membrane of either structure. The glomerular basement membranes near the mesangial regions are frequently wrinkled and present a corrugated, thickened, and contracted appearance. The sclerotic zones in the mesangium are generally hypocellular and contain cellular debris resembling fragments of double-layered cell membranes (Fig. 4–11). The vascular spaces in these regions are compromised by this sclerotic process. The endothelial cell cytoplasm adjacent to the sclerotic zones is thickened,

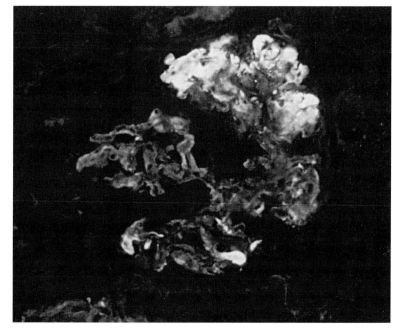

Figure 4–9. Focal segmental glomerulosclerosis. There are large, coarsely granular, local IgM aggregates in the sclerotic areas, as well as less intensely staining deposits in the rest of the mesangial areas. (Immunofluorescence micrograph, ×400.)

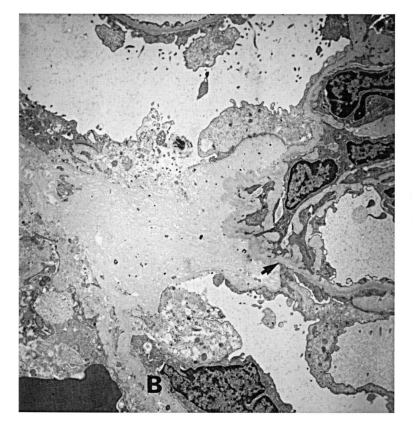

Figure 4–10. Focal segmental glomerulosclerosis. A synechia formsa bridge between the basement membrane of Bowman's capsule *(B)*, and the collapsed glomerular tuft *(arrow)*. (Electron micrograph, ×1500.)

Figure 4–11. Focal segmental glomerulosclerosis. The mesangial matrix and cellularity are increased. The podocytes show complete foot process effacement *(arrows)* and cytoplasmic swelling. (Electron micrograph, ×1600.)

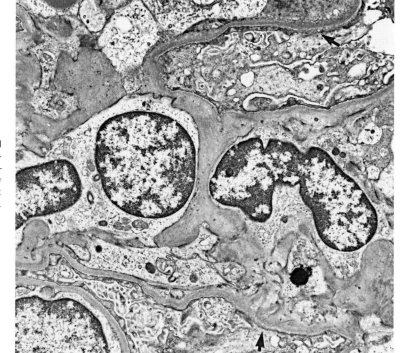

contains many cytoplasmic organelles, and frequently lacks fenestrae.

Prognosis

Although there are few long-term studies in patients with isolated proteinuria and focal sclerosis, the prognosis is quite good in the absence of the nephrotic syndrome. In the presence of the nephrotic syndrome, the prognosis can best be determined by the response to corticosteroids. In children, who have a prompt response, the outcome approaches that in the minimal lesion group. Those who are steroid resistant or steroid dependent may develop progressively worsening renal function. The use of cyclosporine has brought little change in the prognosis, although the preliminary data are quite promising. In adults, Cameron (see textbook list) has reported that approximately one half of patients will develop chronic glomerulonephritis within 10 years. Some investigators have identified a subgroup of these patients who pursue a course of rapid progression to end stage. The glomerular lesions in this group are quite severe, hyalin deposits are conspicuous, and it may be difficult to be sure that the underlying lesion was focal.

COLLAPSING GLOMERULOPATHY

Collapsing glomerulopathy, initially described in patients with HIV nephropathy, was recently reported in several adult patients without evidence of HIV infection or intravenous drug abuse. The disease consists of glomerular capillary collapse of varying severity, with wrinkling of the basement membranes and podocyte hyperplasia and hypertrophy.

The etiology of this syndrome is unknown, but the clinical characteristics differ somewhat from those of the usual form of focal and segmental glomerulosclerosis. It has been reported only in adults, predominantly black men. The clinical manifestations are extremely severe, and most patients present with severe hypertension and a full-blown nephrotic syndrome. Anorexia and fever are often associated with these symptoms, but so far tests for AIDS have been negative in these patients. Other systemic symptoms may also accompany the renal symptoms, such as diarrhea, dyspnea, arthalgias, and rash. The search for viruses other than HIV has been negative. The outcome is very poor, and most patients reach end-stage renal failure within 15 months, regardless of therapy. Thus the presentation is quite similar to that of HIV nephropathy.

Histology

Light Microscopy

The principal lesion is glomerular capillary collapse, which can be segmental or diffuse but usually affects large areas of the glomeruli (Fig. 4–12). The basement membranes are massively wrinkled, and there is gradual oblit-

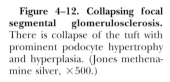

Figure 4–12. Collapsing focal segmental glomerulosclerosis. There is collapse of the tuft with prominent podocyte hypertrophy and hyperplasia. (Jones methenamine silver, ×500.)

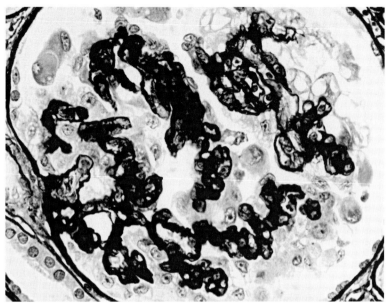

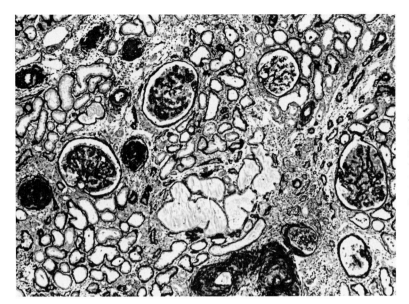

Figure 4–13. Collapsing focal segmental glomerulosclerosis. The collapsed loops completely obliterate the vascular spaces. There is marked hyperplasia of the glomerular visceral epithelial cells, with the formation of synechiae. The tubules are severely affected, with some showing cystic dilatation. (Jones methenamine silver, ×80.)

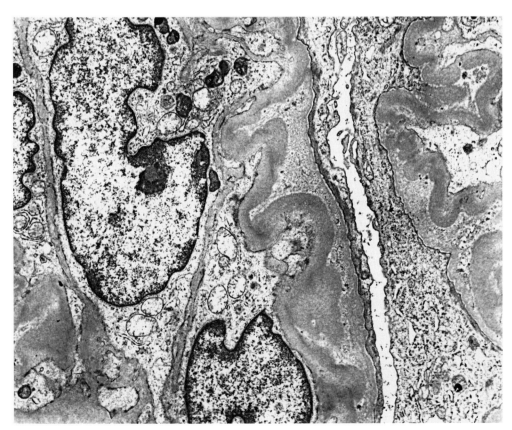

Figure 4–14. Collapsing focal segmental glomerulosclerosis. The tufts are obliterated and the lamina densa is wrinkled. Podocyte hypertrophy and effacement of the foot processes are evident. There are no tubuloreticular inclusions. (Electron micrograph, ×3500.)

eration of the lumina. It is interesting that there is atrophy or even disappearance of the endothelial or mesangial cells, giving the tuft a simplified appearance reminiscent of that seen in ischemic glomeruli. However, distinct visceral epithelial cell abnormalities are present that are not present in chronic ischemic lesions. These epithelial lesions are conspicuous and constitute one of the hallmarks of the disease. They consist of considerable cytoplasmic swelling, large hyalin cytoplasmic droplets, and marked vacuolization of the cytoplasm. In most cases these lesions are associated with podocyte hyperplasia that may resemble crescents, although there is no parietal cell proliferation. In occasional cases, the nuclei are enlarged, hyperchromatic, and irregular in shape and contain large nucleoli.

The nonaffected areas show little or no mesangial sclerosis. Finally, at late stages there is considerable global sclerosis. Another feature that differs from focal sclerosis is that the lesions do not predominate in the vascular pole but are randomly distributed.

Tubular lesions are conspicuous and consist of vacuoles, epithelial atrophy, and considerable dilation with large, proteinaceous casts (Fig. 4–13). The interstitium contains large cellular infiltrates that are particularly rich in leukocytes. Interstitial sclerosis becomes prominent when the lesions progress and is accompanied by severe tubular atrophy. Sclerotic changes are often found in both arterioles and mid-sized arteries.

Immunofluorescence Microscopy

By immunofluorescence microscopy the pattern is that of focal and segmental glomerulosclerosis with patches of C3 and IgM staining.

Electron Microscopy

Electron microscopy largely confirms the light and immunofluorescence microscopic lesions of collapse and wrinkling of the glomerular basement membranes (Fig. 4–14). The pedicels are effaced, and subepithelial spaces are filled with a flocculent, electron-lucent material. Note the absence of deposits. Endothelial tubuloreticular inclusions, so common in AIDS nephropathy, are rarely present.

The visceral epithelial cells contain large cytoplasmic vacuoles or inclusions. In addition, nuclear abnormalities, such as nuclear

inclusions or condensation of nuclear chromatin, are frequent.

SELECTED READINGS

1. Border WA: Distinguishing minimal change disease from mesangial disorders (nephrology forum). Kidney Int 34:419, 1988.
2. Churg J, Habib R, White RMR: Pathology of the nephrotic syndrome in children. A report of the international study of kidney disease in children. Lancet 1:1299, 1970.
3. Cortes L, Tejani A: Dilemma of focal segmental sclerosis. Kidney Int 49:s-57, 1996.
4. D'Agati V: The many masks of focal segmental glomerulosclerosis. Kidney Int 46:1223, 1994.
5. Detwiler RK, Falk RJ, Hogan SL, Jennette JC: Collapsing glomerulopathy: A clinically and pathologically distinct variant of focal segmental glomerulosclerosis. Kidney Int 45:1416, 1994.
6. Habib R: Focal glomerular sclerosis. Kidney Int 4:355, 1973.
7. Jao W, Pollak VE, Noraris SH, et al: Lipoid nephrosis: An approach to the clinicopathologic analysis and dismemberment of idiopathic nephrotic syndrome with minimal glomerular changes. Medicine 52:445, 1973.
8. Korbet SM, Schwartz MM, Lewis EJ: Primary focal segmental glomerulosclerosis: Clinical course and response to therapy. Am J Kidney Dis 23:773, 1994.
9. Schwartz MM, Korbet SM: Primary focal segmental glomerulosclerosis: Pathology, histological variants and pathogenesis. Am J Kidney Dis 22:874, 1993.
10. Schwartz MM, Lewis EJ: Focal segmental glomerular sclerosis: The cellular lesion. Kidney Int 28:968, 1985.
11. Velosa J, Glasser RJ, Nevins TE, Michael AF: Experimental model of focal sclerosis: II. Correlation with immunopathologic changes, macromolecular kinetics and polyanion loss. Lab Invest 36:527, 1977.
12. Whitworth JA, Turner DR, Leibowitz S, et al: Focal segmental sclerosis or scarred focal proliferative glomerulonephritis. Clin Nephrol 9:229, 1978.

MESANGIAL PROLIFERATIVE DISEASE

This category of renal disease is clinically indistinguishable from minimal change. The age, sex, and prior history of this group of patients are identical to those in patients with minimal change. The only feature that may be useful in making a distinction is that these patients may, at onset or soon thereafter, require continuous steroid therapy to maintain their urine protein-free.

This category represents a mixed group of diseases sharing the common features of mild mesangial proliferation, often coexisting with IgM deposits in the mesangial regions. Some researchers do not believe that this is a sepa-

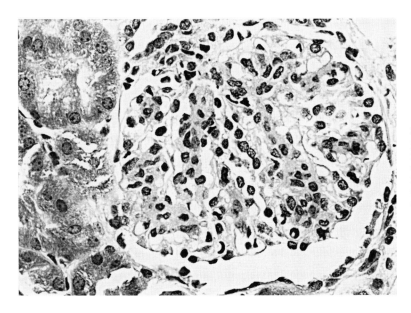

Figure 4–15. Diffuse mesangial hypercellularity in idiopathic nephrotic syndrome. There is a marked, global increase in the number of mesangial cells. The mesangial matrix, tuft lumina, and basement membranes are not affected. (H&E, ×500.)

rate diagnostic entity and group it with minimal change nephrotic syndrome.

Histology

Light Microscopy

The mesangial regions are uniformly but moderately more prominent than normal. This change appears to be principally the result of an increase in the number of cells (Fig. 4–15). Mesangial nodules are not seen, and the glomerular extracellular matrix appears normal in both the mesangial and peripheral basement membrane zones.

Immunofluorescence Microscopy

In contrast to minimal change, in this disease immune deposits are clearly evident. As seen by light microscopy, the lesions are limited to the mesangial regions. Deposits of IgM

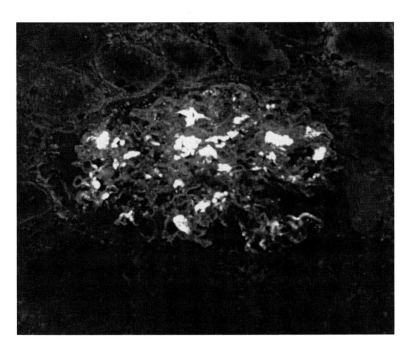

Figure 4–16. Diffuse mesangial hypercellularity in idiopathic nephrotic syndrome. Global, coarsely granular IgM deposits are restricted to the mesangium. (Immunofluorescence micrograph, ×250.)

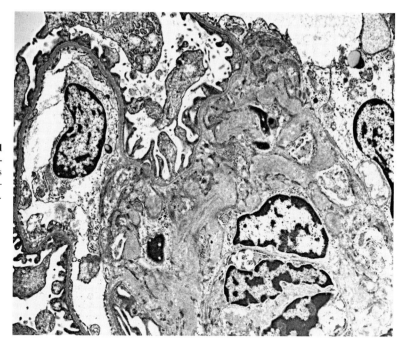

Figure 4–17. Diffuse mesangial hypercellularity in idiopathic nephrotic syndrome. The pedicels are locally effaced, and the mesangial matrix is increased in amount. (Electron micrograph, ×1500.)

and sometimes of C3 are present in each mesangial region, and all glomeruli are affected (Fig. 4–16). In fact, were it not for the immunofluorescence findings, it would be possible to overlook the light microscopic changes and conclude that the disease belongs to the minimal change category.

Electron Microscopy

The visceral epithelial cell pedicels are widened, and in several areas are effaced in a manner approaching that seen in minimal change (Fig. 4–17). Nonetheless, the pattern of the alterations of the pedicels is not as uniform and diffuse as in minimal change. The epithelial cell cytoplasm contains many vacuoles, as well as an increased number of other intracellular organelles. The plasma membranes on the urinary surface show villous transformation.

The mesangial regions contain easily detectable electron-dense deposits within the extracellular matrix. No other changes are visible.

Prognosis

The outcome in this disease is not well established. A number of reports lump these patients together with those who have minimal change. However, in the many series that separate the patients by category, only 30 to 50% of patients with mesangial changes achieve complete remission with steroid therapy. In addition, most investigators agree that this group of patients has an increased risk of developing focal and segmental glomerulosclerosis and subsequent renal functional deterioration.

SELECTED READINGS

1. Border WA: Distinguishing minimal-change disease from mesangial disorders. Kidney Int 34:419, 1988.
2. Brown EA, Upadhyaya K, Hayslett JP: The clinical course of mesangial proliferative glomerulonephritis. Medicine 58:295, 1979.
3. Cohen AH, Border WA, Glassock RJ: Nephrotic syndrome with glomerular mesangial IgM deposits. Lab Invest 38:610, 1978.
4. International Study of Kidney Disease in Children: Primary nephrotic syndrome in children: Clinical significance of histopathologic variants of minimal change and of diffuse mesangial hypercellularity. Kidney Int 20:765, 1981.
5. Southwest Pediatric Nephrology Study Group: Childhood nephrotic syndrome associated with diffuse mesangial hypercellularity. Kidney Int 24:87, 1983.
6. Trompeter RS, Lloyd BW, Hicks J, et al: Long-term outcome for children with minimal change nephrotic syndrome. Lancet 1:368, 1985.
7. Waldherr R, Gubler MC, Levy M, et al: The significance of pure diffuse mesangial proliferation in idiopathic nephrotic syndrome. Clin Nephrol 10:171, 1978.

MEMBRANOUS GLOMERULONEPHRITIS

The term *membranous nephropathy* (also called membranous, epimembranous, or extramembranous glomerulonephritis) designates a morphologic entity characterized by the presence of immune deposits distributed uniformly along the outer aspects of the glomerular basement membranes. This lesion, the most common glomerular pattern observed in adult patients with the nephrotic syndrome, may also be found in association with systemic diseases (e.g., systemic lupus erythematosus), viral hepatitis B or C, toxins such as heavy metals, and exposure to certain drugs such as penicillamine and gold salts (Table 4–2).

Pathogenesis

It is now thought that this glomerular disease results from the formation of immune deposits on the epithelial aspects of the glomerular basement membrane. It has been postulated that antibodies, mostly of the IgG class, react with an antigen present on the podocytes. This conclusion is based on studies of a rat model (Heymann's nephritis). The immune deposits in this model consist of IgG antibodies that have been shown to react with an antigen present on the pedicels of the rat podocyte. Antibody bound to the podocyte membranes induces complement activation, likely via the alternative complement pathway. The presence and nature of a locally synthesized glomerular antigen have not been demonstrated in humans. Proteinuria is a complement-dependent phenomenon and requires activation of the terminal complement components. This activation may lead to oxidant production by the podocytes and result in the alteration in glomerular basement membrane permeability that leads to proteinuria.

The localization of antibodies to the subepithelial space might be predisposed to by antigens that arrive passively and become fixed or "planted" because of the physical characteristics of the antigen. For instance, materials could be localized to the subepithelial space on the basis of charge selectivity. These antigens are responsible for the in situ formation of immune complexes. A potential role for complement in the induction of proteinuria has been demonstrated in several animal models but remains unproved in humans.

Thus the experimental models have shown that membranous glomerulonephritis can occur as the consequence of immune complexes formed locally along the glomerular walls. The antigen has been shown either to derive from the circulation or to be a biosynthetic product of the cells abutting the glomerular basement membrane. The antigens derived from the circulation arrive at the subepithelial site either because of the hemodynamic forces operative within the glomerulus or as a consequence of the size and charge of the antigen, or both. The result is that the number of antigens that can lead to this anatomic localization is quite diverse, and the morphologic pattern is representative but not diagnostic of a particular etiology. For instance, several putative antigens have been suggested to play a pathogenetic role, including DNA in systemic lupus erythematosus. Other antigens have been demonstrated in a few clinical syndromes: thyroid antigens in patients with autoimmune thyroiditis, hepatitis virus–associated antigens (HBsAg, HBe antigen), tumor antigens (carcinoembryonic antigen), parasite or fungal antigens (*Treponema, Schistosoma,* and *Echinococcus*), and antigens belonging to the coagulation cascade.

The exact role that each antigen might play and the frequency of their association with either the underlying disease or with the syndrome of membranous glomerulonephritis remains to be proved, and the etiologic factors

Table 4–2. Membranous Glomerulonephritis

Idiopathic
Secondary to toxins
  Gold
  Bismuth
  Mercury
  Silver
Drug-induced
  Penicillamine
  Nonsteroidal anti-inflammatory agents
  Captopril
Associated with other diseases
  Systemic lupus erythematosus (and mixed connective
    tissue disease)
  Autoimmune thyroiditis
  Sickle cell disease
  Sarcoidosis
  Myasthenia gravis
  Carcinoma
Infections
  Syphilis
  Schistosomiasis
  Filariasis
  Hepatitis B
  Hepatitis C

remain largely undetermined. Thus, this syndrome remains in the category of idiopathic diseases.

Patient Presentation

Membranous glomerulonephritis is the most common entity in adult patients who present with the nephrotic syndrome. It is also present in children but is a less common cause of the nephrotic syndrome. This lesion may spontaneously regress in children, but this outcome is less common in adults.

The proportion of patients with membranous glomerulonephritis in a group of nephrotic adults seems to vary with the geographic location of the survey and with the clinical use of renal biopsy in the evaluation of the nephrotic syndrome. It should be remembered that a significant percentage of patients with membranous glomerulonephritis have an underlying extrarenal disease or have been exposed to toxins. Thus the clinical manifestations of the primary process may overshadow or mask the renal lesion.

Membranous glomerulonephritis is most frequently found after the third decade of life. Proteinuria is more or less constantly present in membranous glomerulonephritis and is often associated with the nephrotic syndrome. Microscopic hematuria and hypertension are also common. Renal failure may occur as the disease progresses but is seldom found as the presenting problem, and this lesion is not a common cause of end-stage renal failure. Serum complement levels are normal, and cryoglobulin levels remain at normal levels in the serum unless there is an associated disease.

Histology

Light Microscopy

The glomeruli are large, and the lesions are homogeneous and diffuse. There is no cellular proliferation. The principal finding is a uniform, diffuse thickening of the peripheral glomerular vascular wall. For this reason, the lesion was initially given the name membranous glomerulonephritis. The other names coined in Europe include extramembranous or epimembranous glomerulonephritis and are better descriptors of the underlying abnormalities. The lesion is almost always restricted to the glomerular basement membranes. Examination of the basement membranes by periodic acid–Schiff (PAS) or silver stains reveals regular subepithelial spikelike projections of the glomerular basement membrane, between which are deposits of proteinaceous material. The overlying visceral epithelial cells are not conspicuous, except for the occasional presence of cytoplasmic protein–containing droplets. As the lesion evolves, the "spikes" progress from being just detectable to becoming progressively larger and eventually occupying the entire subepithelial space as a broad band of extracellular matrix with substantial distortion of the glomerular architecture. This transition has been arbitrarily divided into four stages:

STAGE 1

Light Microscopy. The vascular walls may appear normal by hematoxylin and eosin (H& E) and PAS stains, but fine stippling of a widened subepithelial space may be appreciated by silver stains because the subepithelial deposits are not stained and thus appear as negative images (Fig. 4–18). This change does not affect all vascular loops uniformly, and the change may be missed by light microscopy.

Immunofluorescence Microscopy. However,

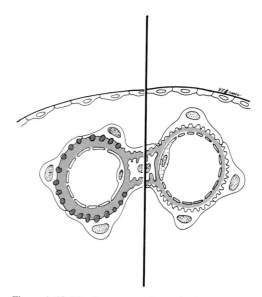

Figure 4–18. Membranous nephropathy. Diagram of the Stage I lesion. There are multiple small subepithelial deposits. The epithelial cells cover both the deposits and the "spikes" of glomerular basement membrane that lie between the deposits. The endothelial cells, the mesangium, and the lumen are not affected.

at this stage, the changes are easily detectable by immunofluorescence microscopy.

Electron Microscopy. The subepithelial deposits are small and indistinct and may appear to be concentrated under the slit diaphragms. The lamina densa often appears normal, and the spikes are not conspicuous. The epithelial cell cytoplasm changes are often quite prominent, with an increased number of cytoplasmic organelles and broadened pedicels containing an accumulation of microfilaments near the deposits (Fig. 4–19).

STAGE 2

Light Microscopy. Diffuse, uniform thickening of the peripheral vascular wall is present in every glomerulus (Fig. 4–20). The peripheral basement membranes are diffusely thickened, and there are uniform, globally distributed subepithelial spikes (Figs. 4–21, 4–22).

Immunofluorescence Microscopy. The deposits are readily apparent in Stage 2 (Fig. 4–23), as they were in Stage 1. They consist of IgG (C3 is present in 20 to 40%) distributed in a regular, granular pattern over the epithelial aspects of the glomerular basement membrane; they are more easily seen at high power to be finely granular (Fig. 4–24). The mesangial regions are unaffected, unless there is an associated systemic disease, such as systemic lupus erythematosus. Granular deposits of IgA and IgM are occasionally found, but they are always in lesser amounts than IgG. Note that the mesangial regions are unaffected.

Electron Microscopy. The subepithelial deposits and the subepithelial spikes are regularly spaced as well as relatively uniform in size and shape. The cytoplasm of the visceral epithelial cells is prominent and contains many organelles. The pedicels are broadened and irregular in width. The mesangial regions remain unremarkable.

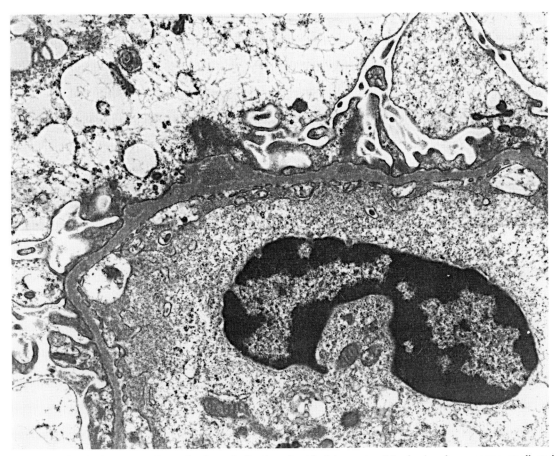

Figure 4–19. Membranous nephropathy, Stage 1. On the subepithelial aspects of the lamina densa, sparse, small, and irregularly shaped deposits are found. (Electron micrograph, ×7100.)

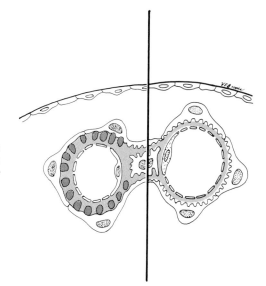

Figure 4–20. Membranous nephropathy. Diagram of the Stage 2 lesion. The subepithelial deposits are larger, and have been partially incorporated within the substance of the thickened glomerular basement membranes.

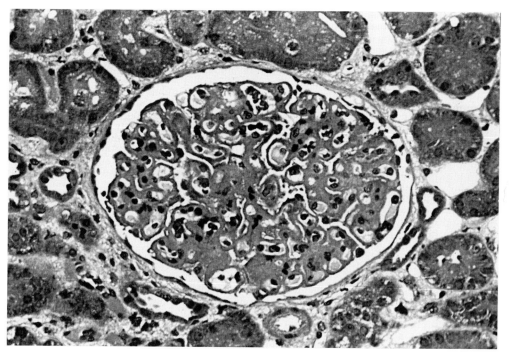

Figure 4–21. Membranous nephropathy, Stage 2. The major histologic change is diffuse thickening of the basement membranes, which gives the impression that the membranes are "stiff." Silver staining is necessary to reveal the spikes and deposits. (H&E, ×300.)

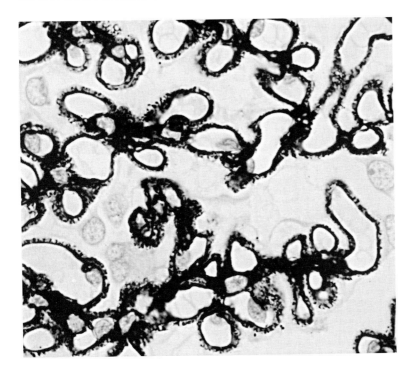

Figure 4–22. Membranous nephropathy, Stage 2. Silver methenamine stain demonstrating well-developed subepithelial spikes that are regular in distribution. (Periodic acid–silver methenamine, ×1000.)

STAGE 3

Light Microscopy. The peripheral glomerular vascular walls are uniformly and diffusely thickened. At this stage, the spikes are thickened and in many regions may have fused. The end result is that there may be an irregularly thickened peripheral basement membrane without clear spike formation (Fig. 4–25).

Immunofluorescence Microscopy. The deposits become progressively larger and more sparsely distributed as they are displaced and incorporated into the increasing quantities of

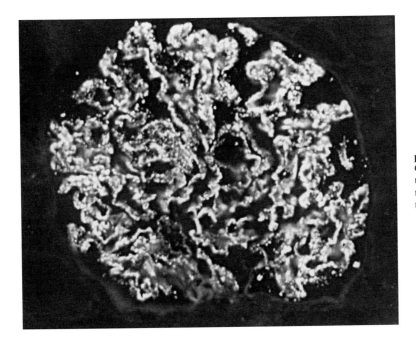

Figure 4–23. Membranous nephropathy, Stage 2 or Stage 3. Granular deposits of IgG covering the epithelial aspect of the basement membrane. (Immunofluorescence micrograph, ×250.)

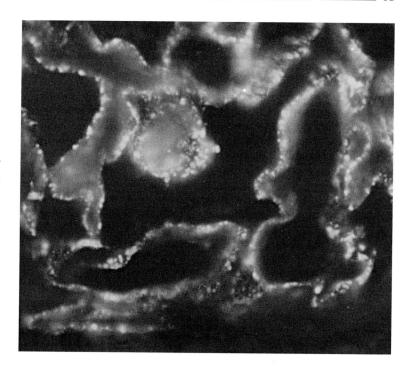

Figure 4–24. Membranous nephropathy, Stage 2. At high-power, the finely granular quality of the IgG deposits are apparent. (Immunofluorescence micrograph, × 1000.)

basement membrane. The deposits may persist in the obsolescent glomeruli.

C4 and C1q are not usually present in idiopathic membranous glomerulonephritis and, if present, warrant a search for systemic lupus erythematosus.

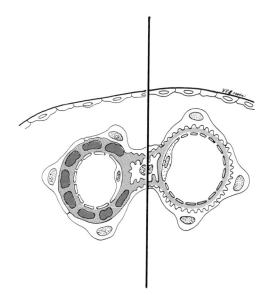

Figure 4–25. Membranous nephropathy. Diagram of the Stage 3 lesion. The deposits are surrounded and partially incorporated within the glomerular basement membranes. The mesangial regions are normal.

Electron Microscopy. The lamina densa is markedly thickened and irregular in contour. Electron-dense deposits are found within the thickened lamina densa as well as on its epithelial aspects. The visceral epithelial cells are similar in appearance to Stage 2, but the pedicels are even more irregular (Fig. 4–26).

STAGE 4

Light Microscopy. Many glomeruli are obsolescent in this stage. The glomeruli remain large even when obsolescent, and the underlying thickened basement membranes may still be appreciated by PAS or silver stains (Fig. 4–27). The nonobsolescent glomeruli are very sclerotic, and the deposits may be difficult to discern. Thus, it may be difficult to determine the nature of the disease except for the fact that the peripheral basement membranes are quite thickened.

Other lesions may be associated with the membranous deposits, especially when the disease progresses. Areas of focal hyalinosis or sclerosis with synechiae may herald progression. In rare instances, crescents, usually segmental and small, have been reported.

The tubules and the interstitium are not affected early in the disease except for evidence of a large glomerular protein leak. Later, as the number of obsolescent glomeruli

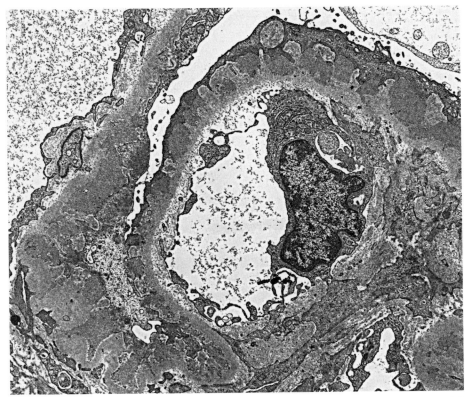

Figure 4–26. Membranous nephropathy, Stage 2 lesion. The deposits are larger and more uniform and lie between large subepithelial spikes of lamina densa. The foot processes are completely effaced. (Electron micrograph, ×7500.)

increases, nephron loss becomes evident because of tubular atrophy and interstitial fibrosis.

Vascular lesions are not a primary feature of this disease but instead parallel the stage of the disease or the age of the patient.

Electron Microscopy. The lamina densa is diffusely and markedly thickened (Figs. 4–28,

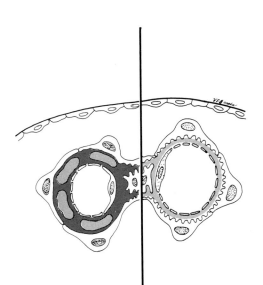

Figure 4–27. Membranous nephropathy. Diagram of the Stage 4 lesion. The basement membranes are massively thickened. The deposits are almost completely incorporated within the lamina densa.

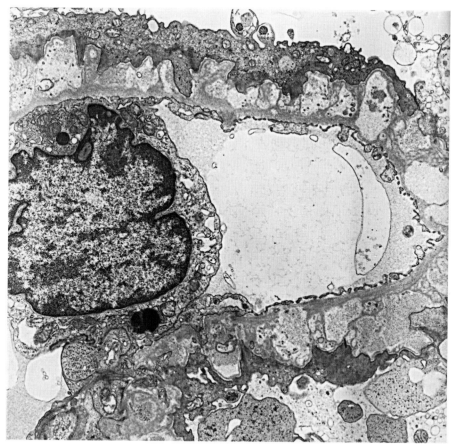

Figure 4–28. Membranous nephropathy, late Stage 4 lesion. Many of the deposits have completely, or partially, disappeared and are replaced by an electron-lucent material. The glomerular basement membranes outline these areas. (Electron micrograph, ×7500.)

4–29). Electron-dense deposits are much less frequently encountered than in Stage 3; they are instead thought largely to disappear, leaving lucent areas within the basement membranes (Fig. 4–29).

Associations with Other Diseases, Drugs, and Toxins

Systemic Lupus Erythematosus
(see Chapter 6)

Membranous glomerulonephritis is present in less than 10% of systemic lupus erythematosus–associated glomerular disease. The epimembranous deposits are most often found in association with deposits in the subendothelial or mesangial spaces and/or with mesangial hypercellularity. The presence of mesangial lesions should lead one to suspect the presence of systemic lupus erythematosus in a biopsy sample thought to represent membranous glomerulonephritis.

Immunofluorescence microscopic examination reveals diffuse, regular, and granular deposits of IgG along the peripheral aspects of the glomerular basement membranes. Deposits may also be found in the mesangial areas, along tubular basement membranes, and along the intertubular capillaries. Complement components are invariably found, and C1q and C4 often codistribute with IgG. Other immunoglobulins, IgA and IgM, may also be conspicuous components of the glomerular deposits.

Rheumatoid Arthritis

The association between rheumatoid arthritis and membranous glomerulonephritis is very tenuous. We, along with others, believe that when membranous glomerulonephritis is

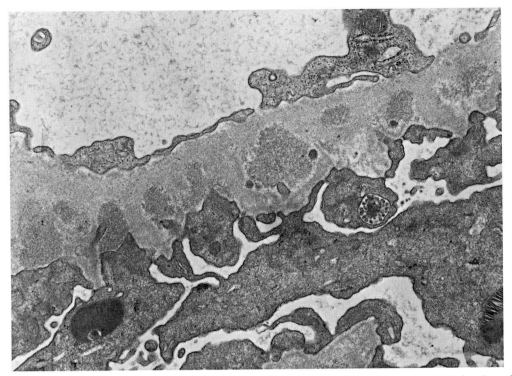

Figure 4–29. Membranous nephropathy, Stage 4 lesion. The basement membranes are markedly, but irregularly, thickened. The electron-dense deposits are surrounded by lamina densa. (Electron micrograph, ×3000.)

found in patients with rheumatoid arthritis, the renal disease is secondary to drug therapy. The drugs most commonly associated with membranous glomerulonephritis in these patients are penicillamine and gold salts.

Infectious and Parasitic Diseases

Membranous glomerulonephritis has been associated with certain viral, infectious, and parasitic diseases. Hepatitis B and C have been incriminated in an increasing number of cases. The bacterial and parasitic diseases most often implicated include syphilis, schistosomiasis, hydatidosis, and filariasis.

Drugs

The occurrence of membranous glomerulonephritis as an adverse reaction to drug therapy is well documented. In general, the clinical course is benign, because the glomerulonephritis most often reverses when the drug is withdrawn. The presence of a free sulfhydryl group is the most common chemical structural correlate (e.g., in antihypertensive agents, penicillamines, and so on), but nonsteroidal anti-

inflammatory agents have also been reported as causal agents.

Heavy metals associated with membranous glomerulonephritis include gold, lead, and mercury. Silver and bismuth have only rarely been reported.

Renal Vein Thrombosis

The occurrence of renal vein thrombosis in patients with membranous glomerulonephritis has been reported to be more common than can be attributed to chance alone. Several findings should lead one to suspect this diagnosis: interstitial edema, dilation of the peritubular capillaries, and the presence of leukocytes in distended glomerular capillaries (Fig. 4–30). These morphologic features are far from specific and should be regarded as nothing more than suggestive unless there are strong clinical reasons to suggest an association.

Prognosis

The prognosis in primary membranous nephropathy has recently been shown to be

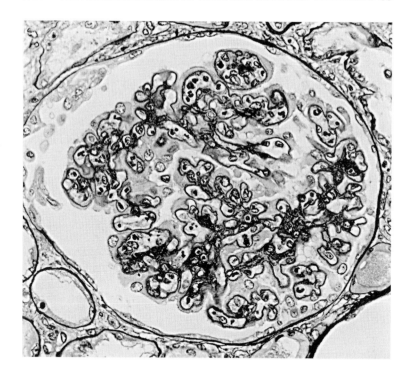

Figure 4–30. Membranous nephropathy, renal vein thrombosis. The basement membranes are uniformly but mildly thickened. The dilated vascular spaces contain marginated neutrophils. There is marked visceral glomerular epithelial cell hypertrophy. (PAS, ×250.)

much more favorable than previously thought. Complete remission of the nephrotic syndrome and, less commonly, of proteinuria may spontaneously occur in nearly 50% of the cases. However, in those patients who do progress, the rate at which renal function declines may be very rapid, with end-stage renal disease being reached in 2 to 5 years. At present, it is not possible to determine which course an individual patient will follow. However, certain features suggest a benign course, including younger age, female sex, absence of the nephrotic syndrome, and the presence of normal renal function and normal blood pressure. In addition, the presence of a spontaneous remission, even if partial or followed by a relapse, signals a benign course. Finally, the presence in the urine of excessive amounts of C5b-C9 complexes (membrane attack) may also be a sign that the patient is at risk of progressive renal function deterioration.

There have been reports that therapy with oral corticosteroids results in amelioration of the nephrotic syndrome, and some groups now use them routinely. Recent reports bring this practice into sharp question. The use of azathioprine has been reported as primary therapy or for its "steroid-sparing" effect, but its use is not currently widespread. A large Italian study suggested that the combined use of corticosteroids and chlorambucil or cyclo-

phosphamide may be the best therapy. However, the protocol is expensive and associated with side effects, and the long-term consequences are not clear. Thus, many groups begin with corticosteroids, and add the other agents if the patient shows signs of progressive renal failure.

The treatment of secondary membranous nephropathy rests solely on treatment of the underlying cause.

SELECTED READINGS

1. Cameron JS, Healy MJ, Adu D, et al: The Medical Research Council trial of short-term high-dose alternate day prednisolone in idiopathic membranous nephropathy with nephrotic syndrome in adults. Am J Med 74:133, 1990.
2. Couser WG: Mediation of immune glomerular injury (Review). J Am Soc Nephrol 1:13, 1990.
3. Doi TM, Mayumi K, Kanatsu F, et al: Distribution of IgG subclasses in membranous nephropathy. Clin Exp Immunol 58:57, 1984.
4. Forland M, Spargo BH: Clinicopathological correlations in idiopathic nephrotic syndrome with membranous nephropathy. Nephron 6:498, 1969.
5. Jennette J, Iskandar S, Dalldorf FG: Pathologic differentiation between lupus and non lupus membranous glomerulopathy. Kidney Int 24:377, 1983.
6. Noel LH, Zanetti M, Droz D, et al: Long-term prognosis of idiopathic membranous glomerulonephritis: Study of 116 untreated patients. Am J Med 66:82, 1979.

7. Ponticelli C, Zucchelli P, Passerini P, et al: Methylprednisolone plus chlorambucil as compared with methylprednisolone alone for the treatment of idiopathic membranous nephropathy. N Engl J Med 327:599, 1992.

8. Schultze M, Donadio JV Jr, Pruchno CJ, et al: Elevated urinary excretion of the C5b-9 complex in membranous nephropathy. Kidney Int 40:533, 1991.

9. Southwest Pediatric Nephrology Study Group: Comparison of idiopathic and systemic lupus erythematosus–associated membranous glomerulonephropathy in children. Am J Kidney Dis 7:115, 1986.

10. Wehrman M, Bohle A, Bogenschutz O, et al: Long-term prognosis of chronic idiopathic membranous glomerulonephritis. Clin Nephrol 31:67, 1989.

MEMBRANOPROLIFERATIVE GLOMERULONEPHRITIS AND DENSE DEPOSIT DISEASE

Membranoproliferative Glomerulonephritis

The term *membranoproliferative glomerulonephritis* refers to a histologic pattern characterized principally by an increased number of intraglomerular cells and thickening of the peripheral glomerular vascular walls. This term, widely used throughout the world, includes both diseases of unknown cause and some associated with systemic and infectious disorders. Membranoproliferative glomerulonephritis, therefore, designates a morphologic pattern that should be integrated within an etiologic context when possible (Table 4–3).

This section reviews the idiopathic forms of membranoproliferative glomerulonephritis. The most common form of secondary membranoproliferative glomerulonephritis is that associated with hepatitis C virus infection, and it is reviewed in Chapter 5. Another term commonly applied to primary membranoproliferative glomerulonephritis is *mesangiocapillary glomerulonephritis*. This name reflects the belief that abnormalities in and of the mesangium are the crucial determinants in the development of the disease process.

Pathogenesis/Classification

There are two major and distinct categories of idiopathic membranoproliferative glomerulonephritis, often referred to as types I and II. These two types are histologically separable, but their clinical features and subsequent course are identical. In the past few years, other histologic subcategories have been proposed, based on minor variants of the two

Table 4–3. Membranoproliferative Glomerulonephritis: Associated Conditions

Autoimmune
  SLE
  Sjögren
  Rheumatoid arthritis
  Complement deficiencies (inherited)
Chronic infections
  Viral hepatitis
    Viral hepatitis B
    Viral hepatitis C (with cryoglobulinemia type II, previously called mixed essential cryoglobulinemia)
  Bacterial
    Bacterial endocarditis
    Infected shunts
    Deep visceral abscesses
    Leprosy
  Protozoal infections
    Malaria
    Schistosomiasis
  Other infections
    Mycoplasma
  Other diseases
    Chronic liver diseases (cirrhosis, alpha$_1$-antitrypsin deficiency)
    Chronic thrombotic microangiopathies (and those in remission)
    HUS/TTP
    Circulating anti-phospholipid (cardiolipin) antibodies
    Radiation nephritis
    Bone marrow transplantation
    Sickle cell anemia
    Polycythemia
    Transplant glomerulopathy
    Paraproteinemia
    Cryoglobulinemia type I
    Waldenstrom macroglobulinemia
    Immunotactoid glomerulopathy
    Light-chain or heavy-chain deposition disease
    Fibrillary glomerulonephritis

major categories. Type III membranoproliferative glomerulonephritis is one of these morphologic variants. It is characterized by the association of mesangial matrix and mesangial cell increase found in type I membranoproliferative glomerulonephritis, with a large number of subepithelial deposits and spikes. We believe that further designations are unnecessary and that there is no need to add further complexity to an already confusing classification in which the histologic nuances do not have etiologic, therapeutic, or clinical outcome correlates.

In other texts, these lesions have been referred to as lobular glomerulonephritis, but this term has been replaced by the descriptor membranoproliferative glomerulonephritis in most recent communications. We therefore provide a detailed description of only two categories: type I, which is associated with splitting of the lamina densa (so-called tram tracks) and glomerular immune deposits; and type II, which is associated with dense, homogeneous deposits of material occupying and expanding the lamina densa of many renal basement membranes. Type III does not differ from type I, save for the presence of the subepithelial deposits and spikes.

Complement abnormalities are frequent in these conditions but are of different types. Patients with dense deposits (type II membranoproliferative glomerulonephritis) often show persistent C3 activation because of the presence of a circulating IgG autoantibody known as C3 nephritic factor. Patients with this factor have marked depression of C3 plasma levels, whereas the early complement components are at normal levels. The nephritic factor is rarely found in patients with type I membranoproliferative glomerulonephritis. The exact role of the complement abnormalities in these diseases is unknown, but some investigators believe that these patients have a complement deficiency that becomes clinically manifest as a glomerulonephritis.

Clarification of the pathogenesis of type II membranoproliferative glomerulonephritis has been complicated by the fact that the biochemical composition of the dense deposits remains unknown.

Both types I and II membranoproliferative glomerulonephritis were initially described in children and, although not restricted to this age group, are much more common therein.

Finally, both types are rare, and their incidence seems to have markedly decreased in the Western world over the past two decades.

Although the pathogenesis is largely unknown, recent publications suggest that hepatitis C may be responsible for a large number of type I membranoproliferative glomerulonephritis cases.

Patient Presentation

Children or adolescents are more frequently affected than adults. The nephrotic syndrome is the most common clinical presentation and is usually accompanied by changes in the urine sediment (red blood cells and red blood cell casts). Occasional patients present with macroscopic hematuria or the nephritic syndrome.

At the time of diagnosis, approximately one half of the patients have a low CH50 and C3

plasma level; C1q and C4 are borderline or slightly depressed in type I membranoproliferative glomerulonephritis and normal in type II. In families with a hereditary deficiency of complement, type I membranoproliferative glomerulonephritis has been reported in the absence of other signs of systemic disease. Finally, some patients with lipodystrophy have been reported to have type II membranoproliferative glomerulonephritis (dense deposit disease).

Histology

Light Microscopy

Type I Membranoproliferative Glomerulonephritis. The most common type of membranoproliferative glomerulonephritis is type I, which is characterized by enlarged, hypercellular glomeruli with a marked increase in extracellular matrix (Figs. 4–31 to 4–33). There often is an infiltrate of neutrophils and mononuclear inflammatory cells, although this is seldom as marked as in acute postinfectious glomerulonephritis.

The mesangial regions are the site of the most intense hypercellularity, as well as a marked increase in matrix (Fig. 4–32). The

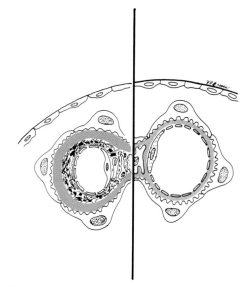

Figure 4–31. Membranoproliferative glomerulonephritis Type I. Note the markedly widened subendothelium that contains deposits, cytoplasmic extensions of adjacent cells, and a second layer of basement membrane beneath the endothelial cell layer. This has been called mesangial interposition, but the exact nature of the cells has not been established. The mesangium contains an increased number of cells as well as deposits.

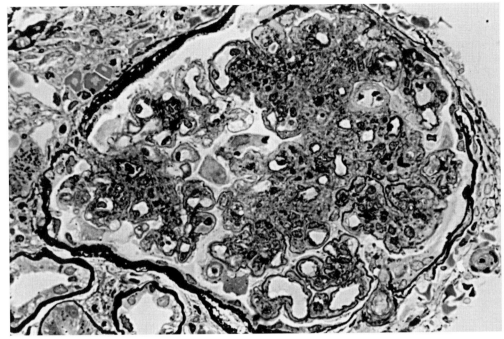

Figure 4–32. Membranoproliferative glomerulonephritis Type I. The architecture of the glomerulus is distorted by the large masses of mesangial matrix, giving it a lobular appearance. There are widespread "double-contoured" basement membranes, the so-called "tram tracks." (PASM, ×400.)

mesangial changes are diffuse and uniform and may result in an almost nodular appearance. The enlarged mesangial regions may impinge on the vascular spaces. This encroachment on the vascular spaces gives the appearance that the mesangium is growing out into the subendothelial region. The term given to this change is *mesangial interposition.*

The lamina densa is diffusely and irregularly thickened and has a double contour configuration (the so-called tram tracks) (Fig. 4–33). The width of the zone between the two lami-

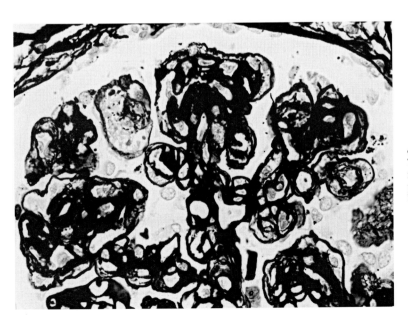

Figure 4–33. Membranoproliferative glomerulonephritis Type I. There is diffuse, global increased mesangial matrix and diffuse duplication of the basement membranes. (PASM, ×500.)

nae of the lamina densa varies widely between and within glomeruli, and irregular profiles of basement membrane may be seen bridging the space, giving it a honeycomb appearance (Fig. 4–33). There may be cytoplasmic elements between the two layers of the lamina densa, and the current belief is that they are derived from macrophages.

Endothelial cells are difficult to see by light microscopy, but they may have a swollen cytoplasm. Subendothelial or intramembranous deposits may occasionally be recognizable.

As this lesion progresses, the hypercellularity becomes less prominent and the matrix increases, resulting in a more lobular appearance. This is the stage that was previously given the name lobular glomerulonephritis. In many cases epithelial crescents may be present, allowing the biopsy sample to be classified as crescentic membranoproliferative glomerulonephritis. When the lesions progress, the capsule becomes multilaminated and thickened, and the remaining tuft undergoes progressive atrophy.

The tubules show no specific lesions but rather reflect the presence of a glomerular protein leak. Thus, there are cytoplasmic hyalin droplets and occasional red blood cells.

The interstitium does not appear to be a primary site of involvement, and lesions in this compartment follow and mirror those in the glomeruli.

The blood vessels are involved only in late stages of the disease.

Type III Membranoproliferative Glomerulonephritis. These lesions differ from those in type I membranoproliferative glomerulonephritis by the presence of large, subepithelial deposits associated with spike formation.

Immunofluorescence Microscopy

Types I and III Membranoproliferative Glomerulonephritis. Deposits are found in the subendothelial and mesangial areas in a coarse, granular pattern along peripheral glomerular basement membranes and in the mesangium. The deposits are found in all glomeruli. C3 is always present and is usually accompanied by lesser amounts of C1q, C4, and properdin (Fig. 4–34). In some cases, C3 is the only immune reactant found in the mesangial areas. However, IgG and IgM usually are also present as heavy, coarse granular deposits in both subendothelial and mesangial areas (Fig. 4–35). IgA deposits are unusual.

C3 may also be detected in Bowman's capsule and tubular basement membranes. Fibrin is often present in the glomeruli in a distribution identical to that of the immunoglobulins. In the absence of C3 deposits, the diagnosis of membranoproliferative glomerulonephritis should be questioned. In type III membranoproliferative glomerulonephritis early complement components are absent.

Electron Microscopy

Type I Membranoproliferative Glomerulonephritis. The characteristic features at the

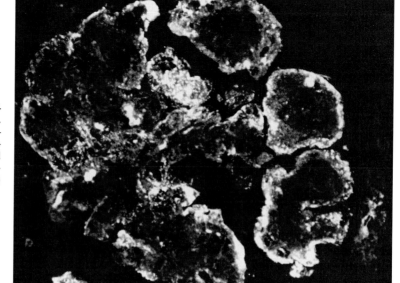

Figure 4–34. Membranoproliferative glomerulonephritis Type I. Nearly continuous, bulky C3 deposits outline the glomerular basement membranes. The mesangial regions are not affected. (Immunofluorescence micrograph, ×400.)

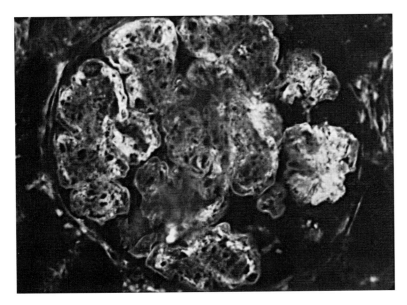

Figure 4–35. Membranoproliferative glomerulonephritis Type I. Large, subendothelial deposits of IgG are distributed in the accentuated lobular pattern. The mesangium and Bowman's capsule contain fewer and less prominent deposits. (Immunofluorescence micrograph, ×250.)

ultrastructural level are deposits and marked distortion of the lamina densa. The deposits are located in both the mesangial and subendothelial regions (Fig. 4–36). The subendothelial deposits are present in one third to one half of the patients and vary considerably in size from loop to loop and among individual patients.

The lamina densa "duplication" is seen to consist of retention of the normal, or native,

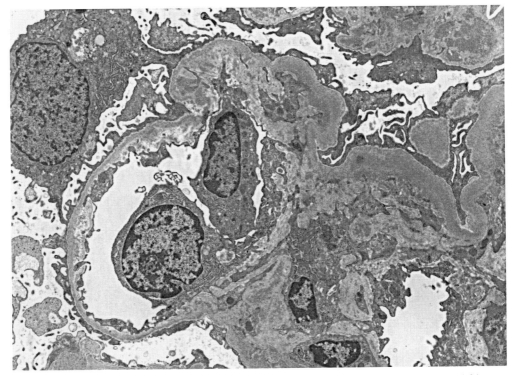

Figure 4–36. Membranoproliferative glomerulonephritis Type I. This early lesion shows partial mesangial interposition and basement membrane duplication. Small electron-dense deposits are present in the subendothelial and mesangial regions. (Electron micrograph, ×2500.)

lamina densa adjacent to the epithelial cells and the addition of new segments of basement membrane beneath the endothelial cell layer (Fig. 4–37). The subendothelial layer is not as regular in thickness as the native lamina densa, and it is quite often discontinuous. Lying between these two layers of lamina densa is a space containing cytoplasmic elements, scattered deposits, and a large amount of flocculent material without definite substructure, often referred to as mesangial interposition. Platelets may be found in the capillary lumina, often in association with fibrin tactoids.

Type II Membranoproliferative Glomerulonephritis: Dense Deposit Disease

Type II membranoproliferative glomerulonephritis is a unique histologic lesion that should not be confused with type I. We and others prefer the term *dense deposit disease.* The glomeruli are enlarged and may be hypercellular, as in type I, but the glomerular basement membrane changes are very specific by each histologic method. The change is a diffuse and regular thickening of the peripheral glomerular basement membranes (Fig. 4–38). The thickening outlines the entire glomerulus, even over the mesangial regions. This histologic change is due to the presence of deposits within the lamina densa and is easily seen on H&E and PAS sections (Fig. 4–39). The deposits may be interrupted or may exist as strings of deposits connected by a thin thread of material, giving them a sausage-shaped contour. These lesions are PAS positive and stain brownish with periodic acid–silver methenamine (PASM) (Fig. 4–40).

The mesangial cellularity is not as marked as in type I, but mesangial sclerosis may be prominent in its late stages. Thus, this lesion may be as lobular in appearance as that of type I.

Epithelial hypercellularity is not often pres-

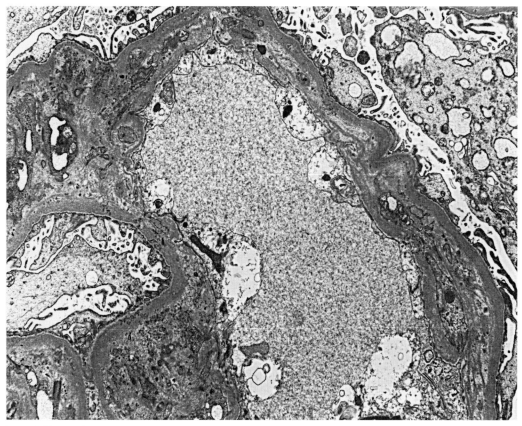

Figure 4–37. Membranoproliferative glomerulonephritis Type I. The duplication of the basement membranes is better seen. (Electron micrograph, ×2800.)

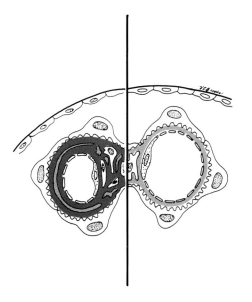

Figure 4–38. Membranoproliferative glomerulonephritis Type II, dense deposit disease. The glomerular basement membrane contains a continuous deposit in this diagram. There is an increase in the number of mesangial cells and in the amount of mesangial matrix.

ent early in the disease, but crescents are frequently seen late in the disease as it progresses rapidly to renal failure.

Similar deposits are found in tubular basement membranes and Bowman's capsule, where they have the same shape and tinctorial characteristics as those in the glomerulus (Fig. 4–39).

Immunofluorescence Microscopy

The immunofluorescence microscopic pattern in membranoproliferative glomerulone-

phritis type II, or dense deposit disease, is unique in both the composition and the distribution of the immunoreactants. Smooth, linear deposits of C3 outline the peripheral glomerular basement membranes (Fig. 4–41). It is important to note that C3 is the only immunoreactant found in these deposits. The deposits are often quite faint and may not be apparent except with high-titer antibodies and an excellent fluorescence light source. In addition to this linear basement distribution of C3, there are also scattered, brightly staining granules of C3 throughout the mesangium.

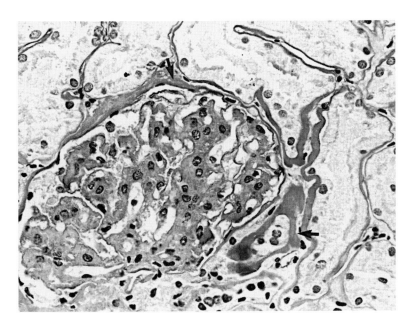

Figure 4–39. Membranoproliferative glomerulonephritis Type II, dense deposit disease. There is an increase in the width of some peripheral basement membranes and deposits in the mesangial matrix. (Bowman's capsule *(arrow)* and the tubular basement membranes *(arrow)* are outlined by conspicuous deposits.) (H&E, ×250.)

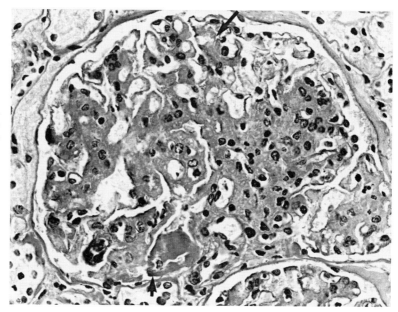

Figure 4–40. Membranoproliferative glomerulonephritis Type II, dense deposit disease. The ribbon-like thickening of the glomerular basement membranes *(arrows)* is associated with mesangial cell proliferation and sclerosis. The mesangium also contains many deposits. (H&E, ×400.)

There is also staining of tubular basement membranes in an irregular fashion (Fig. 4–42).

Electron Microscopy

As noted by light and immunofluorescence microscopy, the deposits within the lamina densa are the most prominent feature (Fig. 4–43). They are strongly electron dense and distort the vascular wall architecture. The deposits underlie the native lamina densa, and segments of newly formed lamina densa are often found between the endothelial cells and the adjacent deposits. Deposits may also be found in Bowman's capsule basement mem-

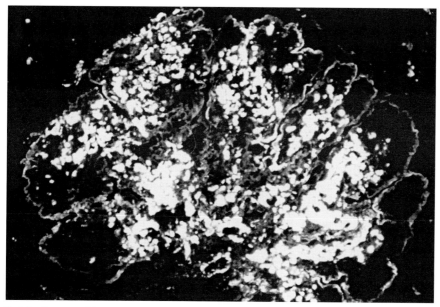

Figure 4–41. Membranoproliferative glomerulonephritis Type II, dense deposit disease. The mesangium contains brightly staining punctate C3 deposits some of which are "ring shaped," and the glomerular basement membranes are faintly stained. (Immunofluorescence micrograph, ×400.)

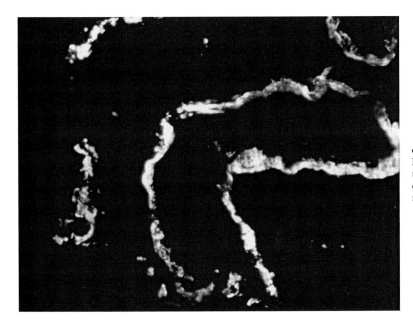

Figure 4–42. Membranoproliferative glomerulonephritis Type II, dense deposit disease. Several tubular basement membranes are outlined by C3 deposits. (Immunofluorescence micrograph, ×400.)

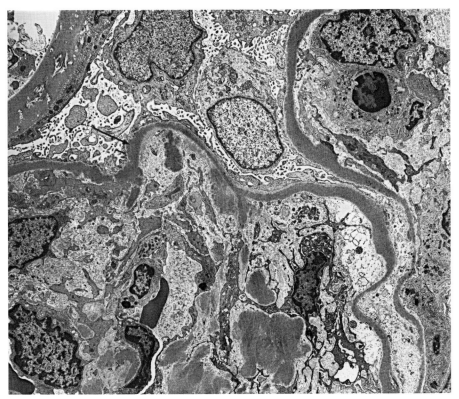

Figure 4–43. Membranoproliferative glomerulonephritis Type II, dense deposit disease. The peripheral glomerular basement membrane is almost completely replaced by dense deposits (arrow). The mesangial matrix also contains multiple "ring-shaped" deposits. (Electron micrograph, ×2000.)

branes, as well as in those of the tubules. In these regions, the deposits are most often segmental and discontinuous. The mesangial regions are expanded principally by an increase in the amount of extracellular matrix. There are few deposits in the mesangium, and the number of cells is not often increased. Mesangial "interposition" is not a common finding.

There may be occasional subepithelial deposits, but they are usually scattered and are not a prominent feature. Visceral epithelial cells show spreading of the pedicels and microvillus formation.

Other Diseases

Type I membranoproliferative glomerulonephritis occurs in widely disparate clinical disorders (see Table 4–3). Lesions that mimic the idiopathic forms have been associated with hereditary complement deficiencies, are occasionally seen in patients with systemic lupus erythematosus, and have been reported in patients with mixed cryoglobulinemia and in some patients with light chain systemic disease (see Chapter 9). In addition, this is a common form of glomerular disease in patients with chronic bacterial infections, viral infections (such as hepatitis C), or parasitic infections (see Chapter 5). It has also been reported in patients with various forms of liver disease, including hepatitis and alcoholic cirrhosis. In the latter, the glomerular immunoglobulin deposits consist mainly of IgA.

It is interesting that the glomerular lesion in patients with hepatitis B appears to be age dependent. In children, the principal lesion is membranous glomerulonephritis, whereas in adults, type I membranoproliferative glomerulonephritis is more typical. The latter may be differentiated from the usual case of type I membranoproliferative glomerulonephritis by the presence of hepatitis B viral antigens in the deposits of some patients.

Prognosis

Type I membranoproliferative glomerulonephritis is thought to be relatively slowly progressive, with 70 to 85% of children and adults remaining free of renal failure in most longitudinal studies. On the other hand, 50 to 60% of patients with type II membranoproliferative glomerulonephritis are in renal failure 10 years after clinical onset. Progression to renal failure is heralded by the appearance of cres-

centic glomerulonephritis in both types I and II membranoproliferative glomerulonephritis.

It has also been stated that the so-called lobular forms progress more rapidly to renal failure, but appropriate clinical trials to test this hypothesis rigorously have not been conducted. Thus, it is likely that cases in this category represent late stages of membranoproliferative glomerulonephritis.

The presence of crescents and of extensive tubulointerstitial lesions is the most reliable predictor of a poor short-term outcome.

Clinical remission independent of therapeutic measures may occur in both types of membranoproliferative glomerulonephritis. This fact, coupled with its declining incidence in the Western world, has made it difficult to evaluate the effectiveness of therapy. However, the use of inhibitors of platelet aggregation, combined with aspirin and steroids, has been stated to be effective in ameliorating the disease process.

Finally, type II membranoproliferative glomerulonephritis very frequently recurs in patients with a renal allograft, whereas this is an infrequent occurrence in patients with type I.

SELECTED READINGS

1. Donadio JV, Slack TK, Holley KE, et al: Idiopathic membranoproliferative (mesangiocapillary) glomerulonephritis: A clinicopathological study. Mayo Clin Proc 54:141, 1979.
2. Habib R, Gubler MC, Loirat D, et al: Dense deposit disease: A variant of membranoproliferative glomerulonephritis. Kidney Int 7:204, 1975.
3. Johnson RJ, Gretch DR, Yamabe H, et al: Membranoproliferative glomerulonephritis associated with hepatitis C virus infection. N Engl J Med 328:465, 1993.
4. Kim Y, Michael AF, Fish AJ: Idiopathic membranoproliferative glomerulonephritis. Contemp Issues Nephrol 9:2337, 1982.
5. Mandelenakis N, Mendoza N, Pirani CL, et al: Lobular glomerulonephritis and membranoproliferative glomerulonephritis. Medicine 50:319, 1971.
6. Ooi YM, Vallota EH, West CD: Classical complement pathway activation in membranoproliferative glomerulonephritis. Kidney Int 9:46, 1976.
7. Rennke H: Secondary membranoproliferative glomerulonephritis. Nephrology Forum. Kidney Int 47:643, 1995.

IgA GLOMERULONEPHRITIS

IgA nephropathy was described by Berger in 1968, and thus its first eponym was Berger's disease. IgA nephropathy was initially recognized because of the unusual immunofluorescence microscopic finding of large mesangial deposits of IgA in patients whose only evidence of renal disease was macroscopic hematuria. In adult patients, the mesangial deposits frequently contained other immunoglobulins (IgM and IgG), and there were associated focal and segmental glomerular lesions (Table 4–4). This disease, described first in Paris, was initially considered benign and thought to be restricted to Europe. It took several years for it to become apparent that IgA nephropathy was not only widespread but, rather than being a benign condition, represented the most common cause of chronic, progressive glomerulonephritis in the Western world and in Asia.

It also became clear that the presence of mesangial IgA deposits as the predominant feature was not restricted to a single disease but that a spectrum of diseases was associated with glomerular deposits of IgA. These included Henoch-Schönlein purpura, systemic lupus erythematosus, and cirrhosis. Because of the diversity of clinical manifestations associated with the presence of mesangial IgA deposits, the use of the term *IgA nephropathy* has remained controversial and tends to obscure the varied types of glomerulonephropathy that share this finding. The other names proposed for this morphologic and clinical entity are mesangial IgA glomerulonephritis, IgA mesangial disease, IgA-IgG nephropathy, and Berger's disease. None is satisfactory, and we must rely on a combination of clinical, laboratory, and morphologic descriptors to arrive at a clear communication of the underlying process. Perhaps this will suffice until the etiology is clarified.

Pathogenesis

The diagnosis relies entirely on the finding of IgA as the predominant immune reactant in the mesangial areas and occasionally along the glomerular basement membranes. It also depends on the exclusion of Henoch-Schönlein purpura, systemic lupus erythematosus, and liver disease on clinical and laboratory grounds.

IgA glomerulonephritis has received considerable attention through multiple clinical and morphologic studies. The clinicopathologic features and geographic distribution of IgA nephropathy are now well defined, but the etiology and pathogenesis remain undefined. A wide variation exists in the frequency with which different countries report IgA nephropathy in the acute phases, but there now seems to be general agreement that it accounts for approximately 10% of all cases of end-stage renal disease. In Europe, it appears to be more common in France, Italy, and Spain. In Asia, the frequency of the disease is high, especially in Japan, where it represents 30 to 40% of all end-stage glomerular diseases. Countries with large African populations seem to have a low incidence of IgA nephropathy. Recently a clustering of IgA nephropathy was found in families, and it was noted that there was a preferential association with some C3 or C4 phenotypes and HLA histocompatibility antigens. Taken together, these data suggest a strong genetic component. One must take this information in the context in which it is presented—namely, that few investigators have performed prospective long-term studies based on renal biopsies, and the appropriate genetic studies remain to be reported.

It is not established, therefore, whether this is a single disease or a group of diseases. Nonetheless, the presence of large deposits of IgA in the mesangium provides a useful way to distinguish this group of patients from those with glomerular aggregates composed princi-

Table 4–4. Focal Proliferative Glomerulonephritis

Etiology	Clinical	Deposits
Idiopathic	Focal proliferative glomerulonephritis	IgA
	Other focal proliferative glomerulonephritides	IgG-IgM
	IgM mesangial glomerulonephritis	IgM-C3
Infectious	Subacute bacterial endocarditis	IgG-IgM
Systemic	Henoch-Schönlein purpura	IgA
	Systemic lupus erythematosus	IgG
	Mixed connective tissue disease	IgG
	Vasculitis	Fibrinogen
	Cirrhosis	IgA
	Mixed cryoglobulinemia	IgM / IgG
Antiglomerular basement membrane	Goodpasture's syndrome (antiglomerular basement membrane)	Linear IgG

pally of other immunoglobulins. It is widely accepted that this is an immune complex disease, based on animal studies that demonstrate that glomerular IgA deposits can be induced by oral immunization. This method of immunization results in circulating IgA immune complexes. The animal studies reinforce suspicions of a similar pathogenesis in humans. Many investigators have noted that in some patients the clinical syndrome follows an upper respiratory tract infection or is exacerbated by the presence of such an event. Some patients have been found to have high levels of circulating IgA complexes, and some have high levels of polymeric IgA. Both these findings remain in the category of interesting observations with uncertain pathogenetic significance, but they leave open the possibility of a role for immunologic factors in the pathogenesis of this disease. It is interesting that some of the circulating complexes contain IgA rheumatoid factor that reacts with autologous IgG. The nature of the antigens present in the circulating immune complexes and the question of whether there is a similar antigen in the mesangial aggregates of IgA remain questions for future research. Possibilities for such antigens include food and viral and microbial antigens. Finally, a defect in either the production of IgA or the clearance of macromolecular IgA has recently been proposed.

Transplantation has also provided some interesting clues about the pathogenesis of this disease. Several patients have developed recurrent IgA nephropathy in their renal allograft. It is important to observe that many such patients have been monitored for extended periods and none have developed a progressive sclerosing disease in the glomeruli of the graft. This suggests that the disease requires both some circulating substance and a kidney that responds by the development of a sclerosing glomerular lesion. This tentative conclusion has received further support from observations on a cadaver kidney that contained mesangial deposits and that was transplanted into a patient who did not have IgA disease. The IgA deposits disappeared from the mesangial regions of the allograft placed into this patient. These data cause speculation that (1) IgA nephropathy might be treated by removing the source of the mesangial IgA aggregates, and (2) that the renal response is the critical factor in the determination of the pathogenicity of the materials that deposit in the mesangium.

Finally, experimental animal models and human renal biopsies suggest that growth factors may play a role. The two most often implicated are platelet-derived growth factor and interleukin-6, although others may also be involved. Nonetheless, it is not clear what role they actually play in the pathogenesis of the lesion.

Patient Presentation

IgA nephropathy may occur at any age but is more common in young adults. There is a male predominance in the Western world, but this does not appear to be the case in Asia. The majority of patients have asymptomatic microscopic hematuria and mild proteinuria and a protracted clinical course. In one third of patients, the hematuria is macroscopic and recurrent and may be associated with flank pain. The hematuric episodes are often immediately preceded (a few hours or days) by an episode of a mild upper respiratory tract virus–like infection. Some patients with mild gastrointestinal flulike symptoms have also been reported. The episodes of hematuria may last for only a few hours and then dissipate. Other patients may develop symptoms of an acute nephritic syndrome, including renal failure, hypertension, edema, and heavy proteinuria. Finally, a small number of patients may have short episodes of acute oliguric renal failure that spontaneously remit.

A benign course is typical in children. Unfortunately, adults most often show signs of significant renal disease by the time the syndrome is diagnosed. Some patients may present with the nephrotic syndrome, but this is not common.

Histology

Light Microscopy

Although the disease was first classified as a focal proliferative glomerulonephritis, it has been recognized that there are multiple histologic patterns, including the absence of detectable light microscopic abnormalities. The most characteristic histologic lesions are focal and segmental mesangial proliferation. In the mild forms, the lesions are minimal, and the glomeruli may appear normal or show minimal increases in the amount of extracellular matrix or the degree of cellularity (Figs. 4–44,

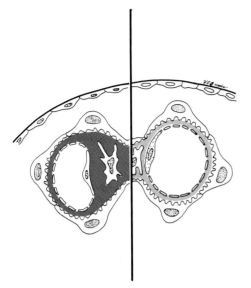

Figure 4–44. IgA nephropathy. Diagram of glomerulus with an increase in the amount of mesangial matrix.

4–45). In addition, these changes may affect only a small number of glomeruli or a small portion of individual glomeruli.

Proliferative and sclerotic lesions of different ages often coexist in the same biopsy specimen. In some patients, polymorphonuclear cells as well as macrophages may be found in the mesangial spaces or the capillary lumina,

usually during acute episodes. Localized crescents may also be found near the foci of mesangial proliferation. Areas of necrosis, and thrombosis if present, are rare and limited and like cellular crescents are more common in biopsies performed early after an acute episode of hematuria (Fig. 4–46). Macrophages are nearly always found in the region of the necrosis. Large crescents with foci of necrosis have been described during episodes of acute renal failure, in which case the diagnosis of Henoch-Schönlein purpura must be excluded on clinical grounds.

Areas of sclerosis involve segments of the glomerular tuft, and in the presence of synechiae, the immediately adjacent Bowman's capsules are frequently thickened and multilaminated (Fig. 4–47). When glomerular basement membrane thickening occurs, it is usually present as irregular, segmental areas of multilamination, in contrast to the diffusely laminated pattern characteristic of membranoproliferative glomerulonephritis. Many or most peripheral glomerular basement membranes appear normal with silver stains. In glomeruli with severe lesions, occasional tram-tracks are seen. The presence of obsolescent glomeruli attests to the chronic nature of the disease.

The mesangial matrix occasionally contains eosinophilic mesangial deposits, often called "fibrinoid," which appear red on trichrome-

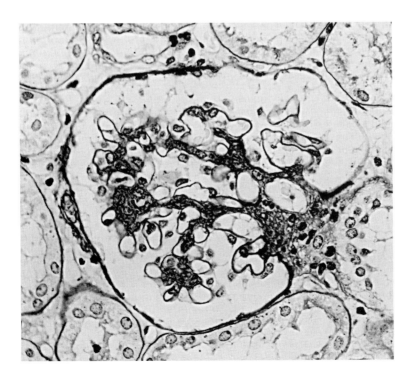

Figure 4–45. IgA nephropathy, mild lesion. The mesangial regions are expanded by a PASM-positive material and a minimum increase in cellularity. Although the glomerular basement membranes are normal, those of Bowman's capsule may be thickened. (PASM, ×400.)

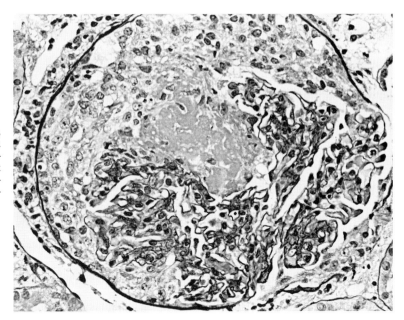

Figure 4–46. IgA nephropathy, severe lesion. There is a large area of fibrinoid necrosis with an adjacent cellular crescent. The rest of the tuft displays mild mesangial hypercellularity. (Jones methenamine silver stain, ×500.)

stained sections. This is a misleading term, because newly formed hyalin also has this appearance. The use of the descriptor *fibrinoid* denotes a more acute process than is ordinarily present in these patients. Therefore, we prefer the use of the term hyalin to describe this material (Fig. 4–48).

Late glomerular lesions are characterized by the development of fibrous crescents (Fig. 4–49).

Tubulointerstitial lesions are often conspicuous and closely parallel the degree of renal functional impairment (see Figure 4–50). Scattered areas of interstitial edema or sclerosis with interstitial inflammatory cell infiltrates predominate around the more severely dam-

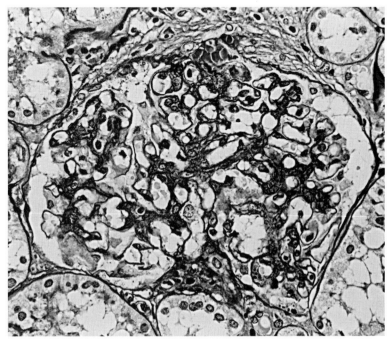

Figure 4–47. IgA nephropathy, chronic lesion. There is diffuse mesangial proliferation and sclerosis with an organized synechia near the urinary pole of the glomerulus, a common finding in organized synechiae. (PAS, ×400.)

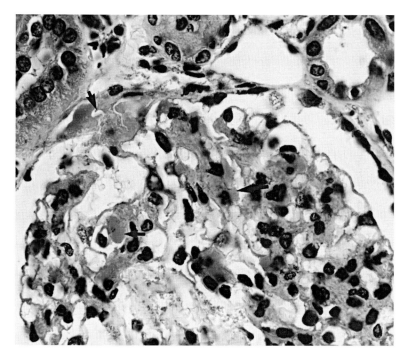

Figure 4–48. IgA nephropathy, moderate lesion. This higher-power view demonstrates glassy mesangial deposits of hyalin *(arrows)* elevating the basement membrane, which is reflected over the mesangium. There is also global mesangial hypercellularity. A small synechia is present *(arrow)*. (H&E, × 630.)

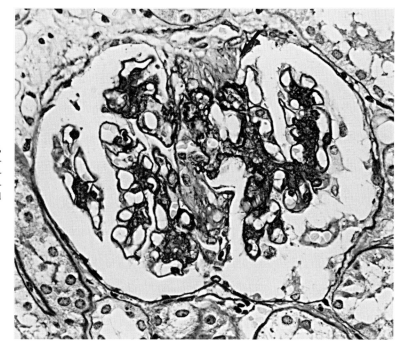

Figure 4–49. IgA nephropathy, severe chronic lesion. There is severe mesangial sclerosis with partial disorganization of the tuft architecture and a large organized synechia *(arrow)*. (PAS, × 400.)

aged glomeruli. In adults, there often are obvious chronic vascular lesions. Red blood cell casts are quite common, especially in patients with macroscopic hematuria.

The World Health Organization working group on classification of glomerular disease has proposed the following categorization:

Class I: Minimal lesion
Class II: Minor changes with small, segmental areas of proliferation (see Figure 4–45)
Class III: Focal and segmental glomerulonephritis with less than 50% of the glomeruli showing obvious changes (Fig. 4–48)
Class IV: Diffuse mesangial lesions with proliferation and sclerosis (Fig. 4–49)
Class V: Diffuse sclerosing glomerulonephritis affecting more than 80% of glomeruli (Fig. 4–50)

Although this classification provides a descriptive framework, many cases cannot be easily categorized using this method.

Immunofluorescence Microscopy

IgA nephropathy, as described earlier, can be accurately diagnosed only by immunochemical methods. Although the light microscopic lesions may be focal, the immunoglobulins are always present in a diffuse pattern by immunofluorescence microscopy.

The single constant finding in this disease is the presence of diffuse deposits of IgA in the mesangium, forming either discrete granules or large aggregates (Fig. 4–51). When large, the deposits may also be found in the subendothelial areas. Uncommonly there are focal, granular subepithelial deposits. IgG codistributes with IgA in more than half the cases, but it is usually present in smaller amounts. The term *IgA-IgG nephropathy* was coined because of the frequent coexistence of these two immunoglobulins in the mesangium. IgM has also been reported in the mesangium of half the patients. C3 is present in most patients and has the same distribution as IgA. C1q and C4 complement components are not commonly present. As in other sclerosing diseases, the membrane attack components may be present.

Fibrinogen deposits, also common, are most often small and inconspicuous. This fact may help in the differentiation of IgA nephropathy from the nephropathy of Henoch-Schönlein purpura because of the prominence of fibrinogen deposits in the latter.

The other immune complex–mediated glomerular disease in which significant IgA deposits are present is systemic lupus erythematosus. IgA deposits may also be found in patients with chronic liver disease.

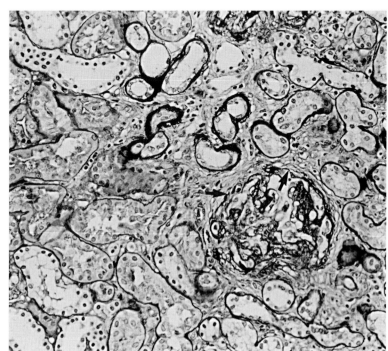

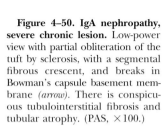

Figure 4–50. IgA nephropathy, severe chronic lesion. Low-power view with partial obliteration of the tuft by sclerosis, with a segmental fibrous crescent, and breaks in Bowman's capsule basement membrane *(arrow)*. There is conspicuous tubulointerstitial fibrosis and tubular atrophy. (PAS, ×100.)

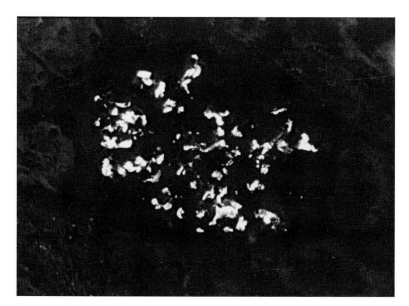

Figure 4–51. IgA nephropathy. The mesangial regions of all glomeruli contain IgA deposits, the typical pattern in this disease. The deposits are globular, restricted to the mesangium, and globally distributed. (Immunofluorescence micrograph, ×250.)

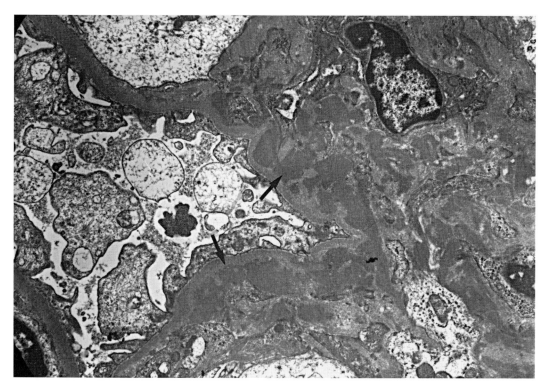

Figure 4–52. IgA nephropathy. Numerous electron-dense deposits *(arrows)* lie within the expanded mesangial matrix, especially near the glomerular basement membranes. The foot processes are relatively well preserved. (Electron micrograph, ×4000.)

Electron Microscopy

The deposits, recognizable as electron-dense granular material, are irregularly spread throughout the mesangial matrix, and some mesangial regions are completely free from recognizable dense deposits. Deposits are not found in the cytoplasm of mesangial cells. The associated mesangial matrix may be expanded, and the number of cells in the mesangium may be increased. The deposits are irregular in size and often lie between the mesangial cells and the adjacent paramesangial basement membrane (Fig. 4–52). Subendothelial deposits are most commonly found adjacent to a mesangial region. Although rare, subepithelial deposits may be noted. They most often are separated from the overlying epithelial cells by a thin layer of electron-dense material resembling basement membrane. The peripheral basement membrane frequently shows thinning and multilamination in patients who have sclerosing lesions by light microscopy. In these areas, there may be localized spreading of the pedicels.

Prognosis

There is no specific treatment for IgA nephropathy, and the natural history is so variable as to make generalizations precarious. As many as 10 to 20% of affected adults develop end-stage renal disease. The most frequent clinical course is thought to be one of slow, progressive deterioration. Various attempts have been made to define the histologic features that predict a poor prognosis. There appear to be none unique to IgA nephropathy, and one must rely on general criteria that are applicable to all other types of severe, progressive glomerular diseases. These include the presence of crescents, abundant sclerosis, severe tubulointerstitial lesions, and advanced vascular lesions. Thus, no single histologic feature or constellation of features provides assistance to the pathologist in predicting which cases of early disease will deteriorate and which will resolve.

SELECTED READINGS

1. Berger J, Hinglais N: Les depots intercapillaires d'IgA-IgG. J Urol Nephrol 74:694, 1968.
2. Beukhof JR, Kardaun O, Schaafsma W, et al: Toward individual prognosis of IgA nephropathy. Kidney Int 29:549, 1986.
3. Clarkson AR, Woodroffe AJ, Bannister KM, et al: The syndrome of IgA nephropathy. Clin Nephrol 21:7, 1984.
4. D'Amico G: Influence of clinical and histological features on actuarial renal survival in adult patients with idiopathic IgA nephropathy, membranous nephropathy, and membranoproliferative glomerulonephritis: Survey of the recent literature. Am J Kidney Dis 20:315, 1992.
5. Emancipator SN: IgA nephropathy: Morphologic expression and pathogenesis. Current concepts in renal pathology. Am J Kidney Dis 23:451, 1994.
6. Galla JH: IgA nephropathy. Perspectives in clinical nephrology. Kidney Int 47:377, 1995.
7. Morel-Maroger LJ, Verroust PJ: Clinicopathological correlations in glomerular diseases. In Jones NF (ed): Advances in Renal Diseases. Edinburgh, Churchill Livingstone, 1975, pp 48–79.
8. Nagata M, Akioka Y, Tsnoda Y, et al: Macrophages in childhood IgA nephropathy. Kidney Int 48:527, 1995.
9. Van Es LA: Pathogenesis of IgA nephropathy. Kidney Int 41:1720, 1992.
10. Yoshikawa N, Ito H, Nakamura H: Prognostic indicators in childhood IgA nephropathy. Nephron 60:60, 1992.

FOCAL SEGMENTAL GLOMERULONEPHRITIS WITHOUT IgA

A number of patients with isolated proteinuria and/or microscopic hematuria have a focal and segmental glomerulonephritis without IgA deposits. Some have isolated C3 deposits and a few have IgG and/or IgM in the mesangium. These biopsy samples remain as a poorly understood entity, and no clinical significance or clear-cut pattern of subsequent behavior has been defined.

CRESCENTIC GLOMERULONEPHRITIS OR RAPIDLY PROGRESSIVE GLOMERULONEPHRITIS

Crescentic glomerulonephritis is the histopathologic term coined to designate an array of severe glomerular diseases that share the common feature of crescents in a large percentage of the glomeruli (Table 4–5). This category of disease is also known as rapidly progressive, subacute, malignant, and extracapillary glomerulonephritis. It is characterized histologically by extensive crescents and clinically by the rapid deterioration of renal function that reaches end stage within a period of days or weeks.

Table 4–5. Crescentic Glomerulonephritis

Light Microscopy	Immunofluorescence Microscopy	Possible Pathogenesis	Association
Crescents / necrosis	Linear IgG Fibrinogen	Antiglomerular basement membrane	Pulmonary hemorrhage
Crescents / proliferation in the tuft	Granular IgG Complement Fibrinogen	Immune complexes	Bacterial infections
Crescents / necrosis	Negative Fibrinogen (?)	ANCA	Systemic symptoms (rash, arthralgias, fever)

ANCA, antineutrophilic cytoplasmic antoantibodies.

This process was first recognized in the early part of the 20th century. The definition, a purely histologic categorization, encompasses several varieties of glomerular disorders characterized by their light microscopic and immunopathologic features. The classification of this group of disorders rapidly evolved after the application of immunopathologic techniques to renal biopsies. Crescents may occur in a large number of glomerular diseases, but the discussion in this chapter is restricted to those diseases in which they constitute the main histologic feature. Crescentic glomerulonephritis in association with systemic diseases is reviewed in other chapters.

Pathogenesis

In the past few years, there has emerged a working classification of crescentic glomerulonephritis based on immunofluorescence microscopic findings. The categories are as follows:

• Glomerulonephritis due to antibodies directed toward glomerular basement membrane antigens (antiglomerular basement membrane)
• Glomerulonephritis due to the deposition or formation of immune complexes in the glomeruli
• Glomerulonephritis in which no immunoglobulins are found in the glomeruli (so-called nonimmune). This group has been subdivided into antineutrophil cytoplasmic autoantibodies (ANCA)-positive (Wegener's granulomatosis and polyarteritis nodosa) and ANCA-negative (the latter probably being very uncommon).

An attempt has been made to relate these findings to a presumptive underlying mecha-

nism, based on animal studies. However, the cause of the disease remains unknown in most patients.

This classification, as will be demonstrated, is of use principally because it provides clinicians with help in determining the treatment approach best suited to each patient.

Crescentic glomerulonephritis (Table 4–5) is an infrequently encountered disease, constituting fewer than 10% in all renal biopsies performed for the diagnosis of glomerulonephritis. Thus, it is difficult for any one group to mount a study of the diagnostic criteria, the pathogenesis and its possible geographic or genetic differences, the best means to treat the various subcategories, and the number of patients in each category. However, the best estimates of the number of patients in each of the categories are as follows:

• Antiglomerular basement membrane antibodies, 20%
• Immune complex, 40%
• Nonimmune, 40%

Antineutrophil cytoplasmic antibodies (ANCA) have been recognized as a serologic marker for pauci-immune glomerulonephritis, with or without evidence of extrarenal disease. The two major types of ANCA are C (cytoplasmic staining) and P (perinuclear staining). C-ANCA antigen is proteinase 3, and P-ANCA antigen is usually myeloperoxidase. P-ANCA is most frequently associated with pauci-immune crescentic glomerulonephritis, whereas C-ANCA is most commonly found in patients with Wegener's granulomatosis.

The mechanism of crescent formation has been the subject of considerable investigation. It was initially assumed that the origin of the cells composing the crescent was exclusively epithelial. Further, these epithelial cells were thought to be derived from Bowman's capsule.

However, early electron microscopic studies pointed out the heterogeneity of cells within the crescent, noting that there were both light and dark cells. The application of cell markers revealed that the crescent was indeed a mixed population of cells and that some were derived from macrophages. One of the early events in the development of crescents is the appearance of fibrin in the urinary space, which is followed by an influx of macrophages into the urinary space. It was suggested that breaks in the glomerular basement membrane, so-called gaps, allowed the passage of both the high-molecular-weight precursors of fibrin and subsequently the macrophages. These two events presage and are thought to induce the proliferation of the indigenous glomerular cells.

The variable cellular composition of the crescent, the multiplicity and variety of the lesions occurring in the underlying glomerular tuft, and the different patterns of immunologic involvement all point to the conclusion that crescentic glomerulonephritis is a syndrome with diverse causes. The common features that draw this group together into one diagnostic category are the presence of large numbers of crescents and a clinical course characterized by abrupt onset and rapid progression to renal failure.

Patient Presentation

Crescentic glomerulonephritis most commonly affects adults, being very uncommon before the age of 30 years. There is a male predominance, especially in the antiglomerular basement membrane variety. This form is also more common in patients with the HLA-DR2 phenotype.

The presenting symptoms may be vague, and the patients often complain of weakness, nausea, and general fatigue. In most instances, the renal disease is characterized by severe, unremitting oliguric or anuric renal failure, which is occasionally heralded by macroscopic hematuria. Hypertension is uncommon and never prominent unless there is severe volume expansion due to sodium retention.

The cause of the disease is completely unknown, for the most part. However, various antecedents have been observed and reported on. Approximately one half the patients have a history of an influenza-like illness preceding the onset of renal symptoms. In this respect, antiglomerular basement membrane disease

has been thought to follow influenza A2 infections, but in most patients, acute and convalescent sera either have not been obtained or have not been informative. Even less well established is a relation between exposure to organic solvents and crescentic glomerulonephritis.

Pulmonary hemorrhage is a complication in almost one third of patients with antiglomerular basement membrane crescentic glomerulonephritis, either at presentation or shortly thereafter. This presentation, in concert with crescentic glomerulonephritis and circulating antiglomerular basement membrane antibodies, has been called Goodpasture syndrome. In these patients, there is a strong correlation between the presence of the antibodies, a history of smoking (or other pulmonary injury), and the presence of pulmonary hemorrhage (see Chapter 6).

The autoantibodies react with the NC-1 region of the type IV collagen of the glomerular basement membrane. This region of the molecule is referred to as the Goodpasture antigen.

Patients with immune complex glomerulonephritis may come to medical attention because of the underlying infectious disease process—for example, with a visceral abscess. Crescentic glomerulonephritis following streptococcal infection is essentially encountered only in children and is very unusual in the United States and Western Europe. Infections such as abdominal abscesses, infected vascular shunts, or sepsis have been associated with crescentic glomerulonephritis and should always be considered because they represent potentially curable causes of crescentic glomerulonephritis.

Patients with nonimmune crescentic glomerulonephritis often present with rash, arthritis, and fever. This triad may lead to confusion between this syndrome and a vasculitis, but it also points out that these disorders may be variants of a unique disease.

Histology

Crescentic glomerulonephritis is one of the renal disorders in which it is imperative that pathologists examine the renal biopsy sample by light and immunofluorescence microscopic techniques and report the results in the shortest interval consistent with accurate interpretation.

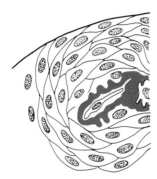

Figure 4–53. Crescentic glomerulonephritis. Diagram shows epithelial cell proliferation and collapse of the glomerulus.

Light Microscopy

Crescentic glomerulonephritis is characterized by the obliteration of Bowman's space by cells (Figs. 4–53, 4–54). The underlying glomerular tuft is compressed and often obliterated. Although there is no agreement about the exact number of crescents required for the diagnosis of crescentic glomerulonephritis, most researchers agree that 80% or more of the glomeruli should be affected. Because this diagnosis carries such a poor prognosis, the pathologist must observe an adequate specimen before this diagnosis is rendered.

The size of the crescent may also have prognostic significance, and it is obvious that glomeruli with large, circumferential crescents represent more severely affected glomeruli than those with more limited involvement.

The cells that form the crescents are often large. Those that have a pale, swollen cytoplasm and a regular oval nucleus are most likely macrophages. They are identifiable as macrophages with the use of monoclonal antibodies to cell surface markers. Occasional mitotic figures may be observed in the smaller, darker cells admixed with the large, clear cells. The latter cells are epithelial in origin. Another unusual pattern is found when the basement membrane of Bowman's capsule has been interrupted. Interstitial cells cross the basement membrane, invading Bowman's space, and form an array of palisading fibroblast-like cells. In this case, as one might expect from the presence of such a large number of collagen-producing cells, the glomerular crescents rapidly organize and the glomeruli become completely and rapidly obsolescent. These are the predominant cell types in the crescents when biopsies are performed at a later time. In addition, neutrophils and red blood cells are frequently observed. It is unusual to find multinucleated cells in the crescent except in patients with Wegener's granulomatosis. In these cases, giant cells and even granuloma formation may be found. Fibrin is often found between cells of the crescent. It is

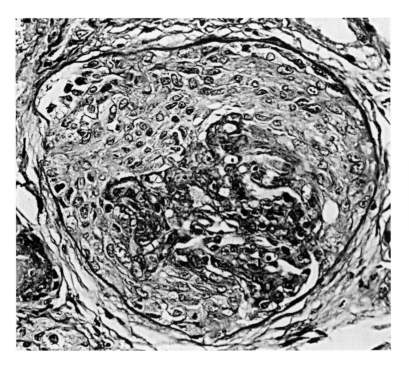

Figure 4–54. Crescentic glomerulonephritis. There is diffuse proliferation of glomerular epithelial cells, which completely occupy the urinary space. The underlying glomerular tuft is compressed and collapsed. (H&E, ×400.)

recognized as strongly eosinophilic areas (Fig. 4–55). Fibrin, present in early cases, disappears soon thereafter. The crescents may contain interstitial cells, if the basement membrane of Bowman's capsule has been breached. This is best seen with silver stains (Fig. 4–54). In this instance, there is continuity between the crescent and a rich periglomerular infiltrate. We believe that this feature is most common in nonimmune crescentic glomerulonephritis and portends a grave prognosis, because it reflects an aggressive inflammatory lesion that repairs by scarring and destruction of the glomerulus.

One interesting and unexplained finding is the frequent observation of a mixture of cellular and partially or completely fibrotic crescents. This would lead one to suspect that the injury may actually be a much more indolent or perhaps recurrent process than the clinical and laboratory data suggest.

The evaluation of the underlying tuft may give precious insight into the underlying pathologic process. Focal and segmental areas of necrosis are often prominent. These are more widespread in the nonimmune form but may also occur in the antiglomerular basement membrane and immune complex varieties. The areas of necrosis involve an ill-defined segment of the tuft, usually in direct contact with the overlying crescent. The necrosis, as with the appearance of fibrin in the crescent, is typical of early lesions. These two findings tend to presage an aggressive fibrotic response. When crescents are extensive, the glomerular tuft is compressed and collapsed. In this case, the glomerular changes may be difficult to identify. An increased number of intraglomerular cells may result from the accumulation of circulating inflammatory cells or the proliferation of endothelial and mesangial cells. As in the examination of the crescent, the use of monoclonal antibodies to inflammatory cell surface antigens has shown that many of the intraglomerular cells are macrophages. Neutrophils and lymphocytes may also be present.

Immunofluorescence Microscopy

Three distinctive patterns may be recognized:

ANTIGLOMERULAR BASEMENT MEMBRANE: LINEAR PATTERN

Deposition of IgG along the glomerular basement membranes in a linear, continuous,

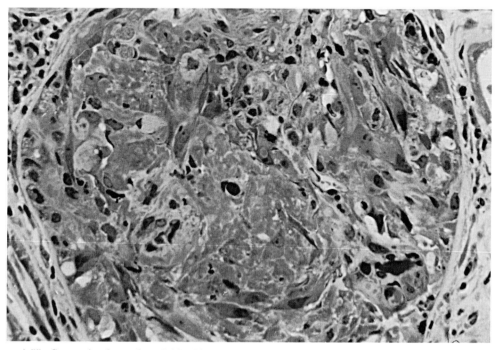

Figure 4–55. Crescentic glomerulonephritis. There is massive fibrinoid necrosis, within a cellular crescent. (H&E, ×500.)

smooth pattern characterizes the antiglomerular basement membrane type of crescentic glomerulonephritis. The linear deposition is diffuse, affecting every loop of each glomerulus (Fig. 4–56). Linear IgG deposition may also occur, to a lesser degree, along Bowman's capsule and along occasional tubular basement membranes. In a few cases in the literature, the antibodies to the glomerular basement membrane are of the IgA class, but IgA and IgM are rarely found in this linear fashion.

In association with IgG, C3 has been detected in a linear but interrupted pattern along the glomerular basement membrane, Bowman's capsule, and tubular basement membranes.

C1q and C4 are not usually present, although there may be some accumulations of these components in areas of sclerosis.

There are only a few circumstances in which the presence of linear deposits of IgG may lead to confusion. First, linear IgG deposits have been found to occur in patients with glomerulosclerosis. This pattern is most commonly seen in patients with diabetes mellitus, but it also occurs in patients with cirrhosis of the liver. However, in both of these circumstances IgG is not the sole immunoglobulin present—IgA, IgM, and albumin are also present in a similar distribution. Of even more importance is the absence of crescents. Detailed studies of these cases have demonstrated that the immunoglobulins are not autoantibodies directed against the glomerular basement membrane.

Finally, linear deposits of immunoglobulins are occasionally present in light chain systemic deposition disease, but, again, the pattern of deposition and the composition of the deposits are different (see Chapter 9). In light chain systemic deposition disease, the deposits clearly predominate around the tubules and glomerular deposits are found in the enlarged mesangial areas. Finally, the deposits are composed of only one type of light chain, mostly kappa, whereas the deposits in antiglomerular basement membrane diease are polyclonal.

Fibrin/fibrinogen deposition is a prominent feature of all types of crescentic glomerulonephritis and parallels the extent of necrotizing areas in the glomeruli (Fig. 4–57). Fibrinogen may also be present within the crescents and in the interstitial tissue. In general, masses of fibrin are more conspicuous in fresh "active" lesions and tend to disappear with progression to chronic lesions.

GRANULAR DEPOSITS: IMMUNE COMPLEXES

Granular deposits of immunoglobulins and complement are found in approximately 40% of patients with crescentic glomerulonephritis. The deposits may be present in the mesangial areas as well as along the endothelial or epithelial aspects of the glomerular basement membrane, in a diffuse or focal pattern. Various combinations of immunoglobulins have been reported, including IgG, IgA, and IgM. They are usually found in association with complement components. Fibrin/fibrinogen

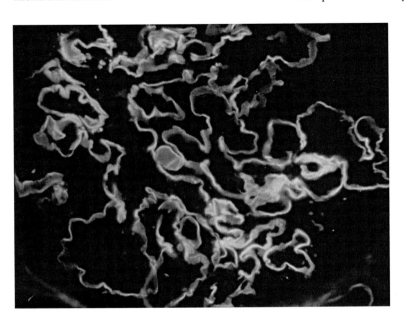

Figure 4–56. Crescentic glomerulonephritis, anti-GBM disease. There are linear IgG deposits along the glomerular basement membranes. (Immunofluorescence micrograph, ×400.)

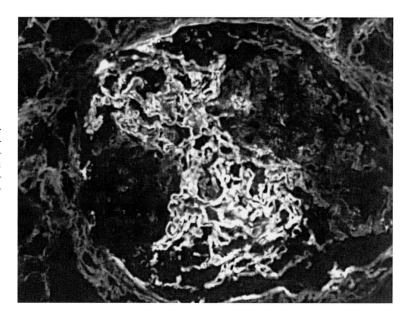

Figure 4–57. Crescentic glomerulonephritis, nonimmune, ANCA-positive. Large masses of the glomerulus contain fibrin/fibrinogen antigen, corresponding to the areas of necrosis. (Immunofluorescence micrograph, ×250.)

deposits invariably are found within foci of necrosis or in fresh crescents.

The appearance and distribution of immune reactants vary with the underlying disease. In biopsy specimens of patients with poststreptococcal glomerulonephritis, only IgG and C3 are found in the small granules scattered over the glomerular tufts. In patients with subacute bacterial endocarditis, the deposits contain IgG and IgM in larger amounts and are largely found within the mesangial and subendothelial areas. The deposits in patients with subacute bacterial endocarditis also contain C3, C4, and C1q. In patients with visceral abscesses, the deposits may contain IgA, associated with IgG and IgM, in both mesangial and subendothelial areas. When IgA is the predominant immunoglobulin and when the deposits predominate in the mesangial areas, in a patient with crescents, the underlying disease may be either IgA disease (see Chapter 4) or Henoch-Schönlein purpura (see Chapter 6). The latter will be associated with its characteristic clinical syndrome.

Finally, there remains a group of patients who have granular immune deposits but in whom no underlying disease can be ascertained.

NONIMMUNE CRESCENTIC
GLOMERULONEPHRITIS

In approximately 40% of patients with crescentic glomerulonephritis, no immune re-

actants can be detected by immunofluorescence microscopic examination. Fibrin/fibrinogen antigens may be present in areas of necrosis or crescents (Fig. 4–57). This group of patients is often considered to represent a variety of vasculitis involving the glomerular vascular bed as its principal target. Patients with ANCA belong to this category.

Electron Microscopy

Biopsy specimens characteristically show collapse of glomerular capillary loops and an increase in the number of cells in Bowman's space, including epithelial cells and cells resembling macrophages. There is widening of the lamina rara interna and swelling of the endothelial cell cytoplasm. Loose masses of proteinaceous material, including recognizable fibrin, are present between the cells composing the crescent.

There may be interruptions of the peripheral glomerular basement membranes through which the cytoplasm of the adjacent endothelial or epithelial cells may protrude. These have been called gaps and are most frequent in areas of necrosis, in marked hypercellularity, and in early crescents. When such gaps are present in the basement membrane of Bowman's capsule, interstitial inflammatory cells or fibroblasts may be seen either traversing these breaks or may be present in large numbers as a component of the cellular crescent lying within the urinary space. If the biopsy is performed later in the course of the disease, the specimen may show the cells separated from one another by extracellular matrix. This matrix is of two varieties. If Bowman's capsule is intact, the intercellular matrix within Bowman's space is composed of homogeneous electron-dense material resembling basement membrane. If the capsular basement membrane has been breached, the matrix contains banded collagen, similar to that found in the interstitium. In both cases, the end result is obsolescence.

Prognosis

Most patients with this group of diseases have severe renal damage at the time of presentation, and the prognosis largely depends on the degree of irreversible glomerular damage.

The development of crescents in any glomerular disease reflects a severe event and bodes a poor prognosis. It is generally accepted that most patients who have circumferential crescents in 100% of their glomeruli uniformly progress to end-stage renal failure without regaining renal function. If the crescents are not diffuse, there is a greater chance of recovery of some renal function with aggressive therapeutic intervention. Patients who have an underlying endocapillary glomerular hypercellularity seem also to have a better chance of recovering renal function.

As in other glomerular disorders, the extent of interstitial fibrosis correlates with the ultimate outcome. Among the other histologic features that may be prognostic indicators is the presence of extensive fibrinoid necrosis. When this is present, rapid and irreversible deterioration of renal function is likely.

Various therapeutic regimens have been applied, but the small number of cases has prevented the establishment of reliable clinical trials. The worst prognosis is generally associated with antibodies against the glomerular basement membranes. Patients with granular immune deposits seem to have a better response to treatment because they often have a treatable form of infectious disease. Recognition of this form of the disease is essential to avoid inappropriate and undesirably aggressive therapeutic approaches.

Treatment protocols are varied and comprise pulse steroids, high-dose methylprednisolone, and/or immunosuppressive drugs. ANCA-positive patients are most frequently treated with intravenous cyclophosphamide. Pooled gamma-globulin therapy has also been proposed, but it is incompletely evaluated. Finally, plasma exchange has been widely used in an attempt to remove the antiglomerular basement membrane antibodies in the plasma.

Relapses may occur in ANCA-positive patients, but they are relatively uncommon in the others. Repeat renal biopsies have been used after the therapeutic trial to determine whether the acute lesions have been ameliorated and whether sclerosis has supervened. This is the only reliable means to determine the amount of fixed renal damage and may provide an estimate of the need and potential for response in any remaining active disease process.

SELECTED READINGS

1. Angangco R, Thiru S, Esnault VLM, et al: Does truly idiopathic crescentic glomerulonephritis exist? Nephrol Dial Transplant 9:630, 1994.
2. Couser WG: Idiopathic rapidly progressive glomerulonephritis. Am J Kidney Dis 2:57, 1982.
3. Jennette JC: Anti-neutrophil cytoplasmic autoantibody-associated disease: A pathologist's perspective. Am J Kidney Dis 18:164, 1991.
4. Jennette JC, Falk RJ, Andrassy K, et al: Nomenclature of systemic vasculitides: The proposal of an international consensus conference. Arthritis Rheum 37:187, 1992.
5. Lerner R, Glassock R, Dixon F: The role of antiglomerular basement membrane antibody in the pathogenesis of human glomerulonephritis. J Exp Med 126:989, 1967.
6. Stejskal J, Pirani CL, Okada M, et al: Discontinuities (gaps) of the glomerular capillary wall and basement membrane in renal diseases. Lab Invest 28:149, 1973.
7. Striker L, Killen PD, Chi E, et al: The composition of glomerulosclerosis. I. Studies in focal sclerosis, crescentic glomerulonephritis, and membranoproliferative glomerulonephritis. Lab Invest 51:181, 1984.
8. Whitworth J, Morel-Maroger LJ, Mignon F, et al: The significance of extracapillary proliferation: Clinicopathological review of 60 patients. Nephron 16:1, 1976.

GLOMERULAR DISEASE OF KNOWN ETIOLOGY

5

BACTERIAL INFECTIONS

Glomerulonephritis Following Streptococcal Infections

Acute glomerulonephritis is the term used to designate glomerulonephritis associated with bacterial infections in sites distant from the kidney. The best example is poststreptococcal glomerulonephritis, which has been considered to be the prototype of an immune complex disease. It is characterized by the development of a diffuse, proliferative glomerulonephritis after a latent period of 8 to 14 days in patients with a streptococcal infection of the upper respiratory tract or skin.

Pathogenesis

Poststreptococcal glomerulonephritis was the first type of nephritis considered to be an immunologic disease. This conclusion was based on the association of circulating immune complexes, a low serum complement level at initiation of the renal lesion, and the finding of immune reactants in the glomeruli. This postulate was further supported by the presence of similar clinical and laboratory observations in patients with serum sickness. Finally, a similar set of findings could be reproduced in experimental animals by eliciting a humoral immune response.

The largest number of cases of acute poststreptococcal glomerulonephritis is now reported from developing countries. This lesion has been almost eradicated from many other regions by the widespread use of antibiotics in the treatment of respiratory tract and skin infections and the institution of proper sanitary conditions.

Patient Presentation

The most common presenting signs and symptoms are hematuria, edema, hypertension, and azotemia. There is a history of a recent infection, often culture-positive for streptococci, in the patient or a family member. An elevated and rising titer to streptococcal antigens establishes the streptococcal infection as the most likely cause of the renal lesion, especially in children. The serum complement levels are low, and circulating antigen-antibody complexes may be detectable during the early phases of the process. The exact pathogenesis of the disease is poorly understood, but factors relating to both the host and the pathogen are important. For instance, several family members may have protein and red blood cells in the urine during an episode of upper respiratory tract infections, but few develop the rest of the symptoms and signs of renal disease. In addition, there are "nephritogenic" strains of streptococci. Finally, a small number of those with acute poststreptococcal glomerulonephritis develop long-term renal sequelae. Beta-hemolytic streptococci are not the only bacteria to be associated with postinfectious glomerulonephritis, but they are the most frequent pathogen.

The renal signs are not always typical. Some patients have only hematuria, and others may have anuria at the clinical onset. Very few have the nephrotic syndrome at the outset, but

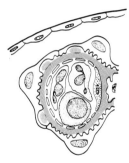

Figure 5–1. Diagram of acute proliferative glomerulone-phritis with subepithelial deposits, proliferation, and exudation.

when present, it portends a poor prognosis. Finally, some have acute oliguric renal failure at the onset.

Histology

Light Microscopy

The glomeruli are the principal site of the lesion and are characteristically large, diffusely hypercellular, and infiltrated with neutrophils (Fig. 5–1). The endocapillary hypercellularity consists of both resident glomerular cells as well as infiltrating mononuclear and polymorphonuclear inflammatory cells. Mesangial and endothelial cells are thought to be the principal glomerular cell types involved in the proliferation. The term *exudative glomerulonephritis* has been used to designate this early lesion,

which leads to almost complete obliteration of the glomerular vascular spaces (Fig. 5–2).

The glomerular basement membranes are not altered, for the most part, although occasional areas of "splitting" (the tram-track lesion) may be observed (Fig. 5–3). In some patients who are examined during the exudative phases of the disease, subepithelial deposits may be visualized (Fig. 5–4). These large subepithelial deposits are seen by light, immunofluorescence, and electron microscopy and have been called humps because of their shape. They are best seen on trichrome-stained sections in paraffin-embedded specimens or on silver stains on plastic embedded sections (Fig. 5–4).

Visceral epithelial cells are not frequently increased in number, although their cytoplasm may be prominent. The presence of marked epithelial proliferation (especially those with diffuse crescents) portends a different prognosis and should be considered as a type of immune-mediated crescentic glomerulonephritis (see Chapter 4).

Within a few weeks after onset of the illness, the glomerular lesions change significantly. The neutrophils disappear, and the number of deposits decreases rapidly. At this stage, the cellular proliferation involves only the mesangial regions. The mesangial matrix may be moderately increased in amount. The glomerular vascular loops again become patent, and the glomerular basement membranes are nor-

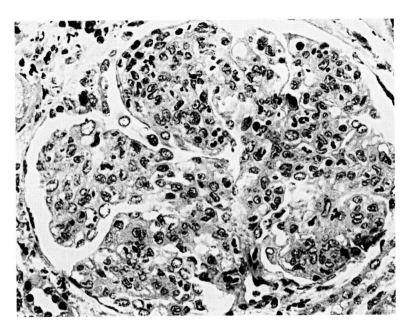

Figure 5–2. Acute poststreptococcal glomerulonephritis. The vascular spaces are occluded by intracapillary proliferation and infiltrating polymorphonuclear leukocytes. (H&E, ×500.)

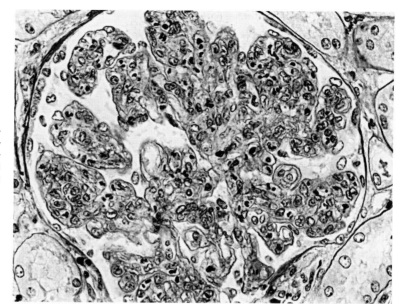

Figure 5–3. Acute poststreptococcal glomerulonephritis. Neutrophils are present within the glomerular tufts. A few tram tracks can be seen. (Jones methenamine silver, ×500.)

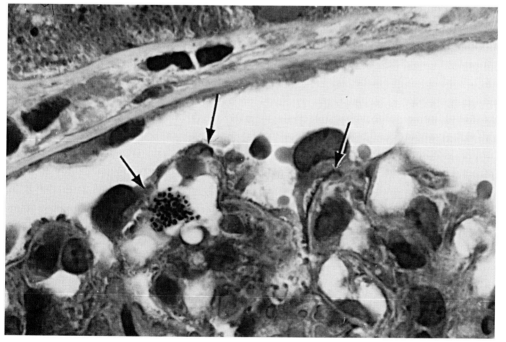

Figure 5–4. Acute poststreptococcal glomerulonephritis. Multiple ''hump-shaped'' subepithelial deposits are present *(arrows)*. (H&E, ×1000.)

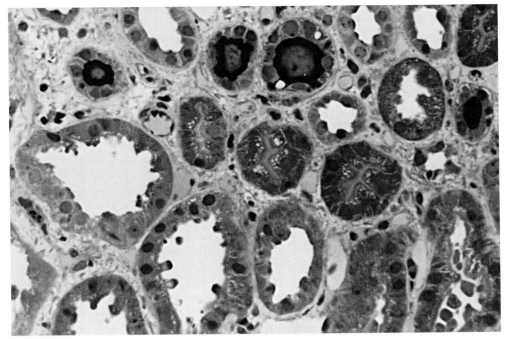

Figure 5–5. Acute poststreptococcal glomerulonephritis. The interstitium is edematous and contains an occasional inflammatory cell. A few red blood cell casts are present. (H&E, ×300.)

mal. At this stage, the lesion is a diffuse mesangial proliferative glomerulonephritis.

The tubules contain many hyalin and cellular casts composed of mixtures of red and white blood cells (Fig. 5–5). Proximal tubular cells may contain protein-laden lysosomes, but necrosis is uncommon.

The interstitium is often widened by edema. Inflammatory cell infiltrates are most prominent except in cases in which there is crescentic glomerulonephritis.

Immunofluorescence Microscopy

The glomerular basement membranes are outlined by small, granular aggregates of IgG and C3 (Fig. 5–6). The deposits are more widely spaced and more irregular in shape than those present in membranous glomerulonephritis. The mesangial regions may also contain granular deposits of immunoglobulins and complement components. IgM may be present, but it is seldom prominent.

Electron Microscopy

The centrolobular regions are filled with cells, and many of the usual anatomic landmarks are not recognizable. There is an increase in the number of endothelial cells, and

their cytoplasm is prominent and filled with organelles. Their usual fenestrated, thin cytoplasm is irregularly thickened (Fig. 5–7).

The mesangial regions are expanded, and their boundaries may be difficult to discern.

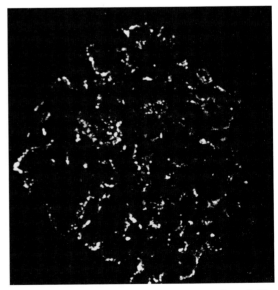

Figure 5–6. Acute poststreptococcal glomerulonephritis. Irregular granular IgG deposits are spread diffusely over the peripheral basement membranes, corresponding to the "humps." (Immunofluorescence micrograph, ×250.)

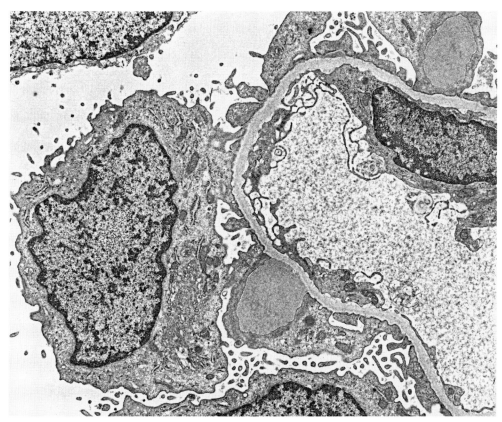

Figure 5–7. Acute poststreptococcal glomerulonephritis. There are two large electron-dense subepithelial "humps." The foot processes are effaced over the deposits, forming a mantle of cytoplasm. (Electron micrograph, ×2200.)

Adjacent mesangial zones often appear to be joined, leaving the impression of the presence of mesangiolysis. Dead cells and cellular debris may be seen, admixed with the increased number of mesangial cells.

The electron-dense deposits on the subepithelial aspects of the glomerular basement membrane are separated from the lamina densa and from the podocytes by a clear zone (Fig. 5–8). The peripheral glomerular basement membrane is otherwise unremarkable.

There are also many deposits within the substance of the mesangial matrix. In the paramesangial area, deposits may be found within the glomerular basement membranes. As noted earlier, the mesangial matrix may be unrecognizable in some areas, and adjacent mesangial areas may coalesce.

The podocytes are prominent, and their cytoplasmic outlines are considerably altered. There is irregular effacement of the pedicels, and many villi are seen on the urinary surface (Fig. 5–8). The number of cytoplasmic organelles is considerably increased, especially in the regions of the pedicels, and the normal dense layer of microfibrils near the glomerular basement membrane is no longer evident (Fig. 5–7).

Prognosis

The immediate prognosis is usually excellent, even when anuria is present at the onset. The exudative response disappears quickly, and the proliferative lesions resolve thereafter. All signs of renal disease disappear in most patients within a few weeks, although in children there may be microscopic hematuria for 1 to 2 years and minimal albuminuria. The prognosis in adults is not as well established, but few cases are reported to progress to end stage, except for those with persistent hypertension.

Glomerulonephritis Due to Other Bacterial Infections

Many bacterial infections have been associated with the development of glomerulone-

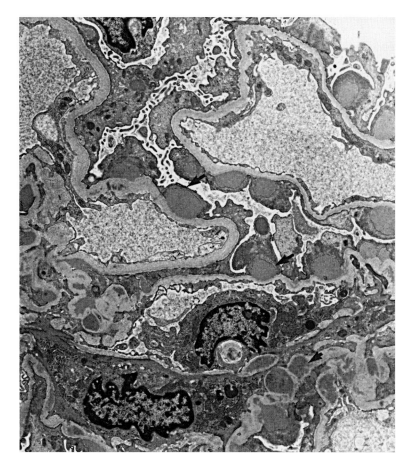

Figure 5–8. Acute poststreptococcal glomerulonephritis. The subepithelial spaces are studded by irregularly spaced deposits *(arrows)*. Smaller deposits are also present in the mesangium *(arrowhead)*. There is extensive effacement of the foot processes and villous transformation of the podocytes. (Electron micrograph, ×2200.)

phritis. In the past decade infections other than streptococcal have become the dominant cause of glomerulonephritis. Apart from the more classic sites, such as shunts or cardiac valves, the skin and viscera are the most common sites of infection. This has resulted in a shift in the peak incidence age to adults, and a worsening of the overall prognosis. In addition, glomerulonephritis due to these causes is more commonly seen in elderly people, in alcoholics, and in immunocompromised adults.

Although the exact cause of the glomerulonephritis remains unproved, it has been assumed that the renal lesions are due to the deposition (or local formation) of immune complexes derived from circulatory components. This supposition is supported by animal studies using protein antigens, but there have been few reports of an identified bacterial antigen in glomerular deposits in humans. The epidemiologic evidence for such a link is clear, however, and most accept the notion that glomerular deposits are related to the infectious agent and the antibody response to it. It is less well documented that the type, titer, or even presence of circulating antigen-antibody complexes is directly related to the renal disease.

The type of glomerular lesions that may be found as a consequence of these bacterial infections covers the spectrum of inflammatory renal diseases. There is some consistency within general categories of infection, allowing positive correlations to be made. These are considered in the following sections.

Acute Endocarditis

Pathogenesis

The renal lesions are due to the formation and/or deposition of immune complexes in the glomeruli.

Patient Presentation

Acute endocarditis is now most frequently seen in drug abusers or patients who have undergone invasive vascular surgery. The patient's condition deteriorates rapidly unless the infection is recognized early and treated effectively. The renal lesions are often not detected or are recognized only by finding a few casts and a small amount of protein in the urine of an otherwise hectically ill patient. Very few patients develop evidence of renal failure.

Histology

Light Microscopy

The glomeruli are diffusely hypercellular, containing a number of intrinsic glomerular cells and leukocytes (Fig. 5–9). Of interest is the fact that the number of neutrophils is often quite small. This stands in sharp contrast to poststreptococcal glomerulonephritis, in which neutrophils are a major component of the hypercellularity at this stage. Localized crescents and synechiae may be present. The glomerular lesion seldom mimics that seen in subacute bacterial endocarditis. The glomerular basement membranes are not thickened, but subepithelial deposits may be recognizable in thin sections stained with periodic acid–Schiff (PAS).

Scattered foci of interstitial infiltrates and tiny foci of tubular necrosis are often seen.

Immunofluorescence Microscopy

IgG and IgM are found in scattered granular deposits along the peripheral glomerular basement membranes and in the mesangium. The most prominent deposits consist of large granules of C3 in the same distribution as the immunoglobulins. When the glomerular lesions are modest by light microscopy, the deposits may be limited to the mesangial regions.

Electron Microscopy

The irregularity of the immune deposits is confirmed by electron microscopy. Quite large but localized electron-dense deposits are seen in the subepithelial and mesangial regions.

Prognosis

The prognosis is excellent if appropriate therapy is instituted early in the course.

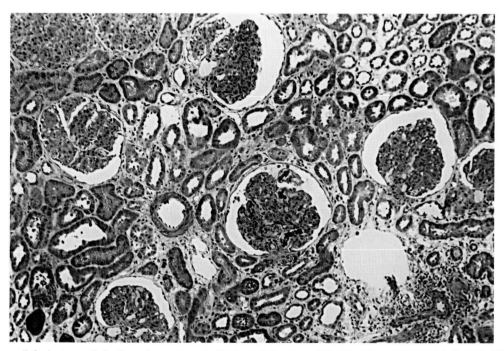

Figure 5–9. Acute postinfectious glomerulonephritis, bacterial endocarditis. The glomeruli are globally and diffusely hypercellular. The interstitium is diffusely edematous and contains many inflammatory cells. (H&E, ×75.)

Subacute Bacterial Endocarditis

Pathogenesis

The renal lesions are due to the formation and/or deposition of immune complexes in the glomeruli. The difficulty in separating an infectious from an immune cause may be a particular problem in patients with repeatedly negative blood cultures, because they may also have plasma findings that contribute to further obfuscation of the true diagnosis. These findings include hypocomplementemia, low titers of antinuclear factors, mixed polyclonal cryoglobulins, and rheumatoid factor. The diagnosis depends on the finding of a positive blood culture and a high level of suspicion.

Patient Presentation

As with acute bacterial endocarditis, this lesion is now most commonly encountered in intravenous drug abusers and patients who have had intravascular operative procedures. The organisms most frequently implicated are streptococci (*Streptococcus viridans*), but valvular infections with staphylococci have also been reported. Whereas patients with acute valvular infections present with a vivid, rapidly progressive illness, those with subacute endocarditis often have a more indolent disease. Renal lesions are much more frequent in the subacute disease, and they become evident within a few weeks after the onset of the intravascular infection. The urine sediment contains red blood cells, white blood cells, and casts containing one or both cell types. Proteinuria is also present. These urine findings suggest an active underlying glomerulonephritis. Renal failure or the nephrotic syndrome is uncommon but may appear if the lesion is not recognized and treated promptly.

The extrarenal signs consisting of fever, rash, splenomegaly, and weakness may lead to the erroneous diagnosis of an autoimmune disease.

Histology

Light Microscopy

The glomerular lesions are initially focal and segmental in most patients. This observation led to the initial, erroneous notion that they were due to emboli derived from the heart valve vegetations. The lesions consist of segmental and focal proliferation coexisting with focal sclerotic (healed) lesions (Fig. 5–10). Diffuse glomerular lesions are present in a smaller number of patients. Both focal and diffuse glomerular lesions may be associated with localized crescents. The crescents and the areas of increased cellularity within the tufts characteristically contain large numbers of macrophages. This unique finding helps differentiate this lesion from other clinical and histologic types of renal disease. After successful treatment and resolution of the lesions, scarred synechiae may be the only residuum (Fig. 5–11).

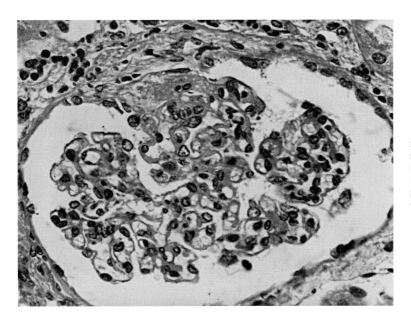

Figure 5–10. Postinfectious glomerulonephritis, subacute bacterial endocarditis. There is segmental sclerosis, with an organized fibrous crescent and mild mesangial hypercellularity. (Masson's trichrome, ×250.)

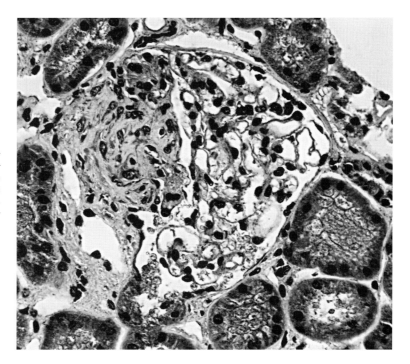

Figure 5–11. Acute postinfectious glomerulonephritis, bacterial endocarditis, post-treatment. There is segmental sclerosis with an overlying organized crescent. The remainder of the tuft is normal. (Masson's trichrome, ×250.)

The interstitium contains multifocal areas of interstitial infiltrate, composed of mononuclear cells.

The blood vessels are usually not involved. Patients with vasculitic lesions have been reported, but this is an exceptional finding.

Immunofluorescence Microscopy

Deposits of IgG, IgM, C3, C1q, and C4 are invariably diffuse, even when the light microscopic lesions appear focal. Those that had focal lesions by light microscopy most frequently have deposits restricted to the mesangium, whereas both mesangial and subendothelial deposits are found in the diffuse lesions.

Electron Microscopy

Electron-dense deposits are present within the mesangial regions. In the diffuse form, deposits are also found in the subendothelial zones, less commonly in the subepithelial areas, and rarely within the substance of the peripheral basement membranes.

Prognosis

If the lesions are promptly diagnosed and treated, the proteinuria and hematuria disap-

pear. It is assumed that the inflammatory glomerular lesions also diminish and ultimately resolve, leaving sclerotic zones. The most severe sequelae are related either to perforation or deformity of a cardiac valve.

Infected Shunts (Infected Intravascular Catheters and Prostheses)

Pathogenesis

The renal lesion is thought to be a consequence of the formation of immune complexes. Thus, plasma levels of complement components are decreased, and circulating immune complexes are present.

Patient Presentation

Infected shunts were first described in children with hydrocephalus who had atrioventricular shunts. Similar lesions have subsequently been reported in patients who have other types of chronic, indwelling intravascular prostheses. The most common bacterium cultured from the prosthesis or blood is *Staphylococcus albus.* These infections often do not come to the attention of the clinical team until some time after the prosthesis has been placed, and often long after the disease has started, because the infection pursues such an indolent course. The renal lesion is recognizable by the presence of significant proteinuria and hematuria. Impairment of renal function is not present early in the course but may appear in the absence of appropriate therapy.

Histology

Light Microscopy

The glomerular lesions are reminiscent of those in type I membranoproliferative glomerulonephritis (also see Chapter 4). There is an increased number of cells within the tuft, composed of macrophages and mesangial cells. Crescents, either local or diffuse, are commonly seen. The peripheral glomerular basement membranes are frequently thickened and duplicated in a diffuse manner.

The interstitium, tubules, and blood vessels do not differ from those in subacute bacterial endocarditis.

Immunofluorescence Microscopy

The glomeruli have diffuse mesangial and peripheral glomerular basement membrane (intramembranous, subendothelial, and less commonly subepithelial) deposits of IgM, C3, C1q, and C4, with a smaller amount of IgG.

No deposits are associated with the tubules or interstitium.

Electron Microscopy

The location of the deposits is confirmed. The architecture of the glomerular basement membrane is even more altered than is appreciated by light microscopy.

Prognosis

As with subacute endocarditis, the signs of renal damage recede and then disappear with appropriate therapy. Patients with severe sclerosing lesions may, however, continue to have proteinuria. Long-term studies on which to gauge the ultimate prognosis are not available, but renal failure is not a common outcome.

Skin, Visceral, and Other Infections

Pathogenesis and Patient Presentation

The lesions are secondary to the presence of deposited immune reactants. Renal failure was present in 56 of 76 in a recent series of patients with bacterial infections that were either uncontrolled, or poorly controlled. The patients had either the acute onset of the ne-

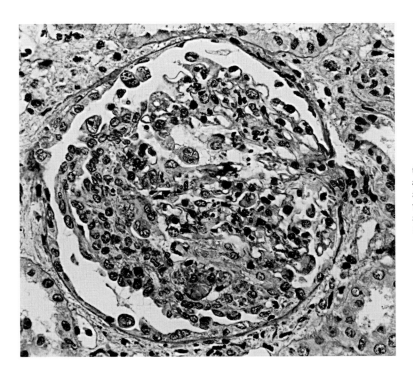

Figure 5–12. Acute postinfectious glomerulonephritis, visceral abscess. There is global mesangial and endovascular proliferation, with infiltrating neutrophils and an organizing segmental crescent. (Masson's trichrome, ×250.)

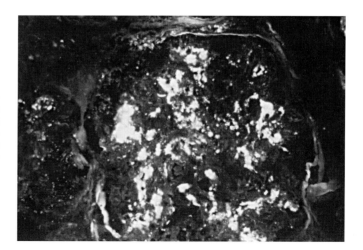

Figure 5–13. Acute postinfectious glomerulonephritis, deep visceral abscess. There are diffuse, large, coarse deposits of C1q in the subepithelial, subendothelial, and mesangial regions. Bowman's capsule also contains deposits. (Immunofluorescence micrograph, ×250.)

phrotic syndrome or acute nephritis. Fourteen required dialysis. The serum complement levels were low in 35%, and multiple infections were present in 25%.

Histology

Light Microscopy

There was endocapillary glomerulonephritis in 58%, mixed endoextracapillary glomerulonephritis in 34%, and membranoproliferative glomerulonephritis in the rest (Fig. 5–12).

Immunofluorescence Microscopy

There were deposits of C3 and/or C1q, and approximately 50% had subepithelial or mesangial deposits of immunoglobulins (Fig. 5–13). In addition, the typical immunofluorescence pattern associated with type I membranoproliferative glomerulonephritis was found in 8%.

Prognosis

Recovery of renal function was not often seen in this group of patients; 20 of 76 recovered normal renal function, 38 had persistent renal disease, and 14 developed chronic renal failure.

SELECTED READINGS

1. Arze RS, Hashid H, Morley R, et al: Shunt nephritis: Report of two cases and review of the literature. Clin Nephrol 19:48, 1983.
2. Beaufils M, Gibert C, Morel-Maroger L, et al: Glomerulonephritis in severe bacterial infections with and without endocarditis. Adv Nephrol 7:217, 1978.
3. Beaufils M, Morel-Maroger L, Sraer JD, et al: Acute renal failure of glomerular origin during visceral abscesses. N Engl J Med 295:185, 1976.
4. Black JA, Challacombe DN, Ockenden BG: Nephrotic syndrome associated with bacteraemia after shunt operations for hydrocephalus. Lancet 2:921, 1965.
5. Boulton-Jones JM, Sissons JGP, Evans DS, et al: Renal lesions of subacute infective endocarditis. Br Med J 2:11, 1974.
6. Gutman RA, Striker GE, Gilliland BC, et al: The immune-complex glomerulonephritis of bacterial endocarditis. Medicine (Baltimore) 51:1, 1972.
7. Kaufmann DB, McIntosh R: The pathogenesis of the renal lesion in a patient with streptococcal disease, infected ventriculoatrial shunt, cryoglobulinemia and nephritis. Am J Med 50:262, 1971.
8. Kim Y, Michael AF: Chronic bacteremia and nephritis. Annu Rev Med 29:319, 1978.
9. Leonard CD, Nagle R, Striker GE, et al: Acute glomerulonephritis with prolonged oliguria. Ann Intern Med 73:703, 1970.
10. Montseny J-J, Meyrier A, Kleinknecht D, Callard P: The current spectrum of infectious glomerulonephritis. Experience with 76 patients and review of the literature. Medicine 74:63, 1995.
11. Morel-Maroger L, Sraer JD, Herreman G, et al: Kidney in subacute endocarditis: Pathological and immunofluorescent findings. Arch Pathol 94:205, 1972.
12. Neugarten J, Gallo GR, Baldwin DS: Glomerulonephritis in bacterial endocarditis. Am J Kidney Dis 3:371, 1984.

VIRAL INFECTIONS

Hepatitis B

Pathogenesis

Among the numerous viral diseases thought to be associated with specific renal lesions, hepatitis B and C are the most extensively documented. Nonetheless, the mechanisms and even the type of renal damage induced by the hepatitis B virus have not been elucidated, and it is not clear whether the association currently described will remain as an established entity.

Hepatitis B antigenemia has been considered to be a pathogenic factor in diseases as diverse as polyarteritis nodosa, membranous glomerulonephritis, and membranoproliferative glomerulonephritis. There appear to be marked geographic variations concerning the incidence of hepatitis B virus infections and the proportion of patients who develop an associated renal disease. In Asia, Africa, and Eastern Europe, essentially all (80 to 100%) of the children with membranous glomerulonephritis are carriers of hepatitis B surface antigen (HBsAg). The number in the United States is smaller (20% of children with membranous glomerulonephritis), but still it represents an important group. In Hong Kong, the percentage of adults who are HBsAg carriers is 30 to 45%, and in the United States and England fewer than 5% are carriers.

It has been generally accepted that the individuals infected with the virus develop circulating immune complexes. Circulating immune complexes are thought to play a major role in the pathogenesis of the many renal lesions associated with hepatitis B virus infection. In fact, the surface (HBsAg), the core (HBcAg), and the e antigen (HBeAg) have all been demonstrated in the glomeruli of hepatitis B carriers with membranous glomerulonephritis. It has been suggested that HBeAg may be the most likely pathogenic antigen, since it is a small molecule and could pass the filtration barrier and is cationic. Both of these characteristics would favor glomerular localization. In addition, membranous glomerulonephritis has been reported to be active when HBeAg is found in the circulation, and it is often quiescent when the antibody to the e antigen appears.

Patient Presentation

The findings vary with the type of renal diseases. Those associated with polyarteritis nodosa and mixed cryoglobulinemia will be described respectively in Chapters 6 and 9. In American children, the hepatitis is often acquired by vertical transmission from siblings; 80% are male and most are black. In adults, most patients are men with a history of drug abuse, homosexuality, acquired immunodeficiency syndrome, or a prior blood transfusion. The liver disease in both adults and children is most often chronic persistent hepatitis.

Hepatitis B surface antigen has most frequently been reported in the serum of children with the nephrotic syndrome and more rarely in nephrotic adults. In these patients, liver symptoms are either absent or not prominent. The renal symptoms in patients who have developed renal disease usually appear after a long delay. Proteinuria is almost always present, and some patients have the nephrotic syndrome, especially those with membranoproliferative glomerulonephritis.

Circulating immune complexes are found in many, and serum complement components are low in 25 to 50% of patients.

Histology

Light Microscopy

Membranous glomerulonephritis and membranoproliferative glomerulonephritis are the varieties of glomerulonephritis most commonly associated with infection with hepatitis B virus (Fig. 5–14) (also see Chapter 4). The lesions do not show any specific features that could differentiate them from their idiopathic counterparts. In addition to membranous and type I membranoproliferative glomerulonephritis, which are by far the most common patterns, other patients have been reported to have endocapillary proliferation and crescentic glomerulonephritis.

Immunofluorescence Microscopy

In patients with membranous glomerulonephritis, deposits of IgG are invariably found in a regular granular pattern along the glomerular basement membranes. This pattern of deposition characterizes the disease. C3 usually codistributes with the IgG. It is interesting that a few patients have been reported to have had mesangial deposits of IgA and IgG in the typical granular membranous pattern.

In membranoproliferative glomerulonephritis, IgG and complement components have always been detected with the coarse granular pattern that characterizes this disease. In addition, most are associated with small deposits of IgM and IgA. The most common pattern is membranoproliferative glomerulonephritis type I, but type III may also be seen. When present, the most common hepatitis B antigen is HBsAg.

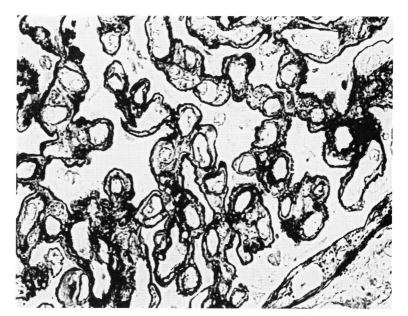

Figure 5–14. Membranoproliferative glomerulonephritis, hepatitis B. There is considerable duplication of the peripheral basement membranes. (Jones methenamine silver, ×800.)

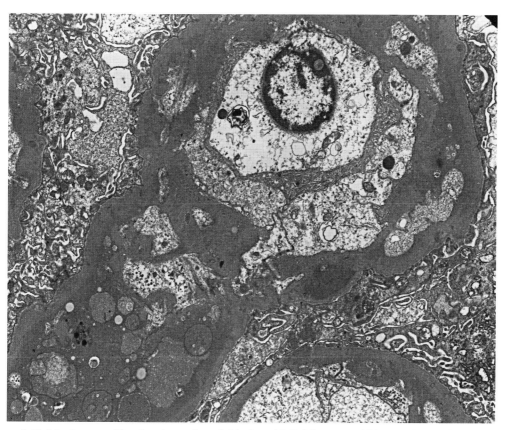

Figure 5–15. Membranoproliferative glomerulonephritis, hepatitis B. The mesangial interposition, subendothelial and mesangial electron-dense deposits, and double-contoured basement membranes are evident. (Electron micrograph, ×2800.)

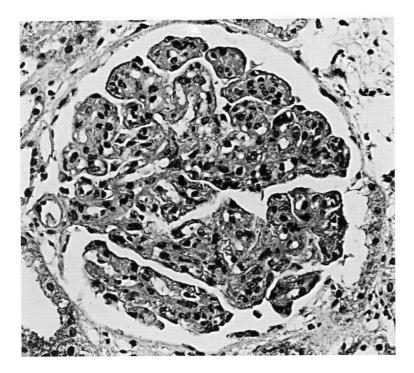

Figure 5–16. Membranoproliferative glomerulonephritis, hepatitis C. There is marked diminution of the vascular spaces due to a global increase in cells, some of which are polymorphonuclear neutrophils. Double-contoured basement membranes and mesangial interposition are visible. (Masson's trichrome, ×250.)

Many researchers have examined biopsy specimens for the presence of hepatitis B–related antigens. These antigens have been demonstrated in membranous glomerulonephritis by some investigators but have not been found consistently. Some early reports claimed the contrary. It seems that the diagnosis of the condition relies more on the association between serologic markers and the clinical association than on the local detection of hepatitis B viral antigens in the glomeruli.

Electron Microscopy

In most cases, the ultrastructural features are not different from those in idiopathic glomerular diseases. Some investigators have described spherical particles of 400 to 600 ang-

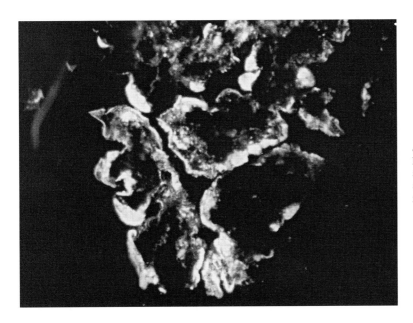

Figure 5–17. Membranoproliferative glomerulonephritis (type 1), hepatitis C. Extensive mesangial and subendothelial C3 deposits are seen. (Immunofluorescence micrograph, ×250.)

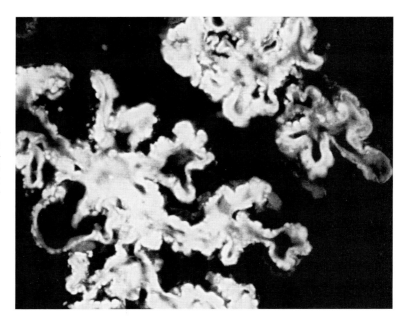

Figure 5–18. Membranoproliferative glomerulonephritis (type 3), hepatitis C. There are subepithelial and subendothelial IgG deposits along the glomerular basement membranes. (Immunofluorescence micrograph, ×250.)

stroms and clear lacunae in the basement membranes (Fig. 5–15).

Prognosis

The disappearance of the carrier state of the virus has been associated with disappearance of proteinuria, especially in children, in whom two thirds undergo a spontaneous remission within a period of 3 years, and progression to end-stage renal disease is rare. The prognosis is less benign in adults, in whom 30% have progressive renal failure in 5 years, and 10% require hemodialysis therapy.

Hepatitis C

This form of hepatitis may be associated with cryoglobulinemic or noncryoglobulinemic membranoproliferative glomerulonephritis. This has led to the speculation that hepatitis C may be generally implicated in membranoproliferative glomerulonephritis, but the most current estimate is that this is probably the case for only 10 to 20% of the cases. Even in those with hepatitis C infections, viral antigen(s) has not been found in the glomerular lesions.

The patients present with proteinuria (sometimes in the nephrotic range), microhematuria, and occasionally red blood cell casts. As with hepatitis B, the patients often have no symptoms of liver disease but have abnormal liver function tests. Serum complement levels are low, and cryoglobulins, circulating immune complexes, and rheumatoid factors are present in most.

The light (Fig. 5–16) and immunofluorescence microscopic findings (Figs. 5–17, 5–18) are those of membranoproliferative glomerulonephritis type I.

SELECTED READINGS

1. Brzosko WJ, Krawzynski K, Nazarewicz T, et al: Glomerulonephritis associated with hepatitis-B surface antigen immune complexes in children. Lancet 2:477, 1974.
2. Collins SB, Bhan AK, Dienstag JL, et al: Hepatitis B immune complex glomerulonephritis: Simultaneous glomerular deposition of hepatitis B surface and e antigens. Clin Immunol Immunopathol 26:137, 1983.
3. Johnson RJ, Couser WG: Hepatitis B infection and renal disease: Clinical immunopathogenetic and therapeutic considerations. Kidney Int 37:663, 1990.
4. Johnson RJ, Gretch DR, Yamabe H, et al: Membranoproliferative glomerulonephritis associated with hepatitis C virus infection. N Engl J Med 328:465, 1993.
5. Southwest Pediatric Nephrology Study Group: Hepatitis B surface antigenemia in North American children with idiopathic membranous glomerulonephritis. J Pediatr 106:571, 1975.
6. Yoshikawa N, Ito H, Yamada Y, et al: Membranous glomerulonephritis associated with hepatitis B antigen in children: A comparison with idiopathic membranous glomerulonephritis. Clin Nephrol 23:28, 1985.

HIV-Associated Nephropathy

Pathogenesis

Acquired immunodeficiency syndrome (AIDS), first described in 1978, is now estimated to affect approximately 20 million people worldwide. The fastest growing incidence and highest prevalence is in sub-Saharan Africa and South and Southeast Asia. It initially appeared that the kidney would be spared, but in 1984 a distinctive sclerosing glomerulopathy was reported in AIDS patients in New York City. Ironically, this report originated from King's County Medical Center in Brooklyn, the same institution that had described the development of focal segmental glomerulosclerosis in intravenous drug abusers, now known as heroin nephropathy, some 10 years before. These initial reports were met with considerable skepticism in West Coast centers where the population of AIDS patients consists predominantly of white homosexuals. From 1984 to 1990, a flurry of additional reports from other urban centers in New York, Miami, Washington, DC, Boston, Newark, Dallas, Los Angeles, Paris, and Milan confirmed the existence of this particularly rapidly progressive form of focal segmental glomerulosclerosis in human immunodeficiency virus (HIV) infected patients and clearly differentiated it from heroin nephropathy.

In a review of over 200 reported cases of HIV-associated nephropathy, 90% of the patients were black, 70% male, and 50% intravenous drug abusers. This racial distribution is particularly striking considering that in the United States, HIV infection is three times more common in whites than in blacks. Even when intravenous drug abusers are excluded from consideration, the black:white ratio is roughly 12:1 among nonintravenous drug abusers with HIV-associated nephropathy. These data indicate a striking black racial predominance in HIV-associated nephropathy independent of intravenous drug abuse and establish the black race as the most important risk factor for nephropathy. Several centers have reported that whites with HIV-associated nephropathy are more likely to have mild focal mesangial sclerosis and mild diffuse hypercellularity.

The incidence of HIV-associated nephropathy in autopsy and biopsy-based studies varies according to patient demographics, biopsy indications, and pathologic criteria for diagnosis. The incidence of focal segmental glomerulosclerosis among AIDS patients at autopsy varies from 1% in a San Francisco–based study to 10% in a Miami-based study. Among 86 HIV-infected patients undergoing renal biopsy at Columbia-Presbyterian Medical Center, 91% had glomerular disease and 9% had tubulointerstitial disease. The most common glomerular lesions were focal segmental glomerulosclerosis (58 patients) and minimal change disease (6 patients), but there was a wide variety of other glomerular lesions. The greater incidence of HIV-associated nephropathy in unselected biopsy series of HIV-infected patients is undoubtedly related to the tendency to biopsy patients with signs of severe glomerular injury. Focal segmental sclerosis accounts for 50% of the glomerular disease in HIV-infected children, and there is a higher incidence of diffuse mesangial hyperplasia and glomerular immune deposits than in HIV-infected adults. The progression to uremia is slower in children than in adults.

Since HIV-associated nephropathy commonly occurs before opportunistic infections are manifest, intercurrent infections do not appear to play a major role in the development of this nephropathy. Glomerular immune deposits are generally not present in HIV-associated nephropathy. Since HIV-associated nephropathy occurs at a stage of HIV infection when the immune system is not yet severely compromised, it is likely that the nature of the host response to viral infection plays a critical role in the development of nephropathy. Proposed mechanisms of HIV nephropathy include the following possibilities, none of which has been proved:

1. Direct renal epithelial (visceral and tubular epithelial) cell injury by virus;
2. Indirect injury by circulating viral products;
3. Indirect injury through cytokines released by infected lymphocytes or monocytes, local or in the general circulation.

Whereas some have suggested that lymphocyte or monocyte-tropic strains of HIV can infect human glomerular endothelial or mesangial cells in vitro, others have failed to confirm these findings. Although viral genome products have been detected by polymerase chain reaction (PCR) in renal biopsies from patients with HIV infection, it is not known whether this is due to contamination by blood cells or is a result of viral infection of renal parenchymal cells. The development of a form of focal segmental glomerulosclerosis resembling HIV-associated nephropathy, recently described in mice transgenic for a HIV gene construct lacking certain structural proteins, suggests that the complete virus may not be required for development of the kidney lesions.

Because a variety of lesions can occur in HIV-infected patients, the term *HIV-associated nephropathy* should be restricted to focal segmental glomerulosclerosis and mesangial cellular changes; it should not be used to describe lesions that fit into other recognized diagnostic categories. For instance, HIV-infected patients may develop an acute postinfectious glomerulonephritis. In this case the correct diagnosis would be acute postinfectious glomerulonephritis in an HIV-infected patient. Because focal glomerulosclerosis often develops in early stages of HIV infection, before overt AIDS, the term *HIV-associated nephropathy* is more accurate than *AIDS nephropathy*.

Patient Presentation

Presenting features include nephrotic-range proteinuria, a bland urinary sediment, and renal insufficiency with rapid progression to renal failure. At Columbia-Presbyterian Medical Center, mean urinary protein excretion at presentation was 6.6 g/24 hours, and mean serum creatinine was 5.4 mg/dl. Most patients in the Center have the nephrotic syndrome, although proteinuria may be decreased in patients with advanced renal failure. Hypertension and edema were relatively uncommon, and the kidneys were enlarged and highly echogenic by ultrasound.

Histology

Light Microscopy

The characteristic histologic finding is focal segmental glomerulosclerosis. Although the morphologic findings mimic those in idiopathic focal segmental glomerulosclerosis, the glomeruli are more often "collapsed," i.e., there is segmental or global retraction of the glomerular basement membranes with decreased or absent vascular lumina (Fig. 5–19). Most often there is no significant increase in mesangial matrix or thickening of the wrinkled glomerular basement membranes, and hyalin deposits are rare. The visceral epithelial cells typically are hypertrophied, with enlarged vesicular nuclei and frequent intracytoplasmic protein resorption droplets. Visceral cell hyperplasia is common, and may mimic cellular crescents. In chronic and advanced lesions, features of segmental and global glomerulosclerosis are found.

Severe tubulointerstitial disease, which often appears out of proportion to the degree of glomerulosclerosis, is an important component of HIV-associated nephropathy. This includes severe interstitial edema, fibrosis and inflammation, tubular degenerative and regenerative changes, and progressive tubular atrophy. The interstitial infiltrate includes lymphocytes (predominantly CD8 positive T cells) as well as plasma cells, monocytes, and B cells. Approximately half of biopsy specimens have many areas of dilated tubules containing abun-

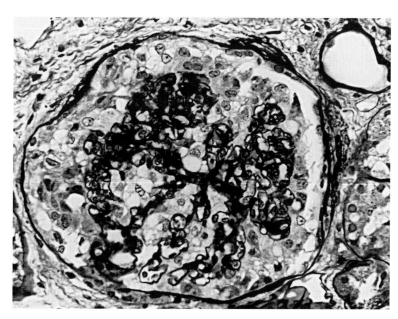

Figure 5–19. HIV nephropathy. The glomerular basement membranes are wrinkled and thickened, and the tuft lumina are effaced. There is marked hyperplasia of epithelial cells in Bowman's space, and the tufts are collapsed. (Jones methenamine silver, ×300.)

dant, loose, proteinaceous casts (Fig. 5–20). This lesion is referred to as microcysts. There also may be focal dilations of Bowman's spaces. The increased tubulointerstitial volume resulting from interstitial fibrosis, edema, and casts probably contributes to the kidney enlargement and hyperechoic appearance on ultrasound examinations.

In some patients the glomerular lesions are restricted to mild, diffuse mesangial hypercellularity. A minority develop a minimal change–like lesion with nephrotic proteinuria and minimal histologic alterations. These mild glomerular lesions appear to be more common in children and white adults. Rarely, these mild mesangiopathies have been reported to evolve into more typical focal segmental glomerulosclerosis on repeat biopsy or at autopsy. The relationship of these purely mesangial lesions to the focal sclerosing lesions within the spectrum of HIV-associated nephropathy remains unclear.

Immunofluorescence Microscopy

There is frequent staining for IgM, C3, and less commonly C1q in areas of collapse or glomerulosclerosis. They may also be uniformly distributed throughout the mesangium. Rarely, patients with a focal segmental glomerulosclerosis pattern on light microscopy are found to have mesangial or glomerular capillary wall immune deposits containing IgG or IgA. The presence of visceral cell cytoplasmic positivity for albumin, IgG, and IgA corresponding to intracytoplasmic protein resorption droplets is a frequent finding and should not be mistaken for glomerular capillary wall immune deposits.

The tubular casts usually stain intensely for albumin, as well as immunoglobulins (IgG and IgA), but not Tamm-Horsfall protein, suggesting nonselective proteinuria.

Electron Microscopy

In the areas of glomerular collapse, there is wrinkling, thickening, and retraction of the glomerular basement membrane, causing narrowing of the vascular spaces (Fig. 5–21). The overlying visceral epithelial cells are hypertrophied with extensive foot process effacement, increased content of organelles, and microvillous transformation. Foot process effacement is generally widespread, affecting nonsclerotic capillaries. Although most specimens lack electron-dense deposits, when present they may be detected in the mesangium or less commonly involving the peripheral glomerular capillary walls, in subendothelial, intramembranous, or subepithelial locations. Endothelial tubulo-reticular inclusions are distinctive and character-

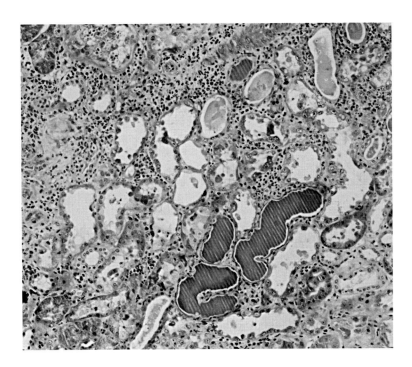

Figure 5–20. HIV nephropathy. The interstitium contains a diffuse inflammatory cell infiltrate composed of lymphocytes and plasma cells. There is marked tubular dilatation (microcysts), associated with tubular atrophy. (H&E, ×200.)

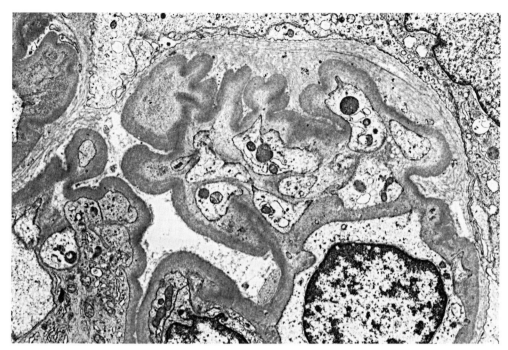

Figure 5–21. HIV nephropathy. The tufts are collapsed, the podocytes are detached, and the vascular spaces are absent. The identity of the cells in the tufts is not clear. (Electron micrograph, ×4000.)

istic features of HIV-associated nephropathy and are present in over 90% of cases. They consist of 24-nm interanastomosing tubular structures located within dilated cisternae of endoplasmic reticulum (Fig. 5–22). These structures are a manifestation of HIV infection and are not specific for the nephropathy. Tubuloreticular inclusions are also commonly observed in the glomerular or vascular endothelial cells of patients with systemic lupus erythematosus as well as with other viral infections. They are particularly large and numerous in the setting of HIV infection, where they may number several per capillary. Other helpful ultrastructural features of HIV-associated nephropathy include granular fragmentation of nuclear chromatin in interstitial and tubular cells, cytomembranous inclusions, cylindrical confronting cisternae, and increased numbers of nuclear bodies in tubular epithelial cells.

Other Glomerular Lesions in HIV-Infected Patients

Increasing numbers of HIV-infected patients have been reported with proliferative glomerulonephritis and variable degrees and intensity of mesangial and peripheral capillary wall deposits containing IgG, IgA, and other immune reactants. IgA nephropathy with elevated serum IgA levels and circulating immune complexes containing IgA idiotypic antibodies has been reported in several patients. Some patients have IgA cryoglobulinemia and hypocomplementemia. In some, the idiotypic antibodies are reactive with IgG or IgM specific for HIV core or envelope proteins. Immune deposits have been eluted from glomeruli and shown to contain HIV core or envelope proteins bound to IgG or IgA. Similar HIV-containing immune complexes have been identified in the serum of these patients.

HIV-infected patients have also been reported to develop hepatitis C–associated membranoproliferative glomerulonephritis and hepatitis B- or C-associated membranous glomerulopathy.

There are an increasing number of reports of hemolytic uremic syndrome or thrombotic thrombocytopenic purpura with renal involvement occurring in HIV-infected patients. The renal biopsy findings are those of glomerular and arteriolar thrombotic microangiopathy (also see Chapter 6). This syndrome is most common in homosexual males, particularly in late stages of HIV infection. There is no clear association with *Escherichia coli* 0157:H7 infec-

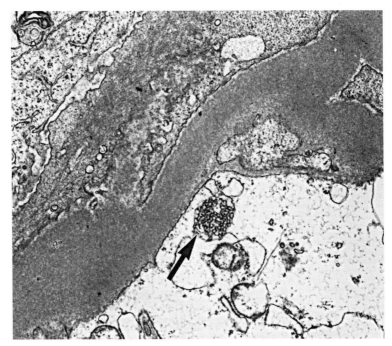

Figure 5–22. HIV nephropathy. Tubuloreticular inclusions are present in the endothelial cell cytoplasm (*arrow*). (Electron micrograph, ×11,000.)

tion or other enteric pathogens. There may be an association with the nephrotoxic potential of some of the newer therapeutic agents.

HIV RNA has been found in megakaryocytes in some patients, suggesting a direct viral infection of platelet precursor cells, with resulting cytopathic effects.

Prognosis

The outcome of HIV-associated nephropathy is universally poor, with an accelerated course to uremia within a few weeks or months, a course much more rapid than in heroin nephropathy or idiopathic focal segmental glomerulosclerosis. At Columbia-Presbyterian Medical Center, the median time from clinical recognition of disease onset to dialysis was 11 weeks, with a small number progressing more slowly over a period of 80 weeks. Patient survival correlated with the stage of HIV infection. Patients in early stages of HIV infection, without opportunistic infection, survived many months on hemodialysis, whereas hemodialysis patients with overt AIDS succumbed to opportunistic infection and cachexia within weeks. Longer patient and renal survival has been reported in patients treated with AZT (zidovudine).

AIDS patients are also prone to development of acute renal failure due to tubulointerstitial injury (unrelated to focal segmental glomerulosclerosis). In a study of 449 AIDS patients at Bellevue Hospital in New York City, acute renal failure occurred at some time during hospitalization in 55% of patients. The etiologic factors included volume depletion in 38%, pentamidine in 17%, amphotericin in 11%, trimethoprim-sulfamethoxazole in 9%, sepsis in 8%, radiocontrast exposure in 4%, and aminoglycoside antibiotics in 2%. Acute renal failure was most common in the preterminal period. At Columbia-Presbyterian Medical Center, acute tubular necrosis was the most common renal pathologic finding at autopsy, affecting 30% of AIDS patients.

SELECTED READINGS

1. Bourgoignie JJ: Renal complications of human immunodeficiency virus Type I. Kidney Int 37:1571, 1990.
2. Carbone L, D'Agati V, Cheng JT, Appel GB: The course and prognosis of human immunodeficiency virus–associated nephropathy. Am J Med 87:389, 1989.
3. D'Agati V, Suh JI, Carbone L, et al: The pathology of HIV-nephropathy: A detailed morphologic and comparative study. Kidney Int 35:1358, 1989.
4. Humphreys MH: Human immunodeficiency virus–associated glomerulosclerosis. Kidney Int 48:311, 1995.

5. Kimmel PL, Phillips TM, Ferreira-Centeno A, et al: Brief report: Idiotypic IgA nephropathy in patients with human immunodeficiency virus infection. N Engl J Med 327:702, 1992.
6. Kimmel PL, Phillips TM, Ferreira-Centeno A, et al: HIV-associated immune-mediated renal disease. Kidney Int 44:1327, 1993.
7. Rao TKS, Filippone EJ, Nicastri AD, et al: Associated focal and segmental glomerulosclerosis in the acquired immunodeficiency syndrome. N Engl J Med 310:669, 1984.
8. Valeri A, Neusy AJ: Acute and chronic renal disease in hospitalized AIDS patients. Clin Nephrol 35:110, 1991.

PARASITIC DISEASES

Although glomerular lesions due to parasitic infestation are unusual in the United States and Western Europe, they represent a major cause of renal disease in developing countries. It is generally considered that parasitic infestation may induce an immune complex glomerulonephritis. Three groups of parasites have been implicated in the development of glomerulonephritis: those that cause malaria, schistosomiasis, and leishmaniasis.

Malaria

Patient Presentation and Pathogenesis

Quartan malaria has been reported to be a cause of an immune complex glomerulonephritis. Patients with quartan malaria have a high incidence of the nephrotic syndrome. They may present with massive edema, pleural effusions, and anasarca. Hypertension and hematuria are uncommon in the early stages of the disease; however, within the first 5 years of the disease, most patients develop decreased renal function that is followed by hypertension. Quartan malaria nephropathy is mainly a disease of childhood.

Although the lesions described later are known as quartan malaria nephropathy and were initially described in areas where quartan malaria was endemic, comparable lesions have been reported in areas where quartan malaria is essentially unknown. Thus, the specificity of the lesion is unknown, and we prefer to use the term *tropical nephropathy*.

Histology

Light Microscopy

The glomerular lesions are characteristic but can be easily overlooked if the pathologist is not familiar with the condition. There is a diffuse alteration of the glomerular basement membranes consisting of a plexiform alteration of the lamina densa. This results in a double layering of the peripheral glomerular basement membranes by silver stain. The lesions may superficially resemble those of membranoproliferative glomerulonephritis, but the glomerular lesions in quartan malaria do not have a proliferative component. In addition to the glomerular basement membrane lesions, segmental areas of glomerulosclerosis are irregularly dispersed within and between glomeruli. The glomerulosclerotic lesions gradually increase in amount and frequency, resulting in end-stage glomerulosclerosis. The peripheral glomerular basement membrane thickening also slowly advances, resulting in obliteration of the vascular spaces.

Immunofluorescence Microscopy

The findings are quite variable. Diffuse deposits of immunoglobulins, including IgG and IgM, may be seen in a mixed pattern of both linear and granular distribution. There are a few reports of malarial antigens in the glomeruli. Complement components are almost always present with immunoglobulin deposits. On the other hand, in patients who have tropical nephropathy and in whom there are no deposits of immune reactants, the etiologic and the pathogenetic linkage of the disease to quartan malaria has been called into question.

Electron Microscopy

The glomerular basement membranes are of irregular thickness and contain lacunae, often filled with electron-dense material. The amount of extracellular matrix in the mesangium is increased, and there is often a subendothelial layer of similar material.

Schistosomiasis

Patient Presentation and Pathogenesis

Schistosoma mansoni has frequently been reported as a cause of renal disease, but infestation with the other schistosomes does not appear to result in renal parenchymal lesions. Renal disease has been well documented only in the hepatosplenic form of *S. mansoni* disease. This is a common parasite in certain

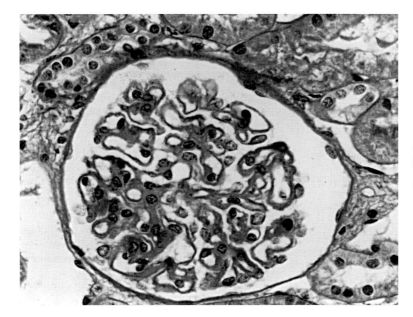

Figure 5–23. Membranous glomerulopathy, filariasis. There is global glomerular basement membrane thickening, without mesangial changes or hypercellularity. (Masson's trichrome, ×250.)

regions of South America, and the renal lesions in Brazil have been well studied. In regions of endemic schistosomal disease, the frequency of glomerular lesions in infected patients has been estimated to be approximately 15%. The cause of the renal lesion has been thought to be the deposition of circulating immune reactants in the glomeruli. In support of this concept are the observations that the patients have circulating immune complexes, and that the glomeruli contain large deposits of immune reactants.

Histology

Light and Electron Microscopy

The glomerular lesions may be identical to those in type I membranoproliferative glomerulonephritis, but focal glomerulonephritis and membranous glomerulonephritis have also been identified.

Immunofluorescence Microscopy

The lesions are similar to that of type I membranoproliferative glomerulonephritis, but the deposits of IgG, IgM, and C3 may be larger. The deposits are mixed—that is, they are both coarse and finely granular.

Filariasis

The filariasis that has most often been reported to be associated with renal disease is loiasis, and the lesion reported is membranous glomerulonephritis (Fig. 5–23).

SELECTED READINGS

1. Andrade AZ, Rocha H: Schistosomal glomerulopathy. Kidney Int 16:23, 1979.
2. Andrade AZ, Andrade SG, Sadifursky M: Renal changes in patients with hepatosplenic schistosomiasis. Am J Trop Med Hyg 20:77, 1971.
3. Hendrickse RG, Adeniyi A: Quartan malarial nephrotic syndrome in children. Kidney Int 16:64, 1979.
4. Kibukamusoke JW, Hutt MSR, Wikls NE: The nephrotic syndrome in Uganda and its association with quartan malaria. Q J Med 36:393, 1967.
5. Martinelli R, Carlos A, Noblat B, et al: *Schistosoma mansoni*–induced mesangiocapillary glomerulonephritis: Influence of therapy. Kidney Int 35:1227, 1989.
6. Morel-Maroger L, Saimot AG, Sloper JC, et al: Tropical nephropathy and tropical extramembranous glomerulonephritis of unknown etiology in Senegal. Br Med J 1:541, 1975.
7. Ngu JL, Chatelanat F, Leke R, et al: Nephropathy in Cameroon: Evidence for filarial derived immune-complex pathogenesis in some cases. Clin Nephrol 24:128, 1985.

DRUG-INDUCED

Heroin-Associated Nephropathy

Glomerular lesions of many types have been reported in drug abusers. The frequency with which one encounters patients with glomerular disease related to drug abuse appears to vary widely among different populations and regions within a country and appears to be declining. At present, most studies in the literature are of patients in the United States. This uneven distribution is far from completely understood. There are many causes of glomerular diseases, other than the drug itself. For instance, intravenous drug abusers are exposed to drugs of widely varying composition and purity, and the means by which they are administered lead to a serious hazard of acquiring infectious diseases. The complications from these causes include infections from unsterile needles and syringes and impurities in the injected materials. For instance, there is a high frequency of subacute bacterial endocarditis in these patients. (For a description of the renal lesions in subacute bacterial nephritis, see the earlier section in this chapter.) In addition, AA amyloidosis is also one of the potential complications of long-term substance abuse. Finally, AIDS occurs with a high frequency in the population who abuse intravenous drugs. Thus, it may be difficult to determine whether the renal disease is due to the effects of the drugs, a viral (HIV) infection, malnutrition, bacterial infection, or some combination of these processes.

Pathogenesis

The term that is used to describe the renal lesion thought to be directly related to heroin abuse is *heroin-associated nephropathy*. This renal lesion occurs exclusively in addicts who inject drugs, either subcutaneously or intravenously. There is no direct evidence that heroin, by itself, causes the renal lesion.

Thus, although heroin is the drug most frequently associated with nephropathy, it is not clear whether the renal manifestations are restricted to this drug or are part of a general, nonspecific response to drug abuse. There is agreement that the most common renal lesion associated with heroin abuse is focal glomerulosclerosis, which often progresses to diffuse glomerulosclerosis. It has become prevalent in areas where drug abuse is endemic and in some metropolitan areas is a major cause of the nephrotic syndrome and end-stage renal failure. The disease seems to affect black males predominantly. It has therefore been speculated that this population may have a susceptibility for the development of sclerosing glomerular diseases that is uncovered by the substance abuse. However, the exact pathogenesis of the lesions remains unknown.

Another cause of glomerular disease in heroin addicts is systemic amyloidosis of the AA type. Amyloidosis occurs in drug abusers who inject the drug subcutaneously, leading to the suspicion that the amyloid disease is secondary to chronic infections in multiple cutaneous sites.

Patient Presentation

Proteinuria is almost always present, and the nephrotic syndrome is very common. Patients who have glomerulosclerosis also have microscopic hematuria. Those with amyloidosis may also present with hypertension. Many patients already have evidence of significant renal failure at the time of presentation, and almost all show rapid and progressive loss of renal function.

Focal Glomerulosclerosis/Collapsing Glomerulopathy

Histology

Light Microscopy

The lesions consist of segmental obliteration of glomerular vascular loops by focal sclerosis (Fig. 5–24). The sclerosis is often accompanied by synechiae. There is seldom evidence of proliferation; rather, there tend to be few nuclei in the areas of sclerosis. The basement membranes near the sclerotic areas are thickened and wrinkled, and the vascular lumina are diminished in size, a picture reminiscent of chronic ischemia. As the lesions progress, larger areas of the glomeruli are affected (Fig. 5–25). Foam cells and large hyalin deposits are often present in the areas of sclerosis. The end result is complete replacement of normal glomerular structures by sclerosis. Bowman's capsule is multilaminated adjacent to the synechiae. The visceral epithelial cells often appear swollen and vacuolated; in some cases, they are increased in number and form localized crescents.

Tubular atrophy and interstitial fibrosis are parallel to the glomerular lesions. Similarly, arteriolar and arterial lesions are often conspicuous.

These lesions are very similar to those seen in idiopathic focal glomerulosclerosis. The one important distinguishing feature in ad-

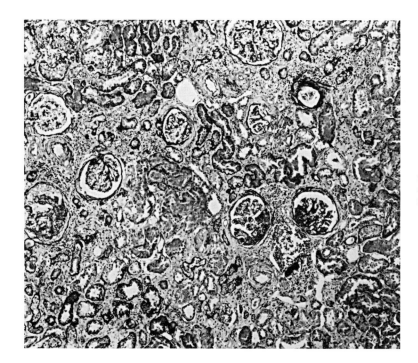

Figure 5–24. Heroin nephropathy. There is focal and segmental sclerosis with foci of severe interstitial fibrosis and tubular atrophy. (PASM, ×40.)

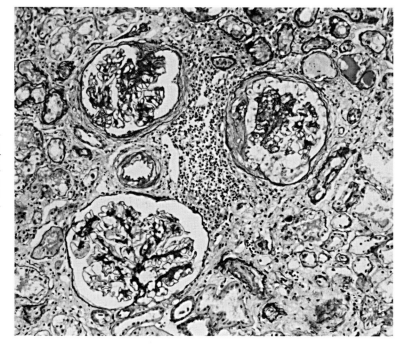

Figure 5–25. Heroin nephropathy. Two glomeruli demonstrate the focal and segmental nature of the lesions. The third is unaffected. The interstitium contains a large cellular infiltrate and marked tubular atrophy and is fibrotic. (PASM, ×100.)

dicts is the presence of considerable wrinkling and thickening of the glomerular basement membranes near the sclerotic zones. This feature has been subcategorized as "collapsing glomerulopathy" (see Chapter 4). Another differential feature is the more frequent presence of extensive interstitial infiltrates and severe tubular atrophy in heroin-associated nephropathy.

Immunofluorescence Microscopy

Large, coarsely granular aggregates of IgM and C3 are found in a segmental distribution corresponding to the areas of glomerular sclerosis. Other immunoglobulins are usually absent. However, there are reports of weak linear deposits of IgG along the glomerular basement membranes, similar to the distribution and intensity reported in some patients with other chronic sclerosing lesions, such as diabetes mellitus.

Electron Microscopy

The glomerular basement membranes are wrinkled and thickened near the sclerotic zones. The pedicels of the podocytes in these areas are partially effaced or detached, similar to the findings in the idiopathic variety of focal and segmental glomerulosclerosis. Electron-dense material resembling immune deposits is not seen, although there often is material resembling hyalin on the endothelial aspect of the glomerular basement membrane and in the vascular spaces, as well as in and abutting the mesangium.

Prognosis

The renal lesions most often relentlessly and rapidly progress to complete obliteration of the glomeruli. Renal failure, requiring renal replacement therapy, is therefore the usual outcome.

Amyloidosis

Amyloidosis of the AA type is the second most common renal pathologic entity encountered in heroin addicts.

Histology

The renal lesions do not differ histologically from those with other underlying diseases that lead to the deposition of AA amyloid (also see Chapter 9). The type of amyloid in the deposits was determined to be AA in these patients by immunofluorescence microscopy.

Prognosis

The development of amyloid deposits in the kidneys is associated with a rapid and progressive loss of renal function. Although the deposition does not appear to be altered or reversed by the interruption of drug abuse, proteinuria markedly abated in one recently reported patient after drug abuse was stopped. The renal amyloid deposits did not visibly decrease in this patient.

Other Lesions

Several other types of glomerular disease have been described in heroin addicts. Some appear to be the consequence of the infectious diseases that are common in addicts, such as subacute bacterial endocarditis. There have also been reports of focal and segmental glomerulonephritis, membranoproliferative glomerulonephritis, and membranous glomerulonephritis. In addition, several reports state that minimal change nephrotic syndrome is common in these patients. The latter reports appeared at a time when the diagnosis of the minimal change nephrotic syndrome included mild, focal sclerotic changes and thus could have represented the early stages of focal glomerulosclerosis.

SELECTED READINGS

1. Cunningham EE, Brentjens JR, Zielezny MA, et al: Heroin nephropathy. A clinicopathologic and epidemiologic study. Am J Med 68:47, 1980.
2. Fillastre JP, Mery JP, Druet P: Nephropathies glomerulaires medicamenteuses. Nephrologie 4:1, 1983.
3. Liach F, Descoeudres CM, Massry SG: Heroin-associated nephropathy: Clinical and histological studies in 19 patients. Clin Nephrol 11:7, 1979.
4. Menchel S, Cohen D, Gross E, et al: AA protein-related renal amyloidosis in drug addicts. Am J Pathol 112:195, 1983.

TOXIN EXPOSURE

Glomerular diseases are a much less frequent complication of toxin exposure than are tubular or interstitial lesions. Unlike many tubulointerstitial diseases, however, the glomerular lesions tend either to remit or to stabilize when the offending agent is removed from the patient's environment. Thus, recognition of this entity may be of considerable clinical importance.

Heavy Metals

Membranous glomerulonephritis is the lesion most frequently described to be associated with prolonged exposure to heavy metals. The following list is in approximate order of reported frequency:

- Gold salts
- Mercury salts
- Silver salts
- Bismuth salts

A small number of patients have also developed a histologic pattern consistent with minimal lesion after exposure to gold salts.

Drugs with a Free Sulfhydryl Group

Penicillamine

In this category, penicillamine is the major drug associated with glomerular disease. Other drugs with a similar structure have been reported, but they are quite rare. Penicillamine has been implicated in the development of several different types of glomerular lesions, but the most common is membranous glomerulonephritis. The lesions are often difficult to detect without careful assessment of the specimen by immunofluorescence microscopy, because often there are few or no basement spikes, and the lesions may be quite irregular in distribution. Much less common is the presence of membranoproliferative glomerulonephritis, and some researchers believe that the presence of epimembranous deposits in these patients, in addition to those in the basement membranes and the mesangial regions, casts the diagnosis of membranoproliferative glomerulonephritis in doubt. Very few patients have been reported to have minimal lesions or focal necrotizing glomerulonephritis. Several patients have been reported to have developed a clinical course resembling that of Goodpasture syndrome, with pulmonary hemorrhage and rapidly progressive renal failure and crescentic glomerulonephritis. One patient had linear glomerular basement membrane deposits of IgG, whereas the rest had granular deposits. Thus, although they all appeared to have an immune-mediated crescentic glomerulonephritis, it was of two different varieties.

Captopril

Very few patients have been reported, but the renal lesion appears to be membranous glomerulonephritis.

Antineoplastic Drugs

Glomerular lesions resembling those present in the hemolytic-uremic syndrome have been reported in patients receiving mitomycin C (see Chapter 6). Occasional patients treated with alpha-interferon have been reported to have developed minimal lesion nephrotic syndrome or focal glomerulosclerosis.

Nonsteroidal Anti-Inflammatory Drugs

Several patients have been reported who have developed the nephrotic syndrome following therapy with nonsteroidal anti-inflammatory agents. The histologic pattern of renal involvement is principally that of interstitial involvement, but it has been reported that in some patients there appears to be effacement of the pedicels. The spreading of the pedicels is not as uniform and diffuse as in minimal lesion nephrotic syndrome, although the patients may have proteinuria. In these cases, the most common agent has been fenoprofen.

Other Drugs

Two other drugs, pyrithioxine and thiopronine, have been reported to be associated with the development of membranous glomerulonephritis. Again, the total number of reported cases is small.

Other drugs have been implicated in the development of proteinuria or a lupus-like syndrome. The following is a list of the most common associations and the general type of histologic lesion reported:

Drug	Lesion
Lithium	Minimal change
Procainamide	Lupus-like
Hydralazine	Lupus-like; ANCA-associated focal segmental necrotizing and crescentic glomerulonephritis
Phenindione	Minimal change
Levamisole	Minimal change
Propylthiouracil	ANCA-associated focal segmental necrotizing and crescentic glomerulonephritis

CIRRHOSIS

The occurrence of glomerular lesions in patients with cirrhosis has been recognized for decades. However, this association has received little attention because the renal lesions seldom require intervention and do not lead to significant sequelae. The most frequent urinary finding is the presence of modest proteinuria and hematuria. The nephrotic syndrome is extremely uncommon.

Pathogenesis and Patient Presentation

Renal lesions have most often been described in patients with alcoholic liver disease. The presence of IgA deposits in glomeruli has suggested that the lesions have an immune complex pathogenesis. In autopsy studies of patients with cirrhosis, it is common to find a wide variety of asymptomatic renal lesions. However, few of these lesions were of significance during life.

Histology

Two histologic patterns have been described, mesangial sclerosis and membranoproliferative glomerulonephritis.

Mesangial Sclerosis

LIGHT MICROSCOPY

Many histologic patterns have been described. The mesangial sclerosis is so characteristic that it has been called hepatic glomerulosclerosis (Fig. 5–26). It may superficially resemble the early changes present in patients with diabetes mellitus, but the peripheral glomerular basement membranes are usually of normal thickness in cirrhotic patients whereas they are nearly always thickened in diabetic patients. Foci of hyalin deposits have been described but are uncommon. Occasionally, crescents may be present. Bowman's capsular basement membrane may be thickened, and obsolescent glomeruli are sometimes present. These changes are most likely not directly related to the hepatic lesion, rather being reflective of a general underlying atherosclerotic process.

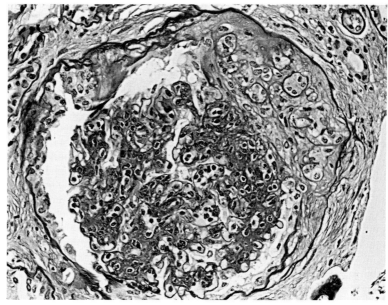

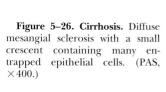

Figure 5–26. Cirrhosis. Diffuse mesangial sclerosis with a small crescent containing many entrapped epithelial cells. (PAS, ×400.)

The interstitium contains patchy areas of fibrosis and tubular atrophy with basement membrane thickening.

Hyalin deposits in small arterioles are a frequent finding.

In summary, the light microscopic changes are relatively mild and nonspecific in many patients, suggesting that there is some mild, chronic renal damage.

IMMUNOFLUORESCENCE MICROSCOPY

Most patients with mesangial changes by light microscopy have mesangial deposits of IgA (Fig. 5–27). The deposits are diffuse, are often quite small, and frequently codistribute with C3. Less commonly, IgG is present in the same distribution as IgA. However, IgG is commonly found in a faint linear pattern, outlining the peripheral glomerular basement membranes. In such cases, IgA and albumin may be found in the same linear pattern. This distribution seems characteristic of sclerotic lesions rather than being specific for cirrhosis, because a similar pattern is sometimes seen in patients with diabetes mellitus.

ELECTRON MICROSCOPY

The mesangial regions are sclerotic, but there are no definable electron-dense deposits. The peripheral glomerular basement membranes are normal, as are the epithelial and endothelial cells.

Membranoproliferative Glomerulonephritis

A small number of patients have been described to have developed a renal lesion resembling membranoproliferative glomerulonephritis after the placement of a portacaval shunt.

LIGHT MICROSCOPY

The light microscopic features are identical to those in patients without cirrhosis and are described in Chapter 4.

IMMUNOFLUORESCENCE MICROSCOPY

The pattern of deposits in membranoproliferative glomerulonephritis associated with cirrhosis is unique. The predominant immunoglobulin found in the mesangial and subendothelial deposits is IgA. The IgA deposits are abundant and diffuse and codistribute with C3. IgG and IgM are present in the same distribution, but in much lesser quantity. Fibrin/fibrinogen deposition is inconspicuous.

The only other clinical syndrome associated with the light microscopic features of membranoproliferative glomerulonephritis and IgA deposits by immunochemical analysis is the Schönlein-Henoch syndrome (see Chapter 6). The major difference between these two entities is the abundance of fibrin/fibrinogen deposits in the Schönlein-Henoch syndrome and their paucity in patients with cirrhosis.

ELECTRON MICROSCOPY

The lesions at the ultrastructural level do not differ from those in other patients with membranoproliferative glomerulonephritis (see Chapter 4).

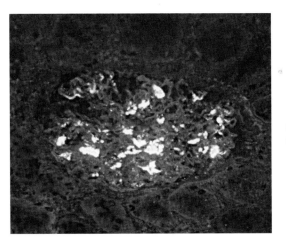

Figure 5–27. Cirrhosis. IgA deposits are evenly distributed throughout the mesangial areas. (Immunofluorescence micrograph, ×250.)

Prognosis

Although the renal lesions are overshadowed by those in the liver, at the present time they may assume more importance as the number of liver transplants increases and patients survive for longer periods. In addition, it will be important to recognize the possibility of pre-existing renal lesions in patients who are recipients of liver transplant and who are being considered for drug therapy that has the potential for renal toxicity.

SELECTED READINGS

1. Berger J, Yaneva H, Nabarra B: Lesions glomérulaires des cirrhotiques. *In* Grunfeld JP, Corvol P (eds): Actualites Nephrologiques de l'Hopital Necker. Paris, Flammarion, 1977, pp 165–176.
2. Bloodworth JMB, Sommers SC: Cirrhotic glomerulosclerosis, a renal lesion associated with hepatic cirrhosis. Lab Invest 8:962, 1959.
3. Callard P, Feldman G, Prandi D, et al: Immune-complex type glomerulonephritis in cirrhosis of the liver. Am J Pathol 80:329, 1975.
4. Manigand G, Morel-Maroger L, Simon J, et al: Lesions glumérulaires et cirrhoses du foie. Note preliminaire sur les lesions histologiques du rein au cours des cirrhoses hepatique, d'apres 20 prelevements biopsies. Rev Eur Etud Clin Biol 15:989, 1970.
5. Neild GH, Gartner HV, Bohle A: Penicillamine-induced membranous glomerulonephritis. Scand J Rheumatol 79:90, 1979.

GLOMERULAR LESIONS IN CHRONIC HYPOXEMIC CONDITIONS

Pathogenesis

Glomerular lesions have been reported in a number of diseases associated with chronic hypoxemia. The spectrum of diseases is large, but cardiac and pulmonary diseases are most commonly associated with this glomerular lesion. Polycythemia may be present, although the renal lesion does not seem to be related to this finding. The pathogenesis of the glomerular lesion is unknown, but the presence of glomerulosclerosis has led some researchers to speculate that the lesions are due to an increase in glomerular vascular hydrostatic pressure.

Patient Presentation

The lesions are most often incidentally noted at autopsy, but some patients may have overt proteinuria. The list of conditions associated with glomerular lesions includes the following:

- Cyanotic heart diseases (especially tetralogy of Fallot)
- Cor pulmonale
- Mitral stenosis
- Severe pulmonary emphysema
- Extreme obesity
- Chronic hemosiderosis
- Polycythemia vera
- Thalassemia

The natural history of the glomerular diseases, their frequency, and their detailed characteristics are not well established. We will provide only those clues that may be useful in suspecting or establishing the diagnosis of these conditions.

Histology

Light Microscopy

The glomeruli appear to be large and congested, and the vascular loops are distended with erythrocytes. This feature is particularly striking because of the fact that the glomeruli do not contain many red blood cells in either normal subjects or patients with most parenchymal diseases. The mesangial matrix may be focally increased in amount, and less frequently the number of mesangial cells may be increased. The peripheral glomerular basement membranes and Bowman's capsule frequently appear thickened and wrinkled.

Inflammatory cells are not evident.

The tubular basement membranes may also be modestly thickened.

Arterial and arteriolar sclerosis may be found.

Immunofluorescence Microscopy

No deposits of immune reactants are found.

Electron Microscopy

The glomerulosclerosis in focal segmental lesions consists of increased mesangial matrix and irregular thickening of the lamina densa of the peripheral glomerular basement membrane.

Prognosis

This is most often an incidental finding; thus the glomerular lesion adds nothing to the patient's course.

SELECTED READINGS

1. Ingelfinger JR, Kissane JM, Robson AM: Glomerulomegaly in a patient with cyanotic congenital heart disease. Am J Dis Child 120:69, 1970.
2. Spear GS: The glomerulus in cyanotic congenital heart disease and primary pulmonary hypertension: A review. Nephron 1:238, 1970.

6

GLOMERULAR DISEASES ASSOCIATED WITH SYSTEMIC DISEASES

SYSTEMIC LUPUS ERYTHEMATOSUS (AND MIXED CONNECTIVE TISSUE DISEASE, POLYMYOSITIS, AND RHEUMATOID ARTHRITIS)

SYSTEMIC LUPUS ERYTHEMATOSUS

Systemic lupus erythematosus (SLE) affects multiple organs, including the kidney, which is a major source of patient morbidity and mortality. Clinical renal disease occurs in approximately 50% of SLE patients, although a much higher percentage might have morphologic changes seen by immunofluorescence and electron microscopy.

SLE patients have a diverse array of autoantibodies, most of which are directed to nuclear components without organ specificity. Antibodies to single-stranded DNA (ss-DNA) are present in about 90% of patients; to double-stranded DNA (ds-DNA) in about 70%; to Smith (Sm) in 30%; to histones in 70%; to ribonucleoprotein (RNP) in 30%; to Ro/SSA in 30%; to La/SSB in 10%; and to proliferation cell nuclear antigen (PCNA) and cyclin in 10%. Some patients also have antibodies to cytoplasmic constituents, including mitochondria, lysosomes, Golgi apparatus, smooth muscle actin, and vimentin or other intermediate filaments. Antibodies to ds-DNA correlate best with active organ system disease and are often detectable in active renal disease. Reduced serum levels of the third and fourth components of complement (C3 and C4) are also frequently used as markers of serologic activity in SLE, and these may return to normal levels following treatment or resolution of disease activity.

Epidemiology and Clinical Features

The prevalence of SLE varies according to the population demographics and racial distribution as well as the clinical criteria used to define SLE. The prevalence of the disease has been estimated at from 4 to 250 cases per 100,000 population, and it is higher among blacks and Asian-Americans than among whites. Whereas SLE occurs in all age groups and both sexes, it is far more common in women of reproductive age (female to male ratio, 8 to 13:1). Its incidence is markedly reduced in childhood and older age populations, in which the female preponderance is no longer evident.

The time at which renal disease appears in SLE patients is varied, although it most often becomes manifest within the first 4 years. Although uncommon, nephritis may be the first manifestation of SLE, especially in those patients with the membranous form of lupus nephritis. The most widely used classification of lupus nephritis is the original World Health Organization classification (Table 6–1). It and a more detailed but less widely used version (modified WHO classification) (Table 6–2) are based primarily on the light microscopy of glomerular lesions, but they also integrate information about the location and distribu-

Table 6–1. Original WHO Classification of Lupus Nephritis

Class I	Normal glomeruli (by LM, IF, EM)
Class II	Purely mesangial disease
	a. Normocellular mesangium by LM but mesangial deposits by IF and/or EM
	b. Mesangial hypercellularity with mesangial deposits by IF and/or EM
Class III	Focal segmental proliferative glomerulonephritis
Class IV	Diffuse proliferative glomerulonephritis
Class V	Membranous glomerulonephritis

LM, light microscopy; IF, immunofluorescence; EM, electron microscopy.

Table 6–2. Modified WHO Classification of Lupus Nephritis

I. Normal glomeruli (by LM, IF, EM)
II. Pure mesangial alterations
   a. Normal by LM, mesangial deposits by IF and/or EM
   b. Mesangial hypercellularity and deposits by IF and/or EM
III. Focal segmental glomerulonephritis
   a. Active necrotizing lesions
   b. Active and sclerosing lesions
   c. Sclerosing lesions
IV. Diffuse glomerulonephritis (severe mesangial, endothelial, or epithelial proliferation and/or extensive subendothelial deposits)
   a. Without segmental lesions
   b. With active necrotizing lesions
   c. With active and sclerosing lesions
   d. With sclerosing lesions
V. Diffuse membranous glomerulonephritis
   a. Pure membranous glomerulonephritis
   b. Associated with lesions of category II (a or b)
VI. Advanced sclerosing glomerulonephritis

LM, light microscopy; IF, immunofluorescence; EM, electron microscopy.

tion of immune deposits as detected by immunofluorescence and electron microscopy (Table 6–3). Use of the WHO classification has greatly improved the reproducibility of diagnosis among individual pathologists, facilitated the communication between clinicians and pathologists, and provided the framework for clinicopathologic and therapeutic studies.

Role of Renal Biopsy

Renal biopsy is not necessary to establish a diagnosis of SLE, but it allows one to define the type, distribution, and severity of the renal lesions. We have shown that renal biopsy provides a more accurate means to guide the choice of treatment and predict prognosis than the urinary sediment or the level of proteinuria and serum creatinine. This is particularly true in patients with severe class IV (diffuse proliferative) lupus nephritis, who may have no clinical renal abnormalities (so-called "silent" diffuse proliferative lupus nephritis). However, renal biopsy is usually reserved for those who have clinical evidence of renal involvement and particularly for those in whom there is a change in hematuria, proteinuria, nephrotic syndrome, or serum creatinine. Repeat renal biopsies are commonly performed to guide treatment. Since lupus nephritis is extremely unpredictable in its ability to reactivate or transform from one class to another spontaneously or following treatment, repeat renal biopsies may be necessary and therapy adjusted according to the change in renal pathologic findings.

Pathogenesis

The pathogenesis of SLE is unknown. Experimental evidence suggests a genetic predis-

Table 6–3. Location and Distribution of Proliferation and Immune Deposits in Lupus Nephritis

	Glomerular Proliferation	Glomerular Deposits by IF and/or EM
Class IIa	None	Mesangial only
Class IIb	Mesangial only	Mesangial only
Class III	Mesangial and focal/segmental endocapillary	Mesangial and focal/segmental subendothelial (+/− sparse subepithelial)
Class IV	Mesangial and diffuse/global endocapillary	Mesangial and diffuse/global subendothelial (+/− sparse subepithelial)
Class V	Mesangial only	Mesangial and diffuse subepithelial

IF, immunofluorescence; EM, electron micrograph.

position that may be modulated by hormonal or environmental factors. In humans, there is a high concordance of SLE (up to 57%) in monozygotic twins and a high familial incidence of autoimmune phenomena. The genetic markers that have been observed with the highest frequency in SLE patients include HLA-DR2, HLA-DR3, HLA-B8, and deficiencies of early complement components, especially C2 and C4A. The importance of environmental factors is underscored by the frequent "flares" of disease activity following exposure to ultraviolet (UV) light. Potential mechanisms by which UV light may promote disease activation include DNA damage, increased binding of anti-Ro and anti-La to keratinocytes, and stimulation of synthesis of inflammatory cytokines. A multiplicity of immunologic derangements have been identified in SLE patients, including B-cell hyperactivity with heightened immunoglobulin production, usually accompanied by reduction in the T-cell suppressor-inducer subset and increased numbers of circulating CD29+ memory helper T-cells. Although the mechanisms that underlie the immunologic manifestations are unknown, the pathogenesis of renal injury seems to be linked to the deposition of immune complexes (ICs) in tissues, either as preformed complexes or by formation in situ.

The physical and local factors that govern the sites of immune complex localization within the glomerulus, tubulointerstitial compartment, and vessels include the amount, size, solubility, charge, avidity, and composition of the immune deposits, as well as their ability to activate complement and generate chemotactic and anaphylatoxic complement fractions. The role of charge may be particularly important in the membranous form of lupus nephritis, in which cationic DNA or histone molecules preferentially bind to negatively charged glomerular basement membrane, permitting planting of antigen with subsequent binding of specific antibody in situ. It is likely that the glomerular response to the immune deposits (i.e., proliferation of indigenous cells, attraction of infiltrating mononuclear or polymorphonuclear leukocytes and platelets, production of toxic oxygen radicals and proteolytic enzymes with endothelial injury and activation of the coagulation pathways, and dysregulated turnover of matrix components) is similar to those operative in other forms of experimental and human glomerulonephritis. The composition of the immune complexes present in the kidney and whether they activate complement before or after tissue deposition are matters of dispute.

Classification of the Renal Lesions

The WHO classification of lupus nephritis is based on glomerular disease, even though the tubular, interstitial and vascular compartments are frequently involved and may make a major contribution to overall disease activity, chronicity, and severity. The accurate classification of lupus nephritis depends on an adequate glomerular sampling, since the lesions may be quite focal and may vary markedly in type, severity, and activity from one glomerulus to another. In addition, examinations by light and immunofluorescence microscopy are required, and electron microscopy may often be helpful. Important features to examine include the distribution of glomerular hypercellularity (mesangial, intravascular (endocapillary), and extraglomerular (extracapillary), the presence or absence of infiltrating leukocytes and necrotizing lesions, the presence of glomerular basement membrane thickening) and the identification of immune deposits (mesangial, subendothelial and/or subepithelial locations). Although immunofluorescence and electron microscopy are the most sensitive techniques for the identification of glomerular immune deposits, the deposits are often large enough to be visible by light microscopy.

Class I (Normal)

There are no glomerular abnormalities by light, immunofluorescence, or electron microscopy. There are few well-documented cases of Class I lupus nephritis, since these patients are not generally referred for biopsy. Although some early series contain examples of Class I lupus nephritis, some lacked studies by immunofluorescence and electron microscopy.

Class II (Purely Mesangial Disease)

Immunoglobulin deposits are always present in Class II. The lesions are subdivided into Class IIa and IIb according to the absence or presence of mesangial hypercellularity (Figs. 6–1, 6–2). In Class IIa, the mesangium is normocellular; however, immune deposits confined to the mesangium can be detected by

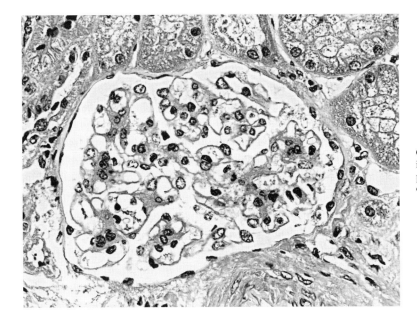

Figure 6–1. Lupus nephritis, Class IIb. The only change visible is segmental, mild mesangial cell proliferation. (Hematoxylin and eosin, ×500.)

immunofluorescence and electron microscopy (Fig. 6–3). In Class IIb, the mesangial immune deposits are accompanied by mild-to-moderate mesangial proliferation, defined as greater than three mesangial cells in mesangial areas away from the vascular pole in 3-μ sections. The mesangial proliferation may vary in distribution from focal to diffuse, may involve the tuft segmentally or globally, and may be accompanied by an increase in mesangial matrix. The presence of any sizeable amount of subendothelial immune deposits warrants a designation of Class III or IV, depending on their distribution and quantity.

Clinical Features

Approximately two thirds of Class IIa patients lack clinical evidence of renal disease. The remaining third have hematuria, leukocyturia, and/or mild proteinuria. Serologic tests such as antinuclear antibodies (ANA), anti-DNA antibody, and serum complements may be positive even if the renal disease is inactive.

In Class IIb patients, approximately one half have an abnormal urinary sediment and proteinuria of less than 1 gram per day. Renal function tests are normal in approximately 80%.

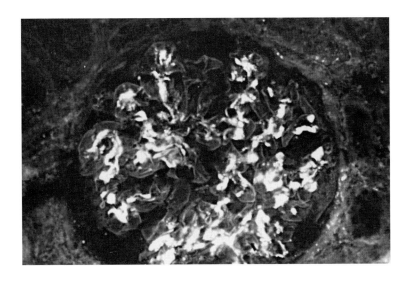

Figure 6–2. Lupus nephritis, Class IIb. The mesangial regions all contain granular IgG deposits. Similar deposits are seen in tubular and Bowman's capsular basement membranes. (Immunofluorescence micrograph, ×250.)

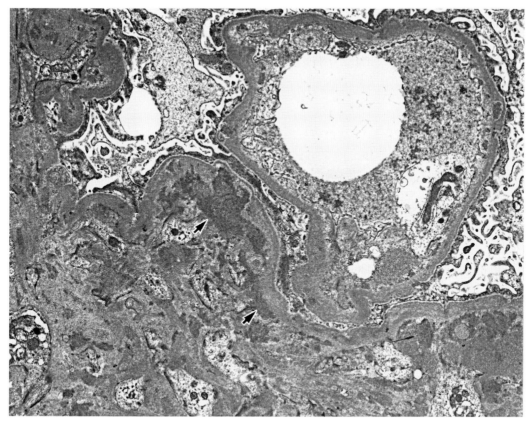

Figure 6–3. Lupus nephritis, Class IIb. There are a large number of deposits in the paramesangial matrix *(arrows).* (Electron micrograph, ×2500.)

Class III (Focal Proliferative)

Light Microscopy

Mesangial proliferation and mesangial immune deposits are most often the background on which the lesions in this class are superimposed. Most consider Class III (focal proliferative) and Class IV (diffuse proliferative) lesions to be qualitatively similar glomerular lesions. Class III and Class IV can be distinguished quantitatively by the arbitrary definition of Class III as endocapillary proliferation involving less than 50% of the total glomerular tufts (of all glomeruli sampled). Class IV is defined as endocapillary proliferation and/or subendothelial deposits involving more than 50% of the total number of glomerular tufts. Some reserve Class III for biopsy specimens in which the endocapillary proliferation is focal and segmental (Figs. 6–4, 6–5). The hypercellularity is composed of endothelial and mesangial cells, as well as infiltrating neutrophils and monocytes.

In Class III, glomerular lesions may vary considerably in activity and chronicity. Therefore, an adequate glomerular sampling is necessary to assess the overall severity and activity. Features of active glomerulonephritis include neutrophil infiltration and necrotizing lesions. *Necrosis* is a term that denotes the presence of intraglomerular fibrin, often associated with pyknosis or karyorrhexis. It is likely that those histologic findings of nuclear "dust," which correspond to apoptosis, result primarily from breakdown of infiltrating neutrophils. It is common to find localized ruptures or breaks in the glomerular basement membrane, best depicted with the periodic acid–Schiff (PAS) or methenamine silver stain, in the areas of necrosis, with overlying cellular crescents. In some cases, there is extravasation of fibrin into the urinary space in the areas of crescents.

Hematoxylin bodies have been thought to be a pathognomonic feature of active lupus nephritis. They are seen in a small percentage of cases (2%) and are usually associated with necrotizing lesions. In hematoxylin and eosin (H&E)–stained sections they are identified as

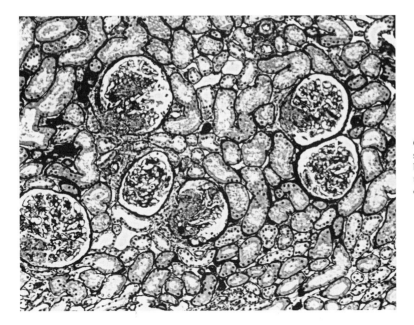

Figure 6–4. Lupus nephritis, Class III. Focal and segmental lesions consist of an increased number of glomerular cells, infiltration with inflammatory cells, and overlying crescents. (Silver stain, ×100.)

rounded, blue, smudgy inclusions, which correspond to naked nuclei that have been altered by binding to ANA, resulting in clumping of the nuclear chromatin.

Subendothelial immune deposits may be so large that they are detectable by light microscopy as glassy, eosinophilic material beneath the glomerular basement membrane. They are best highlighted in trichrome-stained sections, which stain the deposits red and the glomerular basement membrane blue, and in Jones methen-amine silver–stained sections, which delimit the deposits as pink and the glomerular basement membrane as black. If the deposits encircle the entire tuft circumference, they are often referred to as "wire loop" deposits. Subendothelial deposits may be so massive as to protrude into or occlude the tuft lumina, forming "hyaline thrombi" (Fig. 6–6). This is a misnomer, as these structures are not true fibrin thrombi but intraluminal immune deposits with the same composition as that of subendothelial deposits.

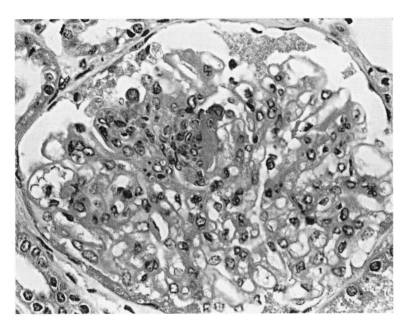

Figure 6–5. Lupus nephritis, Class III. There is segmental endocapillary proliferation, associated with necrosis and nuclear debris and inflammatory cell infiltrates. The other mesangial regions are modestly expanded. (H&E, ×500.)

In Class III lupus nephritis, there often are patchy interstitial infiltrates of lymphocytes, monocytes, and plasma cells. Tubular basement membrane and interstitial and arterial immune deposits may also be identified by immunofluorescence and electron microscopy.

As the renal process becomes more chronic, there is progression to focal and global glomerulosclerosis. Segmental crescents may heal as synechiae between the tuft and Bowman's capsule or as subcapsular fibrous proliferation with focal ruptures of the basal lamina of Bowman's capsule. Tubular atrophy, interstitial fibrosis, and arteriosclerosis are frequently observed in a patchy distribution, predominating around the glomerulosclerotic lesions. These chronic lesions are considered inactive and irreversible.

Immunofluorescence Microscopy

Focal subendothelial and diffuse mesangial immune deposits are detectable by immunofluorescence and electron microscopy in the areas of endocapillary proliferation (Fig. 6–6).

Clinical Features

Approximately 50% of patients with Class III lupus nephritis have an active urinary sediment defined as hematuria and/or leukocyturia. Proteinuria is common, affecting almost two thirds of cases, but approaches nephrotic levels in only a quarter to a third. Renal insufficiency is uncommon, affecting approximately 10% to 25% of patients. Positive ANA and hypocomplementemia are detected at the time of biopsy in approximately two thirds of patients.

Class IV (Diffuse Proliferative)

Light Microscopy

As described, Class IV lupus nephritis is qualitatively similar to Class III lupus nephritis, but the glomerular lesions are more diffuse and global (affecting over 50% of the total glomerular capillaries). Thus these two morphologic expressions of lupus nephritis are part of a disease continuum. All the active features described under Class III may also be detected in Class IV, but they are usually more generalized (Figs. 6–7, 6–8, 6–9). Subendothelial immune deposits are more global and diffuse, paralleling the widespread intraglomerular cell proliferation. In fact, the sine qua non of active Class IV disease is diffuse subendothelial immune deposits. In some patients, the patterns of glomerular proliferation may be more membranoproliferative, with mesangial interposition and duplication of glomerular basement membrane producing "double contours" similar to those seen in idiopathic membranoproliferative glomerulonephritis. In some cases the subendothelial deposits are

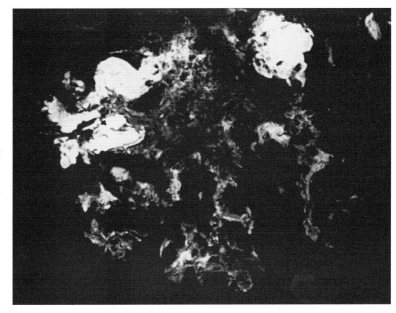

Figure 6–6. Lupus nephritis, Class III. There are very large, coarse endocapillary deposits of IgG, corresponding to the "hyaline thrombi." (Immunofluorescence microscopy, ×250.)

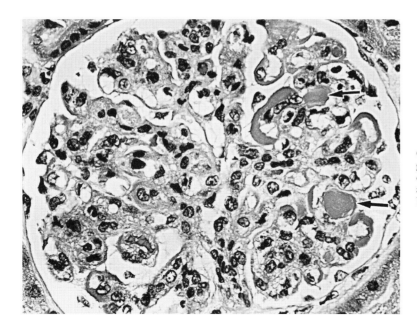

Figure 6–7. Lupus nephritis, Class IV. There is moderate global cellular proliferation, with conspicuous wire loop deposits and intraluminal "hyaline thrombi" *(arrows)*. (H&E, ×500.)

massive, producing diffuse wire loops with only mild mesangial proliferation. In severe cases, diffuse crescents may be present (Fig. 6–9). As in other types of glomerulonephritis, massive crescents carry an extremely poor prognosis.

Interstitial inflammation and tubulointerstitial and vascular immune deposits are most common in Class IV biopsies. As the process becomes chronic, there is progression to glo-

merulosclerosis with fibrous crescents, tubular atrophy, interstitial fibrosis, and arteriosclerosis.

Immunofluorescence Microscopy

In all classes of lupus nephritis, the immune deposits usually contain all classes of immunoglobulin (IgG, IgM, and IgA), although IgG is usually the most intense and the most wide-

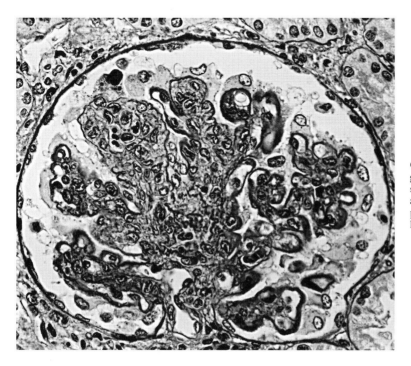

Figure 6–8. Lupus nephritis, Class IV. There is moderate global hypercellularity, with widespread wire loop deposits. There are infiltrating neutrophils. The podocytes appear markedly swollen. (Silver stain, ×500.)

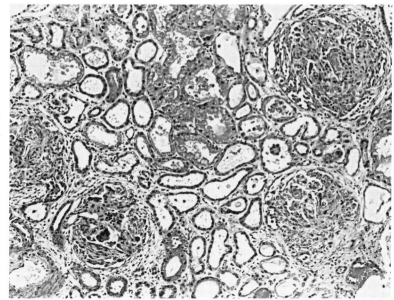

Figure 6–9. Lupus nephritis, Class IV. The glomeruli are diffusely involved with circumferential crescents with compression of the hypercellular tufts, which have compressed vascular spaces. The proximal tubules are dilated, and the epithelium is flattened. There is prominent interstitial edema and infiltrates. (H&E, ×100.)

spread. The deposits in class IV best illustrate the large, granular mesangial and subendothelial deposits (Fig. 6–10).

IgA may be codominant with IgG but, unlike the case in IgA nephropathy, is rarely dominant in intensity. Complement components C1q, C3, and C4 are also readily detectable. Properdin, although not generally tested in routine practice, has been identified in the glomerular immune deposits, suggesting a role for alternative as well as classic complement pathway activation. Fibrinogen and other fibrin-related antigens are detected in areas of necrosis where they are intensely reactive. More generalized, delicate positivity for fibrinogen may also be seen in areas of intraglomerular proliferation lacking necrotizing lesions.

The quality of the glomerular immune deposits by fluorescence is often helpful for proper classification. Mesangial deposits outline the axial regions of the tuft but do not

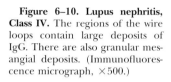

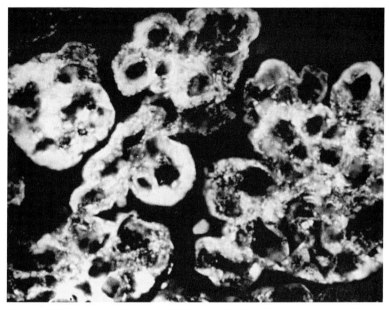

Figure 6–10. Lupus nephritis, Class IV. The regions of the wire loops contain large deposits of IgG. There are also granular mesangial deposits. (Immunofluorescence micrograph, ×500.)

extend into the peripheral loops. Suben-dothelial deposits are often ring-shaped or semilunar, with a smooth outer contour corresponding to the delimiting glomerular basement membrane (Fig. 6–10). Wire loop deposits may be quite thick and massive, and hyaline thrombi appear as globular deposits that may obliterate the lumen. The thrombi also contain immunoglobulin components (Fig. 6–11). Subepithelial deposits tend to be more rounded and granular in texture. Tubulointerstitial deposits may involve the tubular basement membrane itself or extend into the interstitial tissue (Fig. 6–12). Vascular immune deposits may involve both arteries and veins. Granular deposits can be identified in the subendothelial basement membrane and medial perimyocyte basement membranes.

Although ANAs are present in over 98% of patients with SLE, only a minority of renal biopsies display renal nuclear staining by fluorescence microscopy. This ANA tissue reactivity is thought to be an artifact of tissue processing such that circulating ANA binds to exposed nuclei in cryostat sections incubated with antihuman IgG. A possible role for in vivo nuclear binding has also been suggested in some murine models of SLE.

Electron Microscopy

The distribution of immune deposits in mesangial, subendothelial, and subepithelial lo-cations corresponds closely to that detected by immunofluorescence microscopy. Massive deposits are present in all glomerular areas: sub-endothelial, subepithelial, and mesangial (Figs. 6–13, 6–14). Cellular changes are marked, and both nuclear debris and neutrophils are prominent in the vascular spaces. The whole architecture of the glomerulus may be so distorted that it becomes difficult to be sure of the anatomic segment under investigation. As noted for the focal lesions, the deposits may contain structures resembling fingerprints or pseudotubules. Such structures are more frequently observed in this histologic class than in the milder lesions. Although quite distinctive for lupus, these deposits are not pathognomonic since similar organized deposits may be detected in patients with cryoglobulinemic glomerulonephritis. This has led to the proposal that these fingerprint structures may be more common in SLE patients with circulating cryoglobulins, a hypothesis that has not been verified.

Electron-dense deposits may also be detected in Bowman's capsule, tubular basement membranes, interstitial capillary basement membranes, interstitial collagen, and the intima and media of arteries, veins, and arterioles. Tubuloreticular endothelial cell inclusions are a common finding in lupus nephritis (Fig. 6–15). They are 24-nm interanastomos-

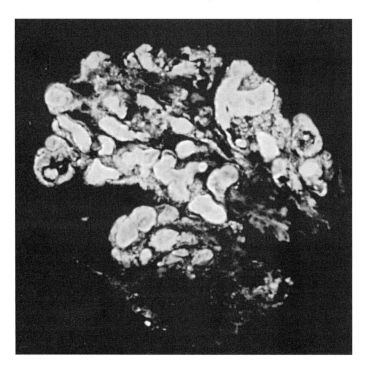

Figure 6–11. Lupus nephritis, Class IV. Massive intracapillary "thrombi" contain IgG. (Immunofluorescence micrograph, ×250.)

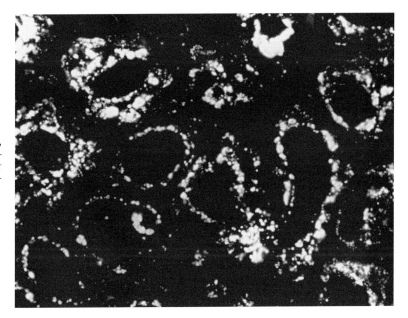

Figure 6–12. Lupus nephritis, Class IV. Numerous granular deposits of IgG outline the tubular basement membranes. (Immunofluorescence micrograph, ×200.)

ing tubular structures located in dilated cisternae of endoplasmic reticulum. They may be found in glomerular, arterial, or interstitial capillary endothelium and can be induced in normal lymphocytes upon exposure to alpha-interferon, and have thus been called "interferon footprints." They are not specific for SLE but are also present in large numbers in human immunodeficiency virus (HIV) or other retrovirus infections.

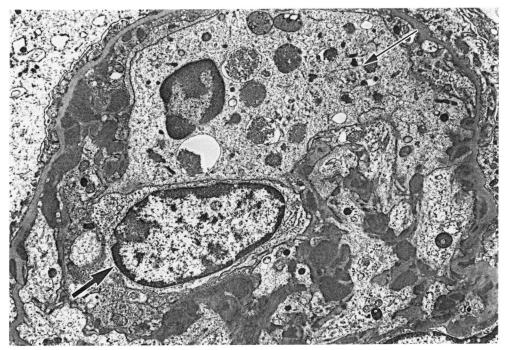

Figure 6–13. Lupus nephritis, Class IV. The vascular space is occluded by endothelial cell swelling *(thick arrow)* and hypercellularity, with infiltrating monocytes *(thin arrow)* containing many phagolysosomes. A small number of subepithelial electron-dense deposits are present as well as mesangial and subendothelial deposits. The podocyte cytoplasm is swollen, and the foot processes are effaced. (Electron micrograph, ×3000.)

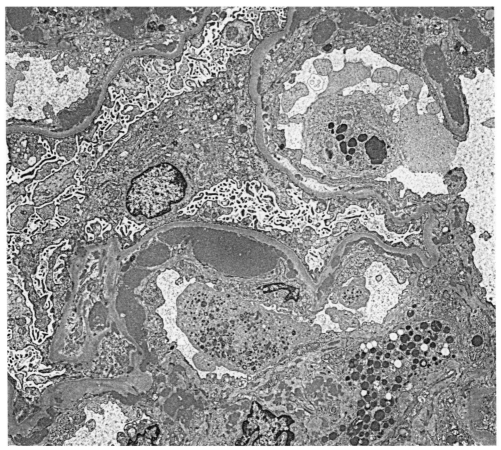

Figure 6–14. Lupus nephritis, Class IV. There are large paramesangial and subendothelial electron-dense deposits (forming wire loops). Several infiltrating monocytes contain lysosomes. The podocytes are hypertrophied and have microvillous transformation. (Electron micrograph, ×2200.)

Clinical Features

The clinical presentation of Class IV lupus nephritis is usually the most severe of all the classes. Up to 75% of patients have active urinary sediment. Over 90% have proteinuria, with the nephrotic syndrome found in approximately half. Because of the insensitivity of serum creatinine determinations, only 50% of patients with Class IV disease have renal insufficiency with elevation of serum creatinine, whereas creatinine clearance may be reduced in up to 75% of patients. Some cases of diffuse proliferative lupus nephritis lack any detectable renal abnormalities. Such examples of "silent" diffuse proliferative lupus nephritis appear to be extremely rare.

Class V (Membranous)

Light Microscopy

Class V lupus nephritis is defined by the presence of diffuse subepithelial immune deposits, producing a membranous pattern (Figs. 6–16, 6–17). In early cases, the glomerular basement membrane may appear normal in thickness by light microscopy, but the presence of numerous small subepithelial deposits is readily demonstrated by immunofluorescence (Figs. 6–18, 6–19) and electron microscopy (Fig. 6–20). In well-established cases, the glomerular basement membranes are seen to be visibly thickened by light microscopy, and spikes may be demonstrable with the Jones methenamine silver stain. Virtually all cases of membranous lupus nephritis have coexistent mesangial immune deposits, often accompanied by varying degrees of mesangial hypercellularity. In pure membranous lupus nephritis Class V, intraglomerular proliferation is absent. If coexistent intraglomerular proliferation and subendothelial deposits are present, a designation of mixed Class V and III or Class V and IV lupus nephritis is warranted,

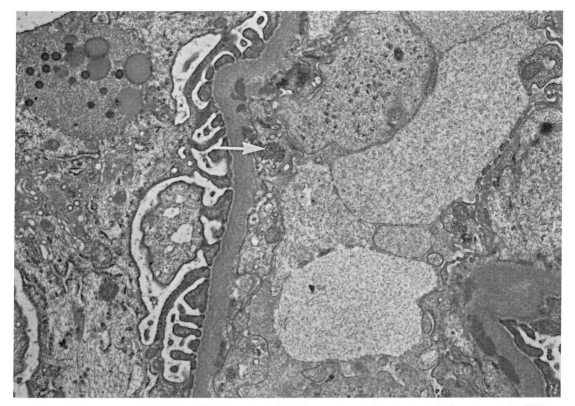

Figure 6–15. Lupus nephritis, Class IV. The endothelial cells contain tubuloreticular inclusions *(arrow).* (×3200.)

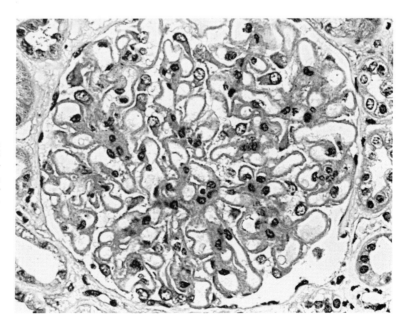

Figure 6–16. Lupus nephritis, Class V. There is global, uniform thickening of the glomerular basement membranes. There is mild, segmental mesangial cell proliferation and sclerosis. (H&E, ×500.)

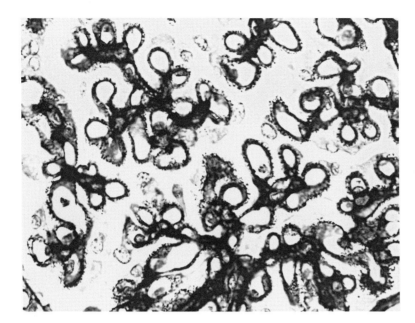

Figure 6–17. Lupus nephritis, Class V. Extensive subepithelial basement membrane spikes are noted. (Silver stain, ×1000.)

depending on the extension of the associated lesions. Because scattered small focal subepithelial deposits may also be found in examples of Class II, III, or IV lupus nephritis, the term *membranous lupus nephritis Class V* should be reserved for cases in which the subepithelial deposits predominate.

Clinical Features

Proteinuria is detected in virtually all patients with Class V lupus nephritis, with the nephrotic syndrome in 90%. Renal insufficiency affects approximately 10% of cases, and it correlates most closely with chronic tubu-

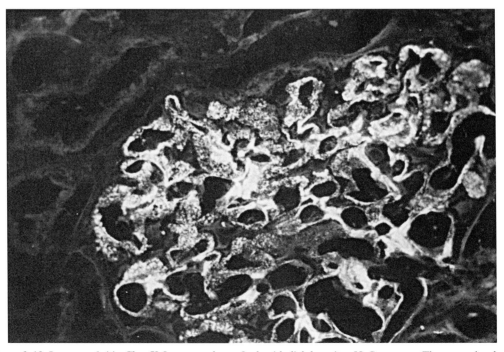

Figure 6–18. Lupus nephritis, Class V. Large numbers of subepithelial deposits of IgG are seen. There are also deposits in the mesangial and subendothelial regions. (Immunofluorescence micrograph, ×400.)

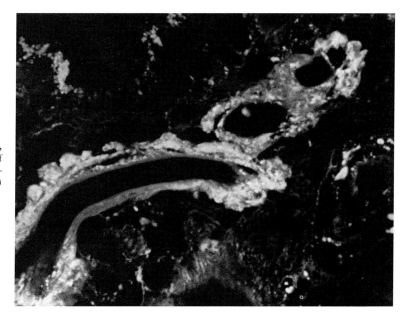

Figure 6–19. Lupus nephritis, Class V. Note vascular deposits of IgG in the small arteries. (Immunofluorescence micrograph, ×250.)

lointerstitial damage. Some patients develop renal involvement before serologic or systemic features of SLE are manifest. In these patients, the presence of mesangial hypercellularity, mesangial immune deposits, and endothelial tubuloreticular inclusions is often helpful in distinguishing membranous lupus nephritis from idiopathic membranous glomerulopathy. Renal vein thrombosis is a serious complication of Class V lupus nephritis, it occurs in 10 to 50% of cases (depending on detection methods). Clinically, renal vein thrombosis

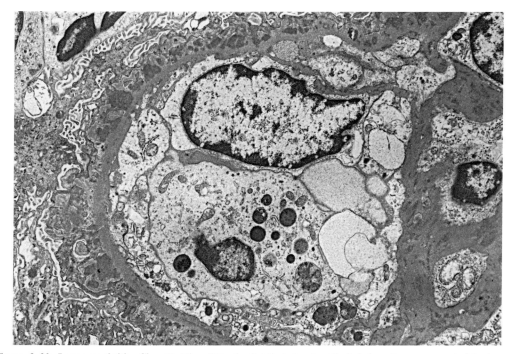

Figure 6–20. Lupus nephritis, Class V. The diffusely distributed subepithelial deposits are separated by basement membrane spikes and vary widely in their size and shape. Deposits are also present in the expanded mesangium. (Electron micrograph, ×3000.)

may be silent, or it may be heralded by the development of flank pain or the new onset of hematuria or pulmonary embolus. The possibility of superimposed renal vein thrombosis should be considered in any biopsy of membranous lupus nephritis with diffuse interstitial edema, neutrophil margination in glomerular capillaries, or interstitial microhemorrhage (see Chapter 5). Histologic features of chronic injury in renal vein thrombosis include interstitial fibrosis and tubular atrophy out of proportion to the degree of glomerulosclerosis.

Class VI (Advanced Sclerosing)

Histology

The modified WHO classification includes a sixth class in which there is advanced chronic disease affecting all renal compartments. The glomerulosclerosis, tubular atrophy, interstitial fibrosis, and arteriosclerosis may be so advanced as to be near end-stage. In these cases, it may be difficult to identify the etiology of the advanced renal disease, except by the identification of sparse residual immune deposits in glomerular, tubulointerstitial, or vascular sites. The few nonsclerotic glomeruli may demonstrate residual hypercellularity.

Clinical Features

Class VI is characterized by severe renal insufficiency with variable (usually subnephrotic) proteinuria and inactive urinary sediment. Hypertension is quite common. Lupus serologies may be active in spite of the inactive and advanced glomerular lesions.

Vascular Lesions

A variety of vascular lesions have been reported. The most common is the presence of immune deposits in the intima and/or media of arterioles, arteries, and veins (Fig. 6–19). These are visible by immunofluorescence and electron microscopy but not by light microscopy. They are most common in Class III and IV lupus nephritis but may occur in Class II and V as well. They are usually clinically silent and do not affect prognosis.

In rare cases of severe lupus nephritis, Class IV deposits are found in arterioles that contain immune deposits admixed with fibrin and fibrinoid deposits, and these usually lack an inflammatory component. These lesions, termed *lupus vasculopathy*, carry an extremely poor prognosis and are most common in active Class IV lupus nephritis, often associated with severe hypertension.

A few patients with lupus nephritis develop *thrombotic microangiopathy*, similar to the lesions seen in patients with hemolytic-uremic syndrome (HUS). Fibrin thrombi are detected in glomeruli, small arteries, and arterioles. Subacute lesions may be identifiable as arterial mucoid intimal edema. By electron microscopy, products of coagulation sometimes appear as subendothelial flocculent, relatively lucent material. Thrombotic microangiopathy may occur in a subset of SLE patients with circulating lupus anticoagulant. Similar lesions have also been reported in patients with a HUS-like syndrome in the absence of identifiable lupus anticoagulant. These lesions carry a poor prognosis and are important to identify in renal biopsy samples because patients may benefit from the use of anticoagulation or plasmapheresis.

An extremely rare finding in lupus nephritis is true *necrotizing vasculitis* of the inflammatory type, indistinguishable from that described in patients with polyangiitis/polyarteritis. In fact, some have evidence of systemic vasculitis. Possible overlaps with antineutrophil cytoplasmic antibody (ANCA)–associated syndromes have not been well studied because of the rarity of this complication of SLE. Most clinicians advocate aggressive immunosuppressive therapy for this vasculitis, similar to that for polyarteritis nodosa.

Activity and Chronicity Indices

Because active features represent acute and thus potentially treatable lesions, whereas chronic features are considered irreversible, renal biopsy specimen interpretation should include a detailed assessment of the activity and chronicity as a guide to treatment and prognosis. A variety of indices have been proposed for the purpose of providing a more quantitative estimate of these active and chronic changes. The most widely utilized is the index proposed by Morel-Maroger and modified by Austin and associates (referred to as the "NIH index")(Table 6–4).

There are six features of activity, including degree of intraglomerular proliferation, wire loop subendothelial deposits, glomerular neu-

Table 6–4. Activity and Chronicity Index in Lupus Nephritis*

Index of Activity (0–24)	
Endocapillary hypercellularity	(0–3)
Leukocyte infiltration	(0–3)
Subendothelial hyalin deposits	(0–3)
Fibrinoid necrosis/karyorrhexis	(0–3) × 2
Cellular crescents	(0–3) × 2
Interstitial inflammation	(0–3)
Index of Chronicity (0–12)	
Sclerotic glomeruli	(0–3)
Fibrous crescents	(0–3)
Tubular atrophy	(0–3)
Interstitial fibrosis	(0–3)

*According to Morel-Maroger[10] and Austin.[4]

trophilic infiltration, glomerular necrosis (karyorrhexis, pyknosis, or fibrinoid necrosis), cellular crescents, and interstitial inflammation. Each feature is graded on a scale of 0 (absent), 1+ (mild), 2+ (moderate), or 3+ (severe). Necrosis and cellular crescents are weighted double (multiplied by 2) because of their greater significance. The individual scores for each of the six histologic features are summed to give the final activity index (scale, 0 to 24). In a similar way, the chronicity index (scale, 0 to 12) is derived by adding individual semiquantitative scores (0 to 3+) for each of the four histologic features of glomerulosclerosis, fibrous crescents, tubular atrophy, and interstitial fibrosis.

Although there is considerable controversy about the validity and reproducibility of the activity and chronicity indices in guiding treatment and determining prognosis, most clinicians and nephropathologists agree that these indices provide a rough estimate of the potential reversibility of the glomerulonephritis. For example, highly active Class III or Class IV lupus nephritis should be treated more aggressively than minimally active glomerulonephritis or scarred, chronic glomerulonephritis. Activity and chronicity indices are particularly valuable when repeat biopsies have been performed on an individual patient, to monitor response to therapy, potential reactivation, or transformation in class.

Prognosis

The primary value of the WHO classification of lupus nephritis derives from its usefulness in guiding treatment and determining prognosis.

The prognosis of mesangial proliferative lupus nephritis (Class II) is excellent (with 5-year renal survival greater than 90%) provided there is no transformation to a more severe class. Because of its favorable prognosis and the potential side effects of immunosuppressive treatment, therapy is not directed to the renal disease in Class II lupus nephritis but only to the systemic manifestations of SLE.

The prognosis of Class III lupus nephritis is variable, depending on its severity. Cases with a small percentage of glomeruli affected by intraglomerular proliferation and lacking necrosis may be treated with steroids alone, whereas more severe Class III cases are usually handled like Class IV lesions, with more aggressive immunosuppression. The 5-year renal survival is 85 to 90%.

Class IV lupus nephritis has been the most extensively studied in series of patients with SLE. Patients with Class IV lupus nephritis have the worst prognosis (5-year survival, 60 to 90%) and represent the group most likely to benefit from aggressive therapy. Whereas early treatment protocols in the 1950s and 1960s consisted of corticosteroids alone, improved renal survival has been achieved in recent decades by the use of more aggressive immunosuppressive regimens, including high-dose intravenous or oral corticosteroids in conjunction with monthly intravenous cyclophosphamide. Other treatment protocols have used steroids together with oral cyclophosphamide, azathioprine, nitrogen mustard, cyclosporine, and plasmapheresis. Repeat renal biopsy samples following treatment have revealed a remarkable ability of immune deposits to undergo resorption accompanied by resolution of intraglomerular proliferation.

The prognosis of Class V lupus nephritis is less well characterized. Five-year survivals range from 70 to 90%, indicating a poorer prognosis than originally thought. Treatment protocols for membranous lupus nephritis vary from steroids alone to more aggressive therapies including combination cytotoxic agents such as steroids and cyclophosphamide or cyclosporine. The subgroups of membranous lupus nephritis with severe unremitting nephrotic syndrome, high chronicity, or overlap with more severe proliferative (Class III or IV) lupus nephritis carry a poor prognosis.

Transformations of lupus nephritis from one class to another may occur in 10 to 40% of patients. Virtually all types of transformations have been reported. The most common is transformation from Class III to Class IV, which may reflect only a disease continuum rather than transformation. Other common transformations include Class II to Class III or IV, and Class III or IV to Class V, especially following treatment. Transformations may be heralded by a sudden change in the activity of the urinary sediment or the severity of proteinuria. Repeat renal biopsies are extremely helpful to document transformations and guide adjustments in therapy.

SELECTED READINGS

1. Appel GB, Cohen DJ, Pirani CL, et al: Long-term follow-up of lupus nephritis: A study based on the WHO classification. Am J Med 83:877, 1987.
2. Appel GB, Pirani CL, D'Agati VD: Renal vascular involvement in systemic lupus. J Am Soc Nephrol 4:1499, 1994.
3. Appel GB, Silva FG, Pirani CL, et al: Renal involvement in systemic lupus erythematosus (SLE): A study of 56 patients emphasizing histologic classification. Medicine 57:371, 1978.
4. Austin HA, Boumpas DT, Vaughan EM, Balow JE: Predicting renal outcomes in severe lupus nephritis: Contributions of clinical and histologic data. Kidney Int 45:544, 1994.
5. Austin HA, Muenz LR, Joyce KM, et al: Prognostic factors in lupus nephritis. Contribution of renal histologic data. Am J Med 75:382, 1983.
6. Austin HA, Muenz LR, Joyce KM, et al: Diffuse proliferative lupus nephritis: Identification of specific pathologic features affecting renal outcome. Kidney Int 25:689, 1984.
7. Bohannon LL, Bennett WM: Silent lupus nephritis—an overview. Int Med 5:73, 1984.
8. Churg J, Sobin LH: Renal disease: Classification and Atlas of Glomerular Diseases. World Health Organization. Tokyo, Igaku-Shoin, 1982.
9. Jennette JC, Iskandar SS, Dalldorf FG: Pathologic differentiation between lupus and non-lupus membranous glomerulopathy. Kidney Int 24:377, 1983.
10. Morel-Maroger L, Mery J, Droz D, et al: The course of lupus nephritis: Contribution of serial renal biopsies. Adv Nephrol 76:118, 1976.
11. Pirani CL, Olesnicky L: Role of electron microscopy in the classification of lupus nephritis. In Hayslett JP, Hardin GA (eds): Advances in Systemic Lupus Erythematosus. New York, Grune and Stratton, 1982, p 54.
12. Pollak VE, Pirani CL: Renal histologic findings in systemic lupus erythematosus. Mayo Clin Proc 44:630, 1969.
13. Schwartz MM, Kawala KS, Corwin HL, Lewis EJ: The prognosis of segmental glomerulonephritis in systemic lupus erythematosus. Kidney Int 32:274, 1987.
14. Schwartz MM, Lan S-P, Bonsib SM, et al: Clinical outcome of three discrete histologic patterns of injury in severe lupus glomerulonephritis. Am J Kidney Dis 13:273, 1989.
15. Silva FG: The nephropathies of systemic lupus erythematosus. In Rosen S (ed): Pathology of Glomerular Disease. New York, Churchill Livingstone, 1983, p 79.
16. Tan EM, Cohen AS, Fries JF, et al: The 1982 revised criteria for the classification of systemic lupus erythematosus. Arthritis Rheum 25:671, 1982.

MIXED CONNECTIVE TISSUE DISEASE

A group of patients present with manifestations that seem to overlap those of systemic lupus erythematosus, scleroderma, and polymyositis. These patients have circulating antibodies to extractable nuclear antigen (ribonuclear trypsin-sensitive antigen) in the absence of the Sm antigen. Renal lesions are uncommon, and when present are mild. In the few reported cases in which a renal lesion was present, the glomerular lesions have been of a wide variety of histologic types, the most common being focal and diffuse mesangial proliferation as well as membranous glomerulonephritis. Mild proteinuria is often the only sign of renal involvement, and rare patients develop the nephrotic syndrome. In the very rare patient who develops hypertension, the vascular lesions resemble those in scleroderma (see later in this chapter). Interstitial lesions are probably more common than previously thought, but this may be due to medications.

POLYMYOSITIS AND DERMATOMYOSITIS

Renal lesions are very uncommon in patients with polymyositis and dermatomyositis, but their exact incidence is not known. In those few cases in which urinary sediment abnormalities have occasioned a renal biopsy, the glomeruli have shown a mild, focal, mesangial proliferative and/or sclerotic lesion. Immunofluorescence microscopic examination of these biopsy specimens revealed granular deposits of IgG, IgM, IgA, and complement. Electron microscopic examination confirmed the presence of deposits in the mesangium and their absence in other sites.

RHEUMATOID ARTHRITIS

Patients with rheumatoid arthritis seldom have renal lesions related to the primary disease. AA amyloidosis may complicate longstanding disease. Almost all the other renal lesions reported in these patients are due to a complication of therapy. The following list includes the common causes of renal disease associated with rheumatoid arthritis, some of which are clearly related to therapy:

1. Renal lesions directly related to rheumatoid arthritis
   a. Amyloidosis
   b. Glomerular lesions
      (1) Mesangial enlargement due to increased matrix; hypercellularity is less common
      (2) Granular deposits of IgM; occasionally there are deposits of IgA and C3
   c. Vasculitis (rare)
2. Renal lesions associated with therapeutic agents used to treat rheumatoid arthritis
   a. Gold salts: membranous glomerulonephritis
   b. Penicillamine: membranous glomerulonephritis
   c. Nonsteroidal anti-inflammatory drugs: minimal change and acute interstitial nephritis
   d. Analgesics: chronic interstitial nephritis (see Chapter 13 for a description of the lesions associated with these agents)

ANKYLOSING SPONDYLITIS

The renal disease in these patients is mostly due to the presence of amyloid deposition, 4 to 16% in most series. In those few patients with hematuria (4 to 5%), the renal lesions consist of mesangial deposits of either IgA or IgM. Isolated C3 deposits were seen in 1 of 116 patients in one series.

SELECTED READINGS

1. Lai KN, Li PKT, Hawkins B, et al: IgA nephropathy associated with ankylosing spondylitis: Occurrence in women as well as in men. Ann Rheum Dis 48:435, 1989.
2. Sellars L, Siamopoulos K, Wilkinson R, et al: Renal biopsy appearances in rheumatoid disease. Clin Nephrol 20:114, 1983.

GOODPASTURE SYNDROME

Goodpasture syndrome is characterized by the association of crescentic glomerulonephritis and acute pulmonary disease (often with massive hemorrhage). Long after its first description, it was recognized that this syndrome was often accompanied by circulating antibodies that react with glomerular (and other) basement membranes. At present, the term *Goodpasture syndrome* is reserved for those patients with all three components—that is, crescentic glomerulonephritis, pulmonary involvement, and circulating antiglomerular basement membrane antibodies. Patients who have the circulating antiglomerular basement membrane antibody but do not have pulmonary disease are best termed as having *idiopathic antiglomerular basement membrane glomerulonephritis*. Because there are other forms of crescentic glomerulonephritis and these may have pulmonary involvement, it is imperative that the renal biopsy specimen be examined by immunofluorescence microscopy, paying special attention to the presence and distribution of glomerular immunoglobulin deposits.

Pathogenesis

See Chapter 4.

Patient Presentation

Goodpasture syndrome is more common in men and is frequently preceded by a flulike illness. Despite attempts to document viral infection, either by culture or by change in serum antibody titers, the association with a viral agent remains unproved. Similarly, a small number of case reports suggest a relationship between solvent exposure and this syndrome. Again, the evidence in humans does not support such a conclusion, and the disease cannot be reproduced in experimental animals.

The antibodies are directed against the nonhelical portion (NC-1 domain) of the α-3 chain of type IV collagen molecules in the glomerular basement membrane. This antigen has now been isolated and studied in detail and has been called the Goodpasture epitope. This antigen is common to all patients with this syndrome and is lacking in patients with Alport syndrome, even though the majority of patients with this syndrome have defects in other type IV collagen α-chains (see Chapter 7).

A small amount of epidemiologic data are available on this syndrome. As noted previously, it is most common in men and in whites. Although it is found in all age groups except young children, it is most common between the second and fourth decades of life. There appears to be a seasonal incidence, peaking in spring or summer, and many pathologists with referral renal biopsy practices have commented on the fact that the outbreaks tend to be geographically localized.

Pulmonary hemorrhage is a serious complication. It is essentially restricted to patients who are smokers or who are exposed to pulmonary injury. The pulmonary lesion begins early in the disease course and may precede the renal symptoms.

Hypertension is not often severe, unless there is marked fluid overload.

Macroscopic hematuria and loin pain may be the first signs of the syndrome and cause the patient to consult a physician. Shortly thereafter, oliguria or anuria becomes evident. The urine sediment is filled with casts of all types, cellular compositions, and sizes (the so-called telescope urine sediment). The amount of protein per unit volume is large, but because patients are often severely oliguric, the 24-hour urine protein excretion may not be greatly elevated.

Not all patients with circulating antiglomerular basement membrane antibodies and linear IgG deposits develop pulmonary lesions and are thus placed into the diagnostic category of idiopathic antiglomerular basement membrane glomerulonephritis. In general, these patients are over 50 years of age and the sex distribution is equal. In addition, myalgias and gastrointestinal symptoms and gross hematuria and oliguria are more common than in Goodpasture syndrome.

Histology

Light Microscopy

The classic lesion is a crescentic glomerulonephritis (Figs. 6–21, 6–22). The glomerular tufts are collapsed, and a large mass of cells occupies Bowman's space. It should be recognized, however, that a spectrum of glomerular lesions may be associated with this syndrome, and the renal lesions may not be as severe as those in the pulmonary tract. Thus, the glomerular crescents may be irregular in distribution and severity, with some glomeruli occupied by crescents and others with focal epithelial cell lesions. The only caveat is that we have seen a few patients whose initial biopsy revealed rather modest lesions and who devel-

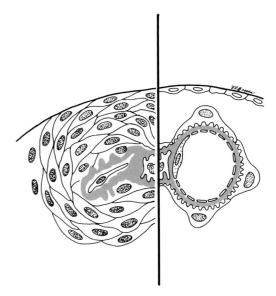

Figure 6–21. Diagram of **diffuse epithelial cell proliferation**.

oped a severe glomerular disease shortly thereafter. Characteristically, the lesions appear to be at a similar stage, which reflects the fact that it is an acute disease.

There are rarely proliferative intraglomerular changes. In fact, the presence of proliferation or exudation within glomerular tufts should raise the question of some other process. In the most severe cases, necrosis of the tuft may be conspicuous.

Bowman's capsule remains intact in many cases. When it is interrupted, the crescent resolves only by sclerosis. Thus there may be prognostic significance in determining the state of its integrity, because it is thought that some cellular crescents may resolve with appropriate therapy.

Immunofluorescence Microscopy

The diagnosis of Goodpasture syndrome rests entirely on the presence of linear glomerular basement membrane deposits of IgG. Essentially all patients with circulating antiglomerular basement membrane antibody have linear deposits (Fig. 6–23). Note, however, that some patients with linear glomerular basement membrane deposits of IgG have either low or undetectable levels of serum antibodies. The immunofluorescence findings are also important to rule out other causes of crescentic glomerulonephritis, such as antigen-antibody complex diseases, nonimmune glomerulone-

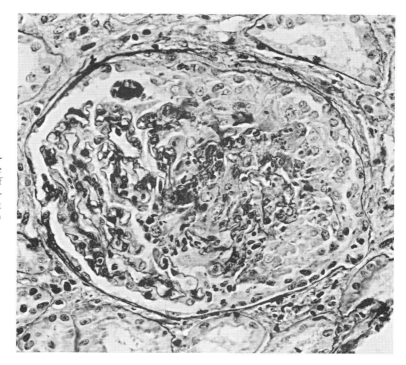

Figure 6–22. Goodpasture syndrome. A crescent occupies the urinary space. Large amounts of fibrin lie between the cells. Neutrophils are also present. The tuft is not hypercellular. (H&E, ×250.)

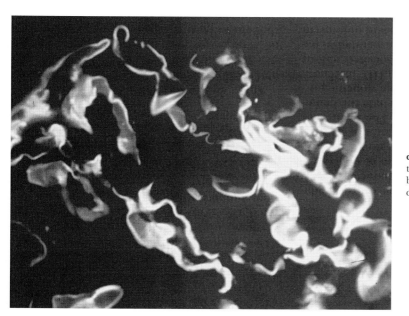

Figure 6–23. Goodpasture syndrome. Linear IgG deposits outline the glomerular basement membranes. (Immunofluorescence micrograph, ×400.)

phritis, and vasculitis (see Chapter 4 and later in this chapter).

The patient's serum can be used to stain frozen sections of normal kidney and lung tissue by the indirect immunofluorescence technique as a preliminary, crude screening test for antiglomerular basement membrane antibodies.

Electron Microscopy

The electron microscopic findings are useful to rule out the presence of immune deposits in those biopsy samples without tissue available for immunofluorescence analysis.

Prognosis

A number of new therapeutic strategies have been introduced in the past decade, including plasmapheresis, high-dose pulse steroids, and cytotoxic drugs. Each form has its proponents, and good results have been obtained when the underlying renal lesions have been early in the course or when the underlying extracellular matrix architecture has been preserved. As mentioned earlier, the disruption of basement membranes bodes a poor therapeutic response. Another indicator of a poor response is the presence of anuria and advanced renal failure at initial presentation.

The serum levels of antiglomerular basement membrane antibodies gradually diminish in most patients. The absolute levels or their persistence is not correlated with the ultimate outcome. Some patients with recurrence of measurable serum antibody levels have been reported, but the significance of this observation is not clear because it does not appear to be related to relapses of the syndrome. Relapses of the syndrome have been reported after bacterial or viral infections. As before, the ultimate outcome depends on the extent of the injury and the response to therapy.

SELECTED READINGS

1. Couser WG: Rapidly progressive glomerulonephritis: Classification, pathogenetic mechanisms, and therapy. Am J Kidney Dis 11:449, 1988.
2. Wilson CB, Dixon FJ: Antiglomerular basement membrane antibody–induced glomerulonephritis. Kidney Int 3:74, 1974.

HENOCH-SCHÖNLEIN PURPURA

Henoch-Schönlein purpura, or anaphylactoid purpura, is a clinical syndrome that has also been called Schönlein-Henoch syndrome. This syndrome predominantly affects children, with 75% of cases occurring in children less than 7 years of age. It has also been reported in adults. The characteristic findings include skin rash, arthralgias, hematuria, and gastrointestinal involvement.

The incidence of nephropathy in Henoch-Schönlein purpura, although quite high, varies widely (from 22 to 66%) among different reports.

During the past few decades, some confusion has been introduced into the literature since the discovery that glomerular IgA deposits were universally present in patients with Henoch-Schönlein purpura. The pattern of glomerular immune deposits is similar to that in IgA glomerulonephritis, leading some investigators to conclude that there are a group of nephropathies linked by the common finding of IgA deposits in the glomeruli. Henoch-Schönlein purpura and IgA nephropathy might therefore represent variants of a similar underlying disorder. Whether this represents an oversimplification or whether there are common pathogenetic factors remains to be proved. There clearly are immunologic abnormalities resulting in glomerular IgA deposits in both disorders, and in occasional reports both diseases have been expressed in family members within a short time frame.

The main argument against a common pathogenetic process is that the two glomerular lesions have a strikingly dissimilar prognosis. The clinical course in IgA nephropathy is one of a slowly progressive loss of renal function in more than one third of the patients, and it is the most common cause of end-stage renal disease due to glomerulonephritis in the Western world. This course of events contrasts sharply with the nephritis in Henoch-Schönlein purpura, in which the overwhelming majority of patients have no long-term renal sequelae. Those who eventually develop end-stage renal failure most often have evidence of severe renal disease at the onset of the clinical syndrome and represent a very small number of those with Henoch-Schönlein purpura.

Pathogenesis

Henoch-Schönlein purpura is often considered a hypersensitivity or leukocytoclastic vasculitis based on the presence of fibrinoid necrosis and IgA deposits in the wall of capillaries of the skin and several other organs. The role of IgA complexes in the causation of this disease has been extensively investigated and has provided the most compelling evidence for a link between Henoch-Schönlein purpura and IgA nephropathy. IgA complexes are present in the peripheral circulation in both IgA nephropathy and Henoch-Schönlein purpura. In addition, both diseases tend to be found in the same geographic areas and affect the same types of patients. Therefore, many investigators believe that Henoch-Schönlein purpura is a multisystem form of IgA nephropathy.

The pathogenesis of the nephritis is unknown, although most investigators agree that the renal disease is somehow related to the presence of circulating IgA complexes. Elevated IgA levels are present in approximately half of the patients. As in IgA nephropathy, it has been proposed that the patients have a defect in the handling of antigens presented to the gastrointestinal mucosa and pulmonary epithelium. It has been suggested that this is the reason for the common association of acute respiratory and gastrointestinal complaints, including allergic responses, in these patients.

The role of genetic factors has yet to be determined, but there have been a few reports of families with Henoch-Schönlein purpura in one member while another had IgA nephropathy.

Patient Presentation

The first signs of renal disease usually appear after an upper respiratory tract infection, but the signs may follow immunizations, drug ingestion, and apparent gastrointestinal viral infections. Hematuria is invariably present and may be macroscopic. Proteinuria, in contrast, is most often moderate. When the nephrotic syndrome is present, the underlying renal lesions are frequently severe, and the few patients thus affected follow a rapidly progressive course to renal failure.

Serum complement levels are usually normal, although circulating immune complexes are a common feature of the acute phase of the disease.

Hypertension may be present. It is interesting to note that patients may have multiple episodes of the syndrome, with each episode having the same benign outcome.

The American College of Rheumatology has established four criteria to identify Henoch-Schönlein purpura and differentiate it from other forms of vasculitis: (1) age less than 20 years, (2) palpable purpura, (3) acute abdominal pain, and (4) a tissue biopsy showing neutrophils around arterioles or venules.

Histology

Light Microscopy

The lesions are variable but often consist of very minor changes. To a large extent, the initial glomerular lesions appear to be a reasonable indicator of the long-term outlook, unlike that in IgA nephropathy. The International Study of Kidney Disease in Children suggested a means to classify the lesions into different grades based on the renal biopsy findings. However, renal biopsies are not routinely performed on these patients, because of the well-known benign outcome of the renal disease. Thus, the reports on the renal findings in Henoch-Schönlein purpura must be interpreted in light of the fact that rather than evaluating the entire spectrum of the renal disease, one is viewing only renal biopsy specimens of patients in whom there is a strong suspicion of the existence of lesions that are severe and unusual.

The classic description of the glomerular changes in Henoch-Schönlein purpura is focal and segmental glomerulonephritis, often associated with tiny foci of fibrin deposition (so-called necrotic areas) (Fig. 6–24). These findings are present in only a small number of patients, and the most frequent change is mild-to-moderate mesangial proliferation. Even this finding has been called into question because it has not been subjected to rigorous analysis by morphometric techniques. Thus, one is often left with the impression that mild proliferation is the principal lesion. Neutrophils may occasionally be present in small numbers. The mesangial accentuation has led some investigators to append the designation "mesangial arborization" to the description of the glomeruli.

The glomerular changes in patients with more severe lesions may reveal areas of widespread necrosis of the glomerular tufts, with the formation of thrombi, karyorrhexis, nu-

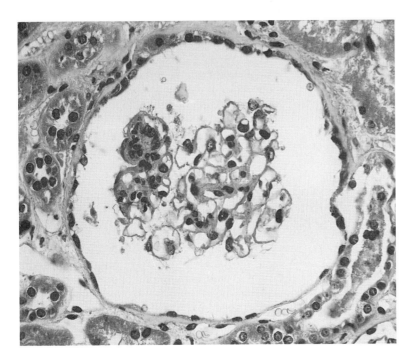

Figure 6–24. Henoch-Schönlein purpura nephritis. Mild lesion showing mild segmental mesangial hypercellularity. (H&E, ×250.)

clear debris, and crescents in the adjacent Bowman's spaces (Figs. 6–25, 6–26). These changes are most often seen in nephrotic patients with macroscopic hematuria. The proportion of glomeruli with crescents has been proposed to be a good indicator of the outcome, with crescent formation in large numbers of glomeruli representing a poor prognosis. In such cases, unlike that in IgA nephropathy, the mesangial proliferation is diffuse and the peripheral glomerular basement membranes may be duplicated, giving them an appearance resembling that of type I membranoproliferative glomerulonephritis. This has been called pseudo-membranoproliferative glomerulonephritis. More rarely, there

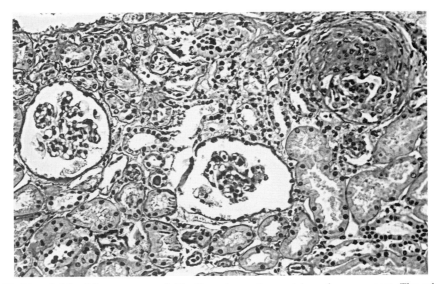

Figure 6–25. Henoch-Schönlein purpura nephritis. One glomerulus contains a large crescent. The other glomeruli appear normal. The interstitium contains a mild infiltrate. The connective tissue surrounding the blood vessel is normal in amount. (Masson's trichrome, ×100.)

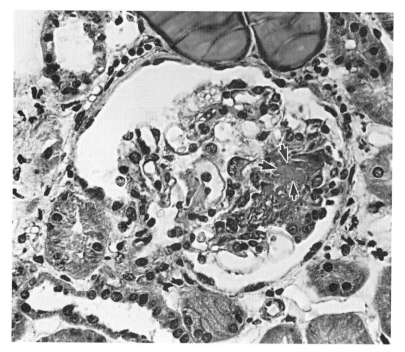

Figure 6–26. Henoch-Schönlein purpura nephritis. A segmental area of necrosis with a small crescent occupies one half of the tuft. The underlying glomerulus shows mild mesangial hypercellularity. Fibrin deposits *(arrows)* are found between the cells of the crescent. (Masson's trichrome, ×250.)

may be diffuse circumferential crescents. Even in these cases, however, the underlying mesangial proliferation is still apparent.

In long-standing disease, areas of glomerular sclerosis replace the necrotic foci, and localized crescents are replaced by fibrous synechiae (Fig. 6–27). The glomeruli ultimately become obsolescent. The tubulointerstitial and vascular lesions parallel the glomerular lesions in the sclerotic stages.

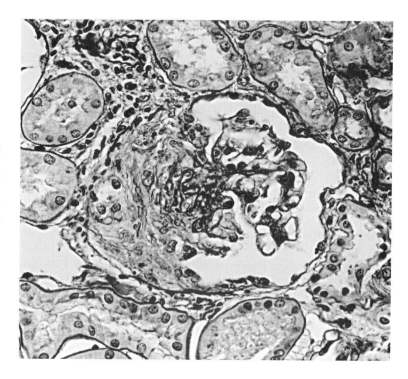

Figure 6–27. Henoch-Schönlein purpura nephritis. There is a sclerosing segmental crescentic lesion, with the rest of the glomerulus showing minimal mesangial sclerosis. Almost half the glomerulus is occupied by mesangial sclerosis and proliferation. (PAS, ×250.)

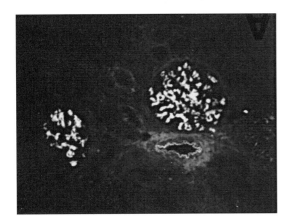

Figure 6–28. Henoch-Schönlein purpura nephritis. Each mesangial region contains large IgG deposits. (Immunofluorescence micrograph, ×100.)

The proposed classification is as follows:

Grade I	Minimal alterations
Grade II	Pure mesangial proliferation
Grade III	Less than 50% crescents
	a. Focal mesangial proliferation
	b. Diffuse mesangial proliferation
Grade IV	50 to 75% crescents
	a. Focal mesangial proliferation
	b. Diffuse mesangial proliferation
Grade V	More than 75% crescents
	a. Focal mesangial proliferation
	b. Diffuse mesangial proliferation
Grade VI	Pseudo-membranoproliferative glomerulonephritis

Immunofluorescence Microscopy

There are diffuse deposits of IgA in each mesangial region, even in those cases in which the glomeruli are essentially normal by light microscopy. The deposits contain IgA in a granular pattern. IgG and C3 codistribute with IgA, and there are small amounts of IgM (Fig. 6–28). There have been several reports on the presence of fibrin/fibrinogen antigens in the mesangial regions, even when there is no evidence of necrosis by light microscopy. Areas of necrosis, of course, contain large masses of material containing fibrin/fibrinogen antigens. In the presence of severe glomerular lesions, large and coarsely granular deposits of IgA and C3 extend along the peripheral glomerular basement membranes (Fig. 6–29). C1q, C4, and other complement components are not often present, although some have reported that beta$_1$-H and properdin may be present in the mesangium. Extraglomerular deposits are not frequent, but there are reports of IgA and C3 along interstitial capillary walls.

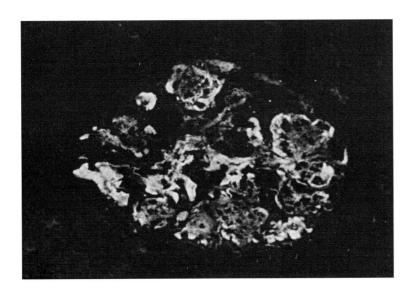

Figure 6–29. Henoch-Schönlein purpura nephritis. Note that these IgG deposits occupy both the subendothelial and mesangial regions of all loops. IgA was also present in the same distribution. (Immunofluorescence micrograph, ×250.)

Electron Microscopy

The mesangial regions contain electron-dense deposits in the extracellular matrix; these are concentrated in the paramesangial areas (Fig. 6–30). In patients with crescents, "gaps" may be seen. Occasional biopsy samples reveal subepithelial, electron-dense deposits.

Prognosis

As noted earlier, most patients with Henoch-Schönlein purpura have some hematuria and thus have a glomerular lesion. However, in the overwhelming majority of such patients, there are no long-term sequelae. Even in patients with focal areas of necrosis or crescents, the prognosis for complete resolution remains excellent. These comments also apply to patients with multiple exacerbations and remissions. Those who have the nephrotic syndrome, impaired renal function, and grade IV to VI glomerular lesions at the outset seem to have a poor prognosis. In these patients the histology appears to provide the most reliable indicator of the future course. There are no long-term trials, but various types of immunosuppressive regimens have been reported in small series, with relatively unpromising results. One small, unconfirmed study suggested that early pred-

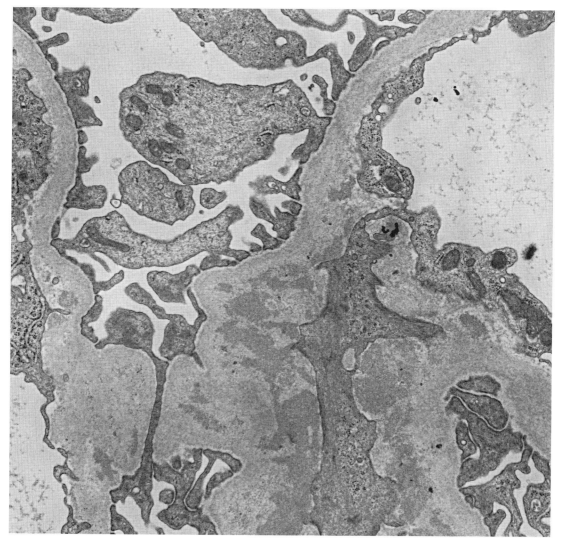

Figure 6–30. Henoch-Schönlein purpura nephritis. The subendothelial space is irregularly widened. The mesangium contains large, electron-dense deposits. (Electron micrograph, ×5000.)

nisolone therapy prevented the development of nephropathy.

SELECTED READINGS

1. Fogazzi GB, Pasquali S, Moriggi M, et al: Long-term outcome of Schönlein-Henoch nephritis in the adult. Clin Nephrol 31:60, 1989.
2. Goldstein AR, White RH, Akuse R, et al: Long-term followup of childhood Henoch-Schönlein purpura. Lancet 339:280, 1992.
3. Levy M, Broyer M, Arsan A, et al: Anaphylactoid purpura nephritis in childhood: Natural history and immunopathology. *In* Hamburger J, Crosnier J, Maxwell MH (eds): Advances in Nephrology. Chicago, Year Book Medical Publishers, 1976, p 183.
4. Meadow SR, Glasgow EF, White RHR, et al: Schönlein-Henoch nephritis. Q J Med 41:241, 1972.
5. Mills JA, Michel BA, Bloch DA, et al: The American College of Rheumatology 1990 criteria for the classification of Henoch-Schönlein purpura. Arthritis Rheum 33:1114, 1990.
6. Niaudet P, Murcia I, Beaufils H, et al: Primary IgA nephropathies in children: Prognosis and treatment. Adv Nephrol Necker Hosp 22:121, 1993.
7. Yoshikawa N, Ito H, Yoshiya K, et al: Henoch-Schönlein nephritis and IgA nephropathy in children: A comparison of clinical course. Clin Nephrol 27:233, 1987.

HEMOLYTIC UREMIC SYNDROME AND THROMBOTIC THROMBOCYTIC PURPURA

The group of diseases of the microvasculature that are histologically characterized by endothelial injury and activation of the coagulation cascade by clinical laboratory examination have been included under the general term *thrombotic microangiopathy*. The syndromes in which these lesions occur include the hemolytic uremic syndrome, thrombocytopenic purpura, postpartum renal failure, HIV infection, systemic sclerosis, and drug-associated lesions (especially in bone marrow transplantation patients treated with cyclosporine and mitomycin C). The development of thrombi is directly correlated with the severity of the injury and is inversely correlated with the outcome. In addition, the outcome depends on the site of renal vascular involvement. The least severe lesions involve only the glomeruli, and the outlook worsens as progressively larger blood vessels manifest injury. The vascular lesions that characterize thrombotic microangiopathy may largely affect the central nervous system (thrombotic thrombocytopenic purpura) or the kidneys (hemolytic uremic syndrome, HUS). The condition has been observed in

acute postpartum renal failure (see Chapter 10) and has been reported as a consequence of mitomycin C and cyclosporine toxicity in bone marrow transplant patients.

Since the hemolytic uremic syndrome and thrombotic thrombocytopenic purpura have overlapping clinical and laboratory features, as well as histologic findings, they are often considered together. However, HUS is much more common in children, whereas thrombotic thrombocytopenic purpura is more common in adults and has more profound central nervous system (CNS) and skin involvement as well as fever.

There are several clinical subgroups of HUS/thrombotic thrombocytopenic purpura:

1. Classic HUS in children following a gastroenteritis with diarrhea (often bloody), and associated with *Escherichia coli* 0157:H7, shigella, salmonella, or pneumococcus.

2. Hereditary HUS. A prostacyclin defect may be present, and the prognosis is poor.

3. HUS associated with pregnancy (see Chapter 10).

4. HUS associated with drugs such as mitomycin C, oral contraceptives, and cyclosporine.

5. HUS associated with other systemic diseases such as scleroderma, systemic lupus erythematosus, malignant hypertension, transplant rejection, HIV infection, or anticardiolipin antibody.

This section is restricted to a discussion of the classic form of HUS.

Pathogenesis

Although the pathogenesis is far from completely elucidated, in the case of the typical diarrhea-associated forms of HUS, the binding of Shiga toxin(s) to endothelial cells is thought to cause injury, resulting in abnormalities of the coagulation system. The endothelial cell injury leads to increased thrombogenicity and leukocyte adherence. Platelets adhere to the damaged endothelium, and after release of various peptides and enzymes, fibrin thrombi form in the glomerular and/or arteriolar lumina.

It is likely that the various syndromes associated with thrombotic microangiopathy have diverse etiologies and that the thrombocytopenia and renal lesions are the end result of the disease process. The rationale to consider these diseases together is that they show comparable lesions, and all appear to be linked to endothelial damage. As stated earlier, the Shiga-like toxins (verotoxins) producing bacteria are major causes of HUS associated with diarrhea. These toxins are produced by *E. coli* 0157:H7 and are similar to the toxins produced by *Shigella dysenteriae* type 1. Lipopolysaccharides and tumor necrosis factor may play an important adjuvant role since they sensitize the cells to the toxins.

Patient Presentation

Thrombotic thrombocytopenic purpura primarily affects young adults, with a female predominance. The disease is characterized by fever, hemolytic anemia, and acute renal failure. Significant hypertension is present in many patients.

HUS is the most frequent cause of renal failure in children. Cases may occur sporadically, or they may be clustered after exposure to contaminated beef products, especially hamburger. The mean age of onset varies from 9 months to 4 years. There have been autosomal recessive (less than 5% of cases) and autosomal dominant forms (very rare, with only 13 families thus far described). While the HUS is most commonly found in children or infants, it may also afflict adults. It may occasionally occur in the absence of hematologic involvement. More than 90% of children with HUS have the diarrhea-associated syndrome.

HUS is triggered by the verotoxin's action on endothelial and red blood cells. A prodrome phase of diarrhea often precedes the renal symptoms. Anemia is always present and is often associated with signs of hemolysis and a decline in haptoglobin levels, the so-called microangiopathic anemia. Schistocytosis is almost constant, and fragmented erythrocytes may be found in glomeruli and arterioles.

Histology

Light Microscopy

There are two varieties of thrombotic microangiopathy: that in which the glomerular lesion predominates and that in which the microvascular lesions also include the arterioles. Although the lesions constitute a continuous spectrum of renal disease, this approach

provides for more consistent evaluation and some prognostic information.

The glomerular loops appear large and fill the urinary space. The most conspicuous abnormality is swelling of the glomerular endothelium, resulting in a marked decrease in the lumen (Figs. 6–31, 6–32). The glomerular basement membranes are multilaminated by silver stain, whereas they have a fluffy appearance with indistinct margins by H&E. Fibrin thrombi are often present and contribute to the severe reduction in the size of the vascular lumen. Fragmented red blood cells may be observed in the lumen. There is a modest increase in the number of mesangial cell nuclei in occasional patients. The mesangial spaces often appear expanded with pale-staining material (mesangiolysis) (Fig. 6–33). However, in patients whose lesions are primarily arteriolar, the principal glomerular change may be wrinkling, collapse, and thickening of the glomerular basement membranes, identical to that observed in ischemic lesions.

Neutrophils and macrophages are rarely found in these glomeruli, in our experience.

In some chronic cases the late lesions resemble those seen in membranoproliferative glomerulonephritis, i.e., duplication of the peripheral basement membranes, mesangial sclerosis and cellular proliferation, and an overall lobular appearance of the glomeruli (Fig. 6–34). However, as the lesions become chronic in patients in whom the primary changes were mostly arteriolar and/or arterial

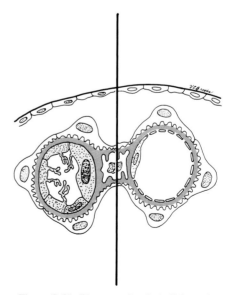

Figure 6–31. Diagram of **endothelial swelling.**

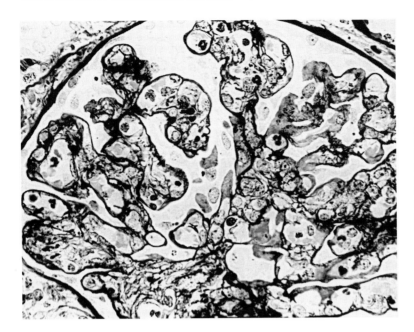

Figure 6–32. Hemolytic-uremic syndrome. There is global endothelial cell swelling and mild proliferation, resulting in a diminution in the size of the vascular space. No inflammatory cells or fibrin thrombi are present. The mesangium has a reticulated appearance, consistent with early mesangiolysis. (Silver stain, ×500.)

changes, the capillary loop widening decreases progressively, to be replaced by areas of segmental collapse with sclerosis of the loops and thickening of Bowman's capsules. This progressive glomerular ischemic lesion is accompanied by an increase in Bowman's space.

The interstitium appears widened by diffuse edema, and there are occasional areas of sclerosis. If the lesions progress and renal failure develops, the interstitial fibrosis may become a major component.

Tubular necrosis is a common finding when biopsies are performed on anuric patients. Mitotic figures may be present in regenerating tubular epithelial cells. Profiles of dilated tubular lumina containing fragmented erythrocytes are occasionally noted.

The degree of vascular involvement is well correlated with the ultimate prognosis. The lesions in patients with little or no arterial damage are much more likely to heal completely than in those with prominent arteriolopathy.

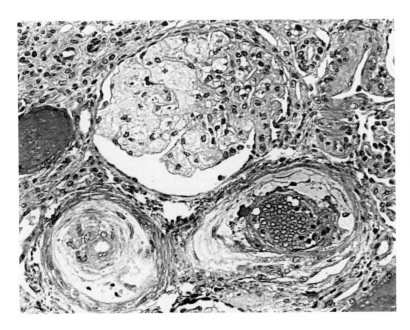

Figure 6–33. Hemolytic-uremic syndrome. The glomerulus is hypocellular, with severe mesangiolysis and endothelial cell necrosis. Two adjacent intralobular arteries have narrowed lumina due to intimal edema and myointimal hyperplasia. There is marked interstitial inflammation, and degenerating red blood cell casts are present in tubules. (H&E, ×300.)

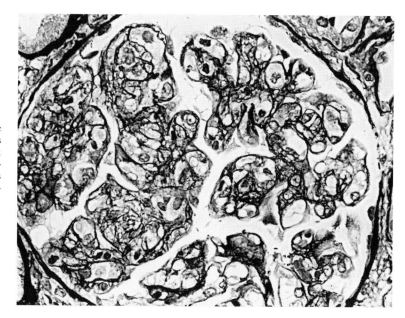

Figure 6–34. Hemolytic-uremic syndrome. This late lesion has membranoproliferative features; basement membranes have a double-contour pattern, and there is endothelial and mesangial cell hyperplasia. (Silver stain, ×500.)

The arterioles may show thrombosis, endothelial swelling, necrosis and/or mucoid change of their walls, and intimal proliferation (Figs. 6–33, 6–35). In the medium-sized arteries, intimal thickening, necrosis, and thrombosis may be observed. These more severe lesions are predominantly found in adult patients. Later the lesions become more sclerotic, particularly in the subintimal zones (Figs. 6–36, 6–37). Some of these arteries may show a mix-

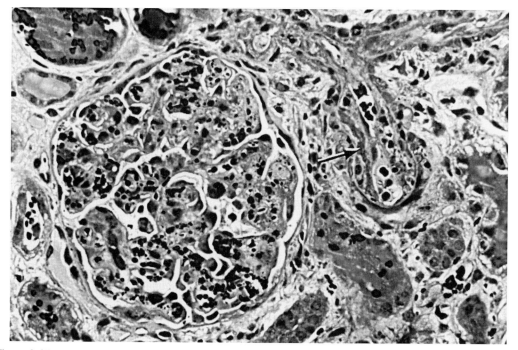

Figure 6–35. Hemolytic-uremic syndrome. The arteriole *(right center)* shows disruption of the media by inflammatory cells and plasma protein deposits *(arrow)*. The lumen is patent, but there are adherent inflammatory cells and the endothelium is swollen. The adjacent glomerulus contains many degenerating cells and aggregates of red blood cells. The vascular spaces are small. (H&E, ×300.)

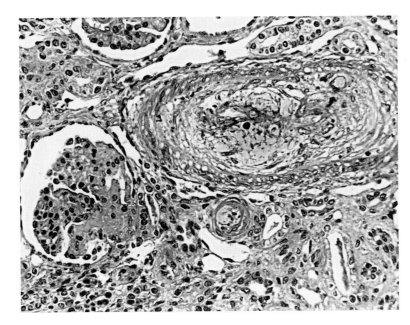

Figure 6–36. Hemolytic-uremic syndrome (late lesion). The glomerulus is severely ischemic and the tufts are collapsed. Both the intralobular artery and the arteriole are occluded by massive intimal edema and mild intimal cell hyperplasia. There is an increase in the external diameter of the blood vessel, but the tunica media is not abnormal in appearance. (H&E, ×300.)

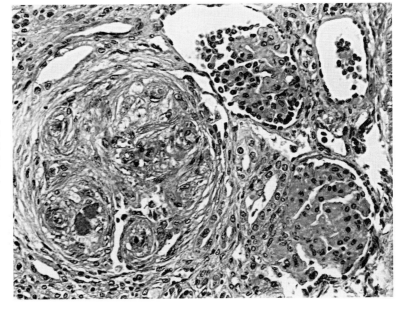

Figure 6–37. Hemolytic-uremic syndrome. This small arteriole is almost completely occluded by an organized thrombus, forming a so-called "glomeruloid body." The adjacent glomeruli show ischemic collapse. (H&E, ×300.)

ture of proliferation and sclerosis, resulting in a picture resembling a glomerulus, the so-called "glomeruloid body" (Fig. 6–37).

Immunofluorescence Microscopy

The immunofluorescence microscopic findings are consistent with the underlying pathogenesis of this group of diseases: immunoglobulins are seldom found, but fibrin/fibrinogen antigens are consistently present in the glomeruli and arterioles (Fig. 6–38). These antigens outline the endothelial lining of the glomeruli and arterioles. This staining pattern affects most glomeruli and all of their segments.

C3 and IgM deposits are occasionally found in the sclerotic areas of advanced cases. These deposits may also be present in the arteries, but these findings have little specificity.

Electron Microscopy

The most characteristic lesion is hypertrophy and swelling of the glomerular endothelium with accumulation of a lucent, fluffy material in both the subendothelial and mesangial regions (Fig. 6–39). The lucent material located between the basement membrane and the endothelium often contains fibrin, fragments of red blood cells, and platelet aggregates or cellular debris. In patients with chronic or persistent changes, a new layer of basement membrane forms on the inner aspect of the original basement membrane, the layers being separated by fluffy, lucent material. The architecture of the basement membrane may thus be severely distorted.

The glomerular vascular loops contain fibrin thrombi and cell debris. Local disruption of the basement membrane with denudation of the endothelium may result in localized aneurysms with dilated vascular loops. The mesangial areas may contain swollen cells with numerous organelles, but proliferation is uncommon. The podocytes show spreading of the pedicels. The arterioles may show lesions mirroring those of the glomeruli—endothelial swelling, lucent material in the subintimal spaces, and intraluminal fibrin thrombi.

Prognosis

The renal outcome in HUS is related to the extent of arterial and arteriolar damage rather than to injury to the glomeruli. Endothelial lesions that are restricted to the glomeruli appear to be much more reversible, usually without residual damage, than those in the arterioles or arteries. Mild cases have an excellent prognosis. At present the mortality rate of severely affected patients is less than 10%. When arteriolar damage is widespread, severe

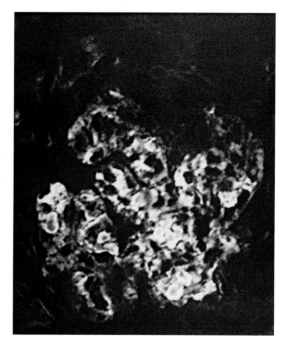

Figure 6–38. Hemolytic-uremic syndrome. Large, irregular deposits of fibrin/fibrinogen lie along the endothelium and occlude some of the lumina in the regions of the "thrombi," and there is also weak staining along the subendothelium. (Immunofluorescence micrograph, ×250.)

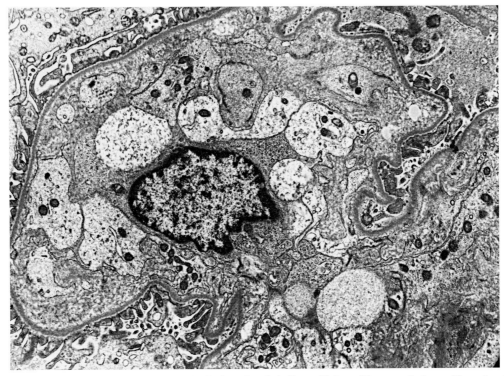

Figure 6–39. Hemolytic-uremic syndrome. The thickened endothelium with loss of fenestrae is shown. The subendothelial space is widened and contains a lucent, flocculent material. (Electron micrograph, ×1500.)

chronic vascular damage rapidly develops and is often accompanied by significant hypertension. In these cases renal failure occurs in 15% of patients. The mortality in thrombotic thrombocytopenic purpura is approximately 30%, a substantial improvement over the prior decades, and it may continue to improve.

New therapies proposed in the past few years aim at the interruption of the coagulation cascade and the inhibition of platelet aggregation. Their effectiveness remains to be established.

SELECTED READINGS

1. Bell WR, Braine HG, Ness PM, et al: Improved survival in thrombocytopenic purpura/hemolytic-uremic syndrome. Clinical experience in 108 patients. N Engl J Med 325:388, 1991.
2. Kaplan BS, Trompeter RS, Moake J: Hemolytic Uremic Syndrome and Thrombotic Thrombocytopenic Purpura. New York, Marcel Dekker, 1992.
3. Loirat C, Sonsino E, Varga-Moreno A, et al: Hemolytic-uremic syndrome: An analysis of the natural history and prognostic features. Acta Paediatr Scand 73:505, 1984.
4. Moake JL: TTP—desperation, empiricism, progress. N Engl J Med 325:426, 1991.
5. Morel-Maroger L, Kanfer A, Solez K, et al: The prognostic importance of vascular lesions in acute renal failure with microangiopathic hemolytic anemia (hemolytic-uremic syndrome). A clinico-pathologic study in 20 adults. Kidney Int 15:548, 1979.
6. Riella MC, Hickman RO, Striker GE, et al: The renal microangiopathy of the hemolytic-uremic syndrome in childhood. Proc Clin Dialysis Transplant Forum 4:112, 1974.
7. Schieppati A, Ruggenenti P, Cornejo RP, et al: Renal function at hospital admission as a prognostic factor in adult hemolytic-uremic syndrome. J Am Soc Nephrol 2:1640, 1992.

SYSTEMIC SCLEROSIS (SCLERODERMA)

The synonyms for progressive systemic sclerosis include *systemic sclerosis* and *scleroderma*. This multisystem disorder belongs to the category of connective tissue disorders. The disease involves multiple organs in a process consisting of disseminated sclerosis affecting all compartments. Prominent vascular lesions typify the renal lesions. They have a major impact on the overall prognosis and are the underlying cause of the progressive loss of renal function. Systemic sclerosis is not rare and has been found in every race.

Pathogenesis

Although the pathogenesis is poorly understood, the most widely accepted postulate is that immunologic mechanisms are involved in the medial smooth muscle and endothelial cell proliferation, the increase in the synthesis of extracellular matrix, and the appearance of inflammatory cells in arteriolar walls. Also in favor of a role for immunologic disturbances is the almost universal presence of plasma antinuclear antibodies and immune complexes, as well as a circulating substance that is toxic for endothelial cells in vitro. It is not known whether the plasma components are markers for the disease or play some role in the pathogenesis of the syndrome.

The vascular lesions result in marked narrowing of the arteriolar lumina. The clinical presentation resembles that of malignant hypertension.

The facts that women are more frequently affected than men and that similar vascular lesions may be found in the postpartum period have led to the speculation that the syndrome may have a hormonal component.

Patient Presentation

The most common presentation is scleroderma (dermal thickening). Renal disease is one of the most serious complications of systemic sclerosis and is reflective of the general state of the vasculature. Thus, renal involvement severe enough to result in an impairment of function indicates advanced and generalized vascular disease. One variety of systemic sclerosis, the CREST syndrome, does not involve the renal vasculature.

Kidney lesions most often become manifest within the first 5 years of the disease. Renal involvement ranges from mild arteriolosclerosis with minimal proteinuria to a malignant hypertensive lesion with glomerular necrosis. The latter presentation, referred to as scleroderma crisis, is associated with thrombotic microangiopathy.

Renal biopsy is not often used in the diagnosis or management of these patients because the course is now well established, and in addition, most patients have malignant hypertension. Thus, renal biopsy could be complicated by severe bleeding.

Histology

Light Microscopy

The glomerular changes are those of endothelial injury resulting in ischemia. The ap-

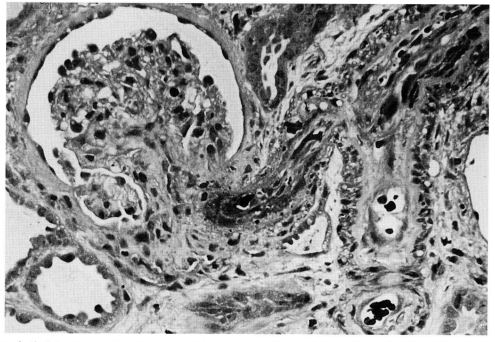

Figure 6–40. Scleroderma. The afferent arteriole is occluded by a fresh thrombus at the hilum. There is fibrinoid necrosis of the wall. The glomerulus is ischemic. (H&E, ×250.)

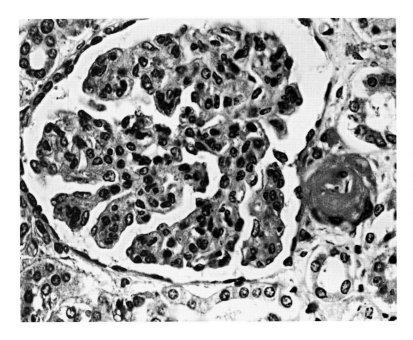

Figure 6–41. Scleroderma. Fibrinoid necrosis of the arteriolar wall has caused thickening and marked luminal narrowing. There is also collapse of the glomerular tuft and mild mesangial hypercellularity. (H&E, ×400.)

pearance of the lesion varies with the stage of the disease. In the acute form, the glomeruli are enlarged, and the individual vascular spaces are distended with red blood cells (Figs. 6–40, 6–41). The number of glomerular cells is not increased, but endothelial swelling is noted (Fig. 6–42). The peripheral basement membranes appear thickened and have indistinct margins, similar to those observed in other disorders associated with thrombotic microangiopathy. One exquisitely acute form, scleroderma crisis, is associated with thrombotic microangiopathy and is characterized by severe necrotizing arteriolar lesions. The glomeruli are often infarcted. The juxtaglomerular apparatus may occasionally be hyperplastic.

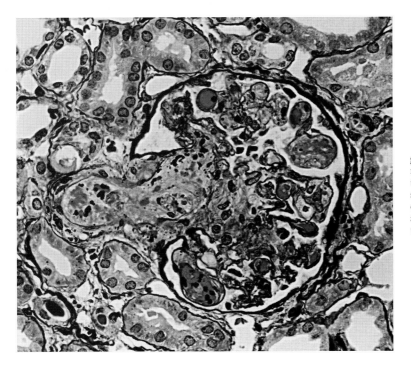

Figure 6–42. Scleroderma. The glomerular vascular spaces are almost completely occluded. The tufts appear to be shrunken and some basement membranes are collapsed *(upper left quadrant)*. The afferent arteriole is filled with a thrombus. (PAS, ×300.)

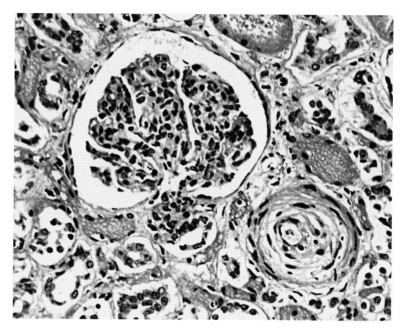

Figure 6–43. Scleroderma. The intralobular artery is severely narrowed by intimal hypercellularity, in a so-called "onion-skin" pattern. The juxtaglomerular apparatus is hypercellular, and the glomerulus is ischemic. (H&E, ×250.)

At later stages, the glomerular basement membranes become progressively wrinkled and thickened and the vascular spaces gradually shrink. At obsolescence, the glomeruli cannot be distinguished from those due to other ischemic diseases.

The tubulointerstitial lesions parallel those in the blood vessels. When the lesions become chronic, wrinkling and thickening of the tubular basement membranes mirror that in the glomeruli.

The vascular lesions are characteristically most prominent in the arcuate and interlobular arteries. They consist of marked thickening of the intima due to proliferation of the endothelial cells and the presence of "mucoid" extracellular matrix substances (Fig. 6–43). The elastic laminae may be duplicated. The medial and adventitial layers are thickened as a result of proliferation of the medial smooth muscle cells and the deposition of extracellular matrix.

The arterioles may also be prominently affected, including necrosis of the wall and proliferation of intimal and medial cells (see Fig. 6–40). In scleroderma crisis, the arterioles may be thrombosed. Those patients with chronic, slowly progressive disease may have arteriolar sclerosis that is not distinguishable from that of essential hypertension.

Immunofluorescence Microscopy

Fibrin/fibrinogen antigens may be present in the glomerular vascular spaces, but immune reactants are not present. The arteries and arterioles may also contain fibrin/fibrinogen antigens in their walls, but IgG, IgA, IgM, IgA, C3, and other plasma proteins may also be trapped within the thrombi. IgM and C3 are most often restricted to the sclerotic zones.

Electron Microscopy

Ultrastructural examination contributes little additional information. The glomerular basement membranes show subendothelial deposits of an amorphous lucent material. The mucoid material in the arteriolar subintimal spaces is electron lucent and may contain profiles of myointimal cells. The small arterioles show concentric layers of basement membranes that are separated by dense granular material.

Prognosis

The course is one of relentless progression of the renal disease to end stage. Angiotensin converting enzyme inhibitor therapy has greatly improved survival in scleroderma crisis, however.

SELECTED READINGS

1. Evans DJ, Cashman SJ, Walport M: Progressive systemic sclerosis: Autoimmune arteriopathy. Lancet 1:480, 1987.

2. Kahaleh MB, Sherer GK, Leroy EC: Endothelial injury in scleroderma. J Exp Med 149:1326, 1979.
3. Lapenas D, Rodman GP, Cavallo T: Immunopathology of the renal vascular lesion of progressive systemic sclerosis (scleroderma). Am J Pathol 91:243, 1978.
4. McCoy RC, Tisher CC, Pepe PF, et al: The kidney in progressive systemic sclerosis. Lab Invest 35:124, 1976.
5. Salyer WR, Salyer DC, Heptinstall RH: Scleroderma and microangiopathic hemolytic anemia. Ann Intern Med 78:895, 1973.

VASCULITIS

Systemic vasculitis comprises a group of diseases characterized by the presence of fibrinoid necrosis and/or acute inflammatory lesions principally affecting the vessel walls. It therefore encompasses a number of disorders that have multisystem involvement. The definition of these diseases is based solely on an aggregation of clinical and pathologic abnormalities, because there currently is no diagnostic laboratory test. It should be remembered that in many immune-mediated glomerular diseases (such as systemic lupus erythematosus, Henoch-Schönlein purpura, or mixed cryoglobulinemia), small arterioles in the kidneys show occasional inflammatory or necrotizing lesions. The presence of these vascular lesions, when they exist as a part of other entities, does not result in their inclusion in the category of vasculitides. The designation *vasculitis* should be reserved for those vascular lesions that include a prominent inflammatory cell component.

Thus the presence of vascular lesions is not sufficient to establish the diagnosis of a vasculitis. This diagnosis is reserved for syndromes in which a vascular lesion is the primary or only lesion in a patient with a multisystem disorder. The kidneys are preferentially affected in these vasculitic disorders and may be the organs that are the main determinant of the overall prognosis. The association between vasculitis and renal disease has been known for several decades, but renewed interest in the early diagnosis and categorization of the renal lesions has been stimulated by the development of effective new therapeutic strategies.

This section is devoted to the renal lesions occurring in the primary systemic vasculitides. These diseases share certain general characteristics:

• Unknown pathogenesis
• Involvement of several organs
• Frequent glomerular involvement
• Rapid course if untreated

A recent consensus conference on the nomenclature of systemic vasculitis developed a categorization that we have modified to focus on the kidney (Table 6–5).

The principal diseases described in this section are microscopic polyarteritis and Wegener's granulomatosis. These diseases are often characterized by the occurrence of necrosis and crescents in the glomeruli and acute inflammatory lesions in the intrarenal vessel walls. A brief description of the other systemic vasculitides is included, as they may occasionally be associated with renal lesions, although much less frequently.

Mixed cryoglobulinemia is described in Chapter 9.

Pathogenesis

It is generally accepted that the systemic vasculitides are caused by immunologic disturbances, but the exact nature and sequence of events leading to the lesions are largely unknown. The three accepted initiating pathways are (1) antibody directed to the vascular wall (principally endothelial cells), (2) immune complex localization, and (3) antibodies directed toward neutrophils (anti-neutrophil cytoplasmic autoantibodies—ANCA), which cause their activation and subsequent adherence to endothelial cells with the induction of endothelial cell injury.

Patients with a polyarteritis nodosa or Wegener syndrome rarely show immunoreactants in their glomeruli, and their plasma complement levels are in the normal range. Recent studies show that antibodies to neutrophil cytoplasmic components are present in the sera of patients with Wegener syndrome. This ob-

Table 6–5. Vasculitides Affecting the Kidney

Large Vessels
Giant cell (temporal arteritis)
Takayasu arteritis

Medium Vessels
Polyarteritis nodosa (macroscopic form)
Kawasaki disease

Small Vessels
Microscopic polyarteritis
Wegener's granulomatosis
Churg-Strauss syndrome
Henoch-Schönlein purpura
Cryoglobulinemic vasculitis

servation may be of help in defining the disease process as well as providing a clue to the pathogenesis of the disease. Finally, the current belief is that nonimmune crescentic glomerulonephritis is a form of vasculitis limited to the kidneys because both crescentic glomerulonephritis and Wegener syndrome have circulating ANCA.

The role of cell-mediated immunity has received more support because of the abundance of macrophages in both glomerular crescents and the vascular wall lesions. This macrophage infiltrate may be so significant that granulomatous lesions may be seen.

Several viral infectious agents have been incriminated in the development of polyarteritis nodosa, especially hepatitis B and cytomegalovirus. The relation between the infection and the vasculitis is not clear, but a substantial number of patients with cryoglobulinemic vasculitis have circulating immune complexes in association with hepatitis C infections.

Polyarteritis Nodosa

General clinical manifestations of polyarteritis nodosa include fatigue, fever, weight loss, myalgias, and arthralgias.

Macroscopic Form of Polyarteritis Nodosa

The macroscopic form of polyarteritis nodosa was originally described by Kussmaul and Maier. There may be few signs of renal disease other than those produced by renal ischemia, except for hypertension, which is an almost universal accompaniment. Acute renal failure in this disease is almost always due to cortical necrosis secondary to widespread involvement of large renal vessels.

HISTOLOGY

Light Microscopy. The likelihood of making a diagnosis of this condition by renal biopsy is small, and biopsy is therefore not indicated except for evaluation of cortical necrosis in the few patients who present with acute renal failure. Nonetheless, if a renal biopsy is performed on a patient who is clinically suspected of having this condition, the sample must be serially sectioned in the search for vascular involvement, because the blood vessel lesions are very segmental and focal in distribution. The lesions are most commonly found in me-

dium-sized arteries (i.e., arcuate, interlobar, and intralobular). The arterial and arteriolar walls contain either localized or circumferential lesions consisting of necrosis and an inflammatory infiltrate (Fig. 6–44). The composition of the infiltrate is most often mixed, but large numbers of neutrophils, macrophages, and lymphocytes are seen. Eosinophils are present in small numbers or are absent. The lesions may be limited to the intima but are seldom restricted to the media or adventitia. The extracellular matrix, including the elastic laminae, may be disrupted in the areas of necrosis. The endothelium often has adherent neutrophils and fibrin thrombi.

Microscopic Form of Polyarteritis Nodosa

Almost all patients with the microscopic form of periarteritis nodosa have glomerular involvement but few have arteritis. The general presenting clinical features are similar to those of the macroscopic form of the disease, except for those related to large vessel occlusion. The renal disease is heralded by signs of an acute, severe glomerular disease. The patients almost always present with hematuria, and the presence of rapidly progressive glomerulonephritis may be the first evidence of the syndrome.

HISTOLOGY

Light Microscopy. The renal lesions in the microscopic form of polyarteritis nodosa are diffuse, in contrast to the focal involvement of the kidney occurring in the macroscopic form. The most common glomerular lesion is fibrinoid necrosis of glomerular tufts. This lesion is usually focal and segmental (Fig. 6–45).

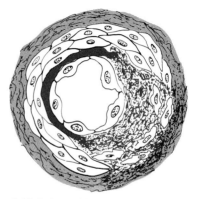

Figure 6–44. Polyarteritis nodosa. Diagram of an artery with **segmental necrosis of the arterial wall.**

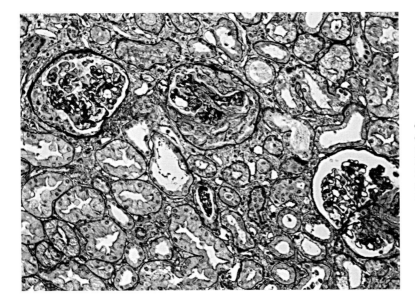

Figure 6–45. Polyarteritis nodosa. All glomeruli contain crescents of varying size. The segmental necrotizing lesion involves one half of the tuft. The glomerulus in the center is collapsed and surrounded by a cellular crescent. (PAS, ×100.)

The extent of the areas of necrosis varies widely within a biopsy specimen and between patients. Crescents are often associated with areas of necrosis, and their number and size parallel that of the necrotic foci (Fig. 6–46). Bowman's capsule may be interrupted, in which case the urinary space is invaded by interstitial cells, and a fibrous crescent rapidly forms (Fig. 6–47). Lesions of diverse age coexist in the biopsy material. Along with the florid crescentic glomerulonephritis may be focal areas of intraglomerular sclerosis and organized synechiae (Fig. 6–48). Intraglomerular proliferation is seldom a conspicuous feature and when pronounced should suggest a search for another cause.

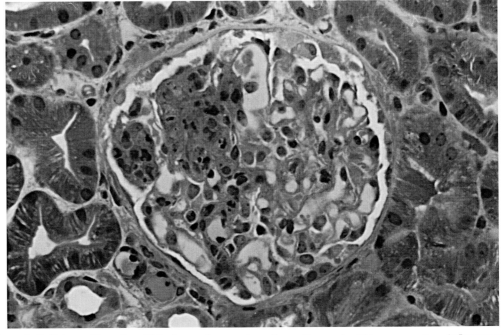

Figure 6–46. Polyarteritis nodosa. This glomerulus contains a focus of necrosis within a crescent, an inflammatory cell infiltrate, and cellular proliferation. (H&E, ×250.)

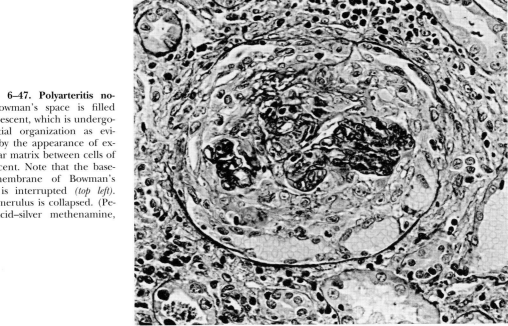

Figure 6–47. Polyarteritis nodosa. Bowman's space is filled with a crescent, which is undergoing partial organization as evidenced by the appearance of extracellular matrix between cells of the crescent. Note that the basement membrane of Bowman's capsule is interrupted *(top left).* The glomerulus is collapsed. (Periodic acid–silver methenamine, ×250.)

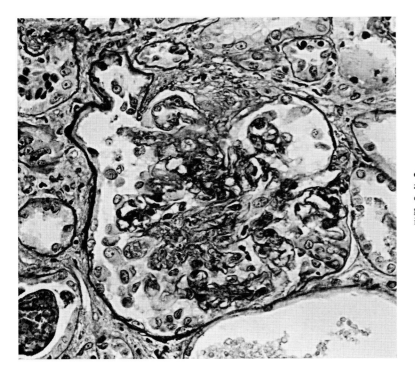

Figure 6–48. Polyarteritis nodosa. This healing lesion contains a small organized (fibrous) synechia (right center). The mesangial matrix is diffusely increased in amount. (PASM, ×250.)

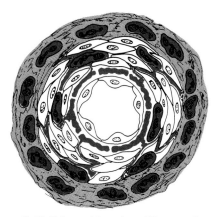

Figure 6–49. Polyarteritis nodosa. Diagram of an **artery with infiltration of the wall by neutrophils.**

The interstitial infiltrate and edema parallel the degree of epithelial cell proliferation, although no specific tubular changes are seen. Later in the disease, tubular atrophy and interstitial fibrosis accompany the glomerulosclerosis.

The general assumption is that middle-sized arteries are not affected in the microscopic form of polyarteritis nodosa; however, our experience is that they may be affected. This is seldom a major feature, but in four of our patients with a necrotizing, crescentic glomerulonephritis an associated inflammatory vascular wall lesion involved the medium-sized arteries (Fig. 6–49). The arteries and arterioles may also be affected by the acute inflammatory process, which consists of necrosis of the wall,

endothelial cell injury, and a dense infiltrate of inflammatory cells (Fig. 6–50).

Immunofluorescence Microscopy. Fibrin is almost invariably found in early lesions. It is localized to circumscribed masses corresponding to the areas of necrosis and crescent formation (Fig. 6–51). Immunoglobulins and complement components are not prominent and when present appear to be a component of the other plasma proteins trapped in the areas of necrosis. They may also be present in small amounts in the areas of sclerosis, but here again, this is a feature common to all sclerosing diseases. There is no convincing evidence of specific deposits in glomeruli or in segments of glomeruli that do not have necrotic foci. Fibrin may be found in the vessel walls as well (Fig. 6–52).

Electron Microscopy. No additional information is obtained by electron microscopy, except for the fact that it confirms the absence of electron-dense deposits, allowing one to differentiate this lesion from an immune complex glomerulonephritis.

Prognosis

The outcome is as variable as the underlying histologic lesions. In the macroscopic form, only a minority of patients develop end-stage renal disease, whereas this is much more common in the microscopic form.

Treatment regimens, including steroids and/or cyclophosphamide, have resulted in a

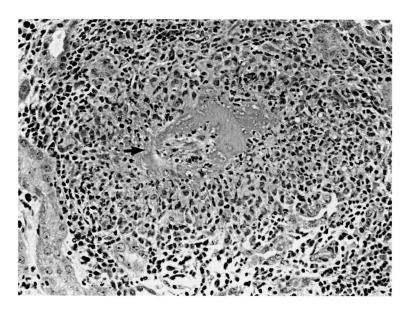

Figure 6–50. Polyarteritis nodosa. The wall of this small artery is invaded by a dense, circumferential vasculitis consisting of an inflammatory cell infiltrate that extends into the perivascular areas and has resulted in complete destruction of the wall (*arrow* showing fibrinoid necrosis around the lumen). (Masson's trichrome, ×250.)

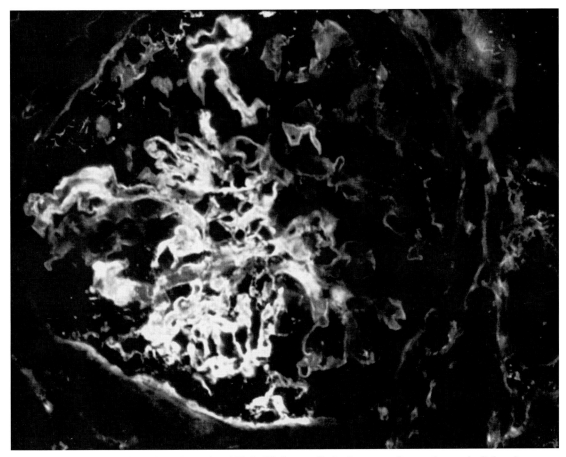

Figure 6–51. Polyarteritis nodosa. Deposits of fibrin/fibrinogen lie in the areas of necrosis seen by light microscopy. (Immunofluorescence micrograph, ×400.)

Figure 6–52. Polyarteritis nodosa. Fibrin/fibrinogen deposits are found within the vasculitic lesions in the wall and lumen of this medium-sized artery. (Immunofluorescence micrograph, ×250.)

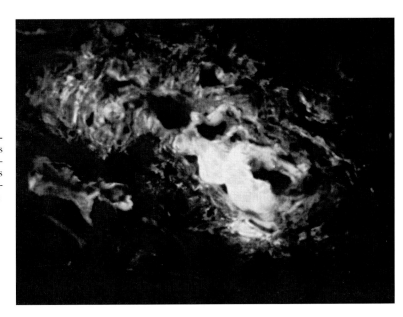

marked improvement of the overall survival in polyarteritis nodosa. However, the renal prognosis in the diffuse crescentic forms of glomerulonephritis remains bleak. The majority of such lesions result in rapid scarring and obliteration of the glomeruli. The small number of such patients has made the performance of clinical trials difficult.

WEGENER'S GRANULOMATOSIS

Wegener's granulomatosis consists of a necrotizing small vessel vasculitis, with characteristic involvement of the upper and lower respiratory tract, accompanied by a necrotizing focal glomerulonephritis. The clinical presentation resembles that of other types of vasculitis and includes fever, anorexia, and weight loss. These symptoms may precede and overshadow those referable to the respiratory tract or the kidneys. This syndrome has been reported in all age groups, including children.

Pathogenesis and Patient Presentation

The renal manifestations may occur at any stage of the disease. Asymptomatic hematuria and proteinuria are the most common laboratory findings, but patients may present with rapidly progressive renal failure.

There are no specific serologic findings. C-reactive protein levels and circulating immune complexes may be elevated, but serum complement levels are almost always normal. These changes are shared with other forms of vasculitis. However, it has recently been observed that the sera of these patients contain antibodies to neutrophil cytoplasmic components particularly proteinase-3. It is of use in establishing the diagnosis of this syndrome.

Histology

Light Microscopy

As in polyarteritis nodosa, a necrotizing glomerulonephritis with crescents is noted. The lesions are focal and segmental in the mild forms, and limited areas of necrosis are seen in the tufts (Fig. 6–53). In the unaffected glomerular segments, the mesangial and vascular spaces appear normal. It is often necessary to obtain serial sections of the biopsy material

in mild forms of the disease, because of its focal nature.

When the lesions are diffuse and severe, most glomeruli are affected, and circumferential crescents and extensive necrosis may be seen (Fig. 6–54). In these cases, the vascular tufts are compressed and collapsed. Bowman's capsule may be interrupted or even completely effaced by the inflammatory cells, which constitute the major cell type of the crescent at this stage of the disease (Fig. 6–55). In these cases, the periglomerular macrophage inflammatory cell process merges with that of the adjacent interstitium, forming what appears to be a periglomerular granuloma. This has been called granulomatous glomerulonephritis. As noted with other forms of crescentic glomerulonephritis in which Bowman's capsule is disrupted, the periglomerular space becomes rapidly replaced with interstitial connective tissue, and the result is an obsolescent glomerulus.

This disease is characterized by exacerbations and remissions. One may therefore find sclerotic lesions and areas of acute inflammation with necrosis occupying the same or adjacent glomeruli.

The interstitium may contain large numbers of inflammatory cells in the regions of glomerular crescents and vascular lesions. In such cases, it is often necessary to apply PAS or silver stains to recognize the underlying normal structures. Granulomatous lesions are seldom seen in the interstitium unless they are contiguous with a similar process involving the blood vessels.

The characteristic vascular lesion of Wegener's vasculitis is a granuloma involving the medial layer of an artery (Fig. 6–56). This is a very focal and segmental lesion, and thus many biopsies may miss such a lesion. Serial sections should be obtained when this diagnosis is entertained. However, the lesions in some patients are those of microscopic polyarteritis.

Immunofluorescence Microscopy

The areas of necrosis always contain fibrin/fibrinogen–related antigens. The glomeruli as a rule contain no immunoreactants, except in localized areas of necrosis and/or sclerosis. In these instances, they most likely represent passive trapping rather than deposition as part of a pathogenetic process. Small deposits of IgM in the mesangium have occasionally been reported.

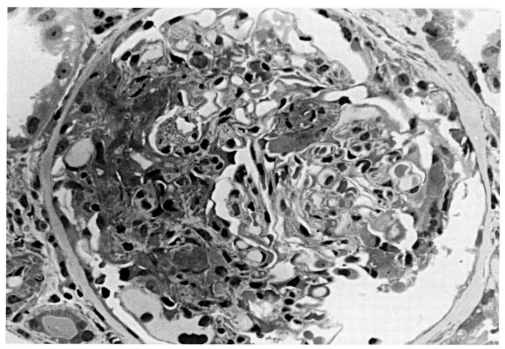

Figure 6–53. Wegeners granulomatosis. Note the irregular involvement of this glomerulus by fibrin deposits and the proliferation of epithelial and intraglomerular cells. The vascular spaces contain a few neutrophils, and there is one small cellular crescent. (H&E, ×300.)

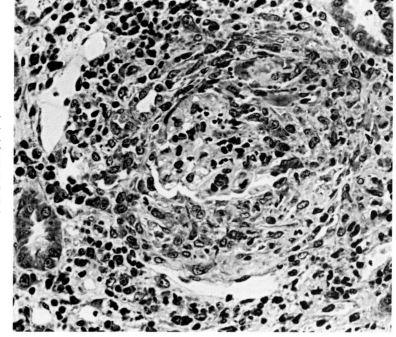

Figure 6–54. Wegeners granulomatosis. The large, circumferential crescent contains many inflammatory cells consisting of neutrophils and monocytes; the infiltrate appears to be in direct contact with the surrounding interstitial inflammation. The tuft is collapsed and contains a few neutrophils. (H&E, ×250.)

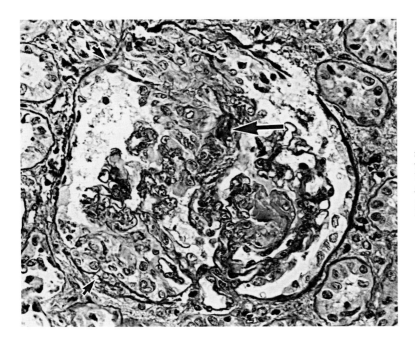

Figure 6–55. Wegeners granulomatosis. Two localized crescents with breaks in Bowman's capsule basement membrane *(small arrows).* A large area of fibrinoid necrosis *(arrow)* lies between glomerular loops. (PAS, ×400.)

Figure 6–56. Wegeners granulomatosis. One arteriolar branch of this small artery is obliterated by a granulomatous inflammatory cell infiltrate that completely effaces the vascular architecture. The media is replaced by a palisading infiltrate of inflammatory cells. Fibrin is also present. (Masson's trichrome, ×350.)

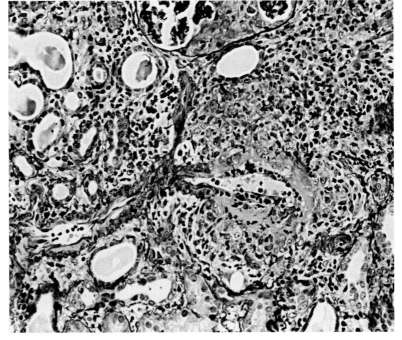

Electron Microscopy

The electron microscopic appearance of the lesions does not add significant new information to that found by light or immunofluorescence microscopy.

Prognosis

The introduction of an effective therapy by Fauci's group at the National Institutes of Health has completely transformed the prognosis in patients with Wegener's granulomatosis. Approximately 80% of the patients respond to therapy with cyclophosphamide and have a prolonged survival time. The glomerular lesions heal rapidly, forming local sclerotic areas. Thus, the ultimate prognosis for renal function depends on the severity and extent of the initial lesions. For this reason, early diagnosis and an aggressive therapeutic posture seem well justified.

OTHER VASCULITIDES

Several other vasculitides may affect the kidneys. Each group comprises only a small number of patients, but each has been proposed as a separate category in the classification of the vasculitides because the group does not fit in the described schema. These will be mentioned very briefly.

Kawasaki's Disease

Kawasaki's disease, also known as mucocutaneous lymph node syndrome, is an acute, multisystemic illness occurring in children. The coronary arteries are the most frequent site of vascular involvement. The vasculature of the kidneys is less commonly involved, but when present, the most prominent lesions are in the mid-sized arteries. Glomerular disease has been described, but it is not clear whether the observed changes are due to vascular lesions affecting the medium-sized arteries or are due to circulating immune complexes. Mild glomerular cell proliferation has been reported, accompanied by granular deposits of C3 and IgM in the mesangium.

Relapsing Polychondritis

Several patients have been described who have a relapsing polychondritis and an associated crescentic glomerulonephritis that is indistinguishable from that in patients with polyarteritis nodosa.

Churg-Strauss Syndrome (Formerly Called Allergic Granulomatosis)

A very small number of patients have been reported to have glomerular lesions similar to those in periarteritis nodosa or Wegener's granulomatosis, with the additional feature of interstitial granulomas that contain many eosinophils. This syndrome is often associated with ANCA. These patients may also have inflammatory lesions of the small arteries and arterioles. Renal lesions are very uncommon in these patients.

Takayasu's Disease

Few renal biopsies have been performed in patients with Takayasu's disease. However, in those studied, the findings consist of mild mesangial prominence with scattered small deposits of immune reactants.

Temporal Arteritis

The renal arteries may occasionally be affected by this relatively common, benign form of arteritis. Rare cases of parenchymal renal disease have been reported in temporal arteritis. One patient had membranous glomerulonephritis, and the relation of the glomerulonephritis to the vasculitis remains conjectural.

Behçet's Disease

Few systematic studies of the kidneys have been performed in patients with Behçet's disease. In the several case reports, sufficient consistency has been observed in the nature of the renal lesions to suggest that there may be an associated renal defect. The most common finding has been mild mesangial hypercellularity, with small deposits of IgG and C3 in the mesangial and subendothelial regions. A few cases with crescentic glomerular lesions and a clinical syndrome of rapidly progressive renal failure have also been reported.

The question of a common pathogenesis

between nonimmune crescentic glomerulonephritis and vasculitis remains open.

SELECTED READINGS

1. Croker BP, Lee T, Gunnells JC: Clinical and pathologic features of polyarteritis nodosa and its renal-limited variant: Primary crescentic and necrotizing glomerulonephritis. Hum Pathol 18:38, 1987.
2. Cupps TR, Fauci AS: The vasculitides. In Smith LH (ed): Major Problems in Internal Medicine. Philadelphia, WB Saunders, 1981, pp 173–202.
3. Jennette JC, Falk RJ: The pathology of vasculitis involving the kidney. Current concepts in renal pathology. Am J Kidney Dis 24:130, 1994.
4. Jennette JC, Falk RJ, Andrassy K, et al: Nomenclature of systemic vasculitides: The proposal of an international consensus conference. Arthritis Rheum 37:187, 1994.
5. Lai KN, Chan KW, Ho CP: Glomerulonephritis associated with Takayasu's arteritis: Report of three cases and review of literature. Am J Kidney Dis 7:175, 1986.
6. Lockwood CM, Jones S, Moss DW, et al: Association of alkaline phosphatase with an autoantigen recognized by circulating anti-neutrophil antibodies in systemic vasculitis. Lancet 1:716, 1987.
7. Ronco P, Verroust P, Mignon F, et al: Immunopathological studies of polyarteritis nodosa and Wegener's granulomatosis: A report of 43 patients with 51 renal biopsies. Q J Med 206:212, 1983.
8. Serra A, Cameron JS: Clinical and pathologic aspects of renal vasculitis. Semin Nephrol 5:15, 1985.

7

HERITABLE DISEASES, PRIMARILY GLOMERULAR

CONGENITAL NEPHROTIC SYNDROME

The appearance of the nephrotic syndrome during the first few months of life is relatively uncommon, and the condition has been called the congenital nephrotic syndrome. The incidence of this disease in Finland is 1 in 8000 newborn infants. It is most often evident shortly after birth, and to fit into this pathogenetic category it must become apparent within the first 6 months of life. The type of underlying histologic lesion in the Western world depends on the patient's genetic background. Patients with a strong genetic linkage are of Finnish extraction and have a macrocystic cortical renal lesion. The others are of various European extractions and have glomerular lesions of two types. The first is restricted to the mesangial regions and, like the microcystic variety, is evident shortly after birth. The second, nonheritable variety consists of the general types of inflammatory or toxic lesions found in older age groups and thus can usually be placed into one of the conventional histologic categories of kidney diseases.

Pathogenesis

Essentially nothing is known of the pathogenesis of the Finnish type of the nephrotic syndrome. However, the disease is kidney specific, since those receiving kidney transplants do not have extrarenal lesions. The glomerular basement membranes have been shown to have a decrease in negatively charged sites, and the proteinuria is glomerular in origin at the outset. The urine protein composition changes to include evidence of a tubular origin, as the renal cysts appear and become the dominant renal abnormality.

The defect has been linked to 19q12-13.1. Although the gene has not been identified, three polymorphic markers have allowed the locus to be restricted to a region encompassing less than 300 kilobases. This finding now allows genetic screening, at least in the Finnish population.

Patient Presentation

The mode of inheritance of the Finnish type is autosomal recessive. The diagnosis can be suspected at birth because of an increased placental size and weight, skeletal abnormalities, and the presence of proteinuria. Afflicted infants are susceptible to infections and have all the serologic abnormalities typical of the nephrotic syndrome. In addition, renal functional impairment becomes evident within the first few weeks and progressively worsens.

The other forms of the nephrotic syndrome that present in the first 6 months of life do not differ in their signs, symptoms, or outcome from those of similar lesions in older children.

Histology

Light Microscopy

Finnish Type, Early. Detailed studies have been made of the renal lesions in these pa-

173

tients. As early as 16 to 24 weeks of gestation, slight dilation of tubules has been noted. This lesion remains the most useful histologic finding in renal biopsies of neonates (Figs. 7–1, 7–2). Microdissection studies reveal that both proximal and distal segments may be involved. A note of caution with respect to this finding is that cystic lesions have been reported in 67 to 75% of most large series, and occasional dilated tubular segments may be seen in other forms of glomerular disease that occur in infants (and adults, of course). Thus, the overall histologic pattern must be evaluated before a diagnosis of the presence or absence of the Finnish type of congenital nephrotic syndrome is made when the lesions are examined during the first few weeks of life. Mesangial proliferation has been described at this stage, but the glomerular changes are usually quite modest and are overshadowed by those in the tubular compartment.

Finnish Type, Late. The cystic lesions progress to involve the entire cortex (see Figures 7–1 and 7–2). The interstitium becomes increasingly fibrotic, and a mononuclear infiltrate is often seen. Again, the glomeruli do not appear to be the primary site of the renal disease, although they may show segmental mesangial proliferation and sclerosis (see Figure 7–2). The lesions in all compartments increase in severity as the syndrome evolves. Because afflicted children are particularly prone to infection, it may be difficult to separate the secondary effects of the patients' overall condition from those due to the underlying genetic defect at this late stage.

Other Types of Renal Disease. This is not a homogeneous group, and the recent epidemic of intravenous drug use in child-bearing women and its accompaniment with human immunodeficiency virus (HIV) even further complicates this picture. However, it is important to differentiate these forms of renal disease from the Finnish type of the nephrotic syndrome in childhood. The histologic lesions in these cases are not different from the expression of the diseases in adults, except for the fact that they are occurring in an infant's kidneys. The main problem in the differential diagnosis is that most observers are unfamiliar with the normal structure of a neonate's kidney. For instance, the glomeruli are normally small, the glomerular basement membranes are thinner than those of adults, the proximal tubules are much shorter than in adults, and so on. Therefore, it may be useful to obtain pediatric consultation in evaluating these lesions.

Immunofluorescence Microscopy

Finnish Type. There is no evidence that an immune component exists in the pathogenesis of this disease. Thus, there are no immune reactants in the kidneys of these patients. Of course, such deposits may develop after infections, but they are not part of the underlying

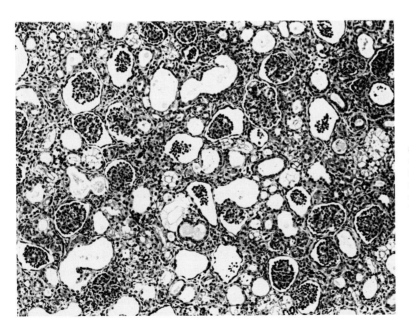

Figure 7–1. Finnish nephrotic syndrome. In this section from an autopsy specimen, the principal abnormality at low power is marked dilation of the tubules and interstitial fibrosis and infiltration. (H&E, ×75.)

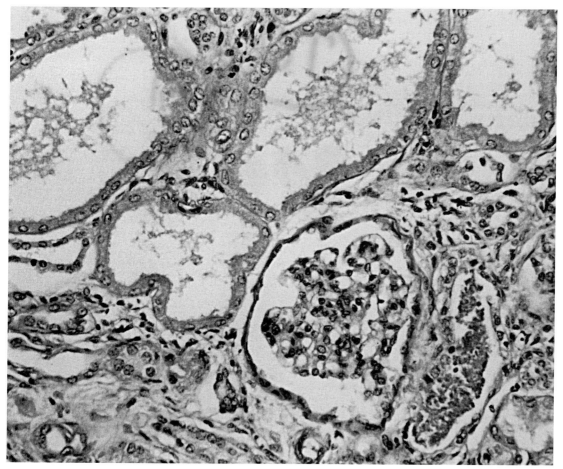

Figure 7–2. Finnish nephrotic syndrome. At higher magnification, the glomerulus is normal, but the tubules have low-lying epithelium and are dilated. The interstitial fibrosis and infiltration are apparent. (H&E, ×300.)

defect. At the late stages, the sclerotic glomerular lesions may also contain C3 deposits. However, this finding is identical to that in other diseases, irrespective of age or disease etiology.

Other Types of Renal Disease. Immune reactants are often found in the glomeruli of these patients. As noted by the light microscopy, they correspond to that expected for the associated clinical and histologic disease.

Electron Microscopy

Finnish Type. At the earliest times of fetal life studied, the glomerular basement membranes have been shown to be prominently altered. The glomerular basement membrane lesion consists of focal splitting of the lamina densa, which is thinner than normal (Fig. 7–3). The overall thickness of the peripheral glomerular wall remains almost normal because of widening of the lamina rara interna and the lamina rara externa. Extensive changes are also noted in the visceral cells, consisting of effacement of the pedicels, microvillus formation, and an increased number of cytoplasmic vacuoles. The mesangial regions are also abnormal, containing an increased amount of extracellular matrix. As the lesions advance, the mesangial sclerosis may become more prominent.

Other Types of Renal Disease. The changes are not homogeneous, reflecting the nature of the glomerular process present. These are described in other chapters. No special features are added by the young age of the patients.

Prognosis

Finnish Type. The nephrotic syndrome appears shortly after birth, and renal function

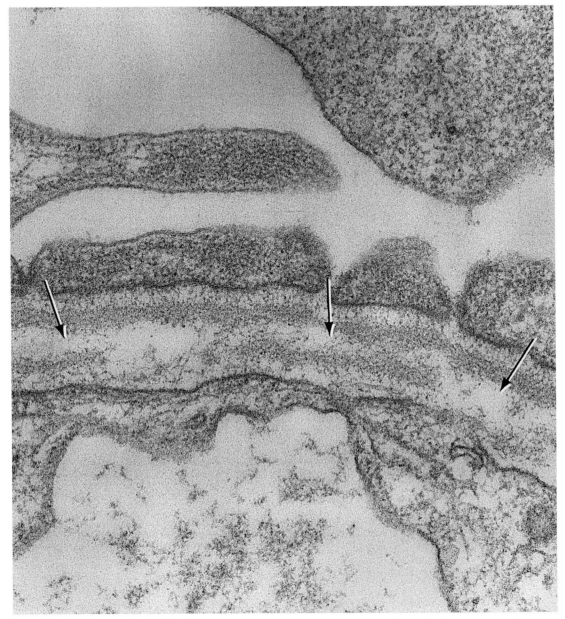

Figure 7–3. Finnish nephrotic syndrome. A small fraction of the peripheral glomerular basement membranes is irregularly duplicated. The space between the electron-dense layers of basement membrane is filled with a flocculent material *(arrows)*. The podocytes are normal. The endothelial cell cytoplasm is thickened in this area. (Electron micrograph, ×30,000.)

progressively deteriorates to end-stage renal disease within the first 3 to 4 years. The most life-threatening complication is sepsis. The nephrotic syndrome is unremitting, and afflicted children are at continuous risk of infections of the body cavities (e.g., pleura, peritoneum, dura). No effective therapy for the nephrotic syndrome has been found, but patients can be managed with renal transplantation, since there are no known extrarenal abnormalities.

Other Types of Renal Disease. The prognosis depends on the cause. If the cause is HIV infection, the outlook is quite poor. On the other hand, if the offending agent can be removed, the prognosis may be quite good. We found that almost two thirds of the patients reach maturity without evidence of significant renal failure. Others report a less optimistic view, but the ultimate prognosis depends on the particular cause of the underlying disease; therefore, it is difficult to make meaningful comparisons between patients or series of patients.

DRASH SYNDROME (WT-1 Gene Defects)

This is a syndrome presenting at birth, consisting of the nephrotic syndrome, Wilms' tumor, and pseudohermaphroditism. The glomerular lesions consist of mesangial widening and sclerosis. The Drash syndrome is associated with specific defects of the Wilms' tumor gene, which is an inhibitor of cell proliferation. Thus, this defect leads to unregulated cell growth in the kidney cortex.

SELECTED READINGS

1. George CRP, Hickman RO, Striker GE: Infantile nephrotic syndrome. Clin Nephrol 5:20, 1976.
2. Habib R, Bois E: Congenital and infantile nephrotic syndrome. Pediatr Nephrol 2:335, 1976.
3. Hallman N, Norio R, Rapola J: Congenital nephrotic syndrome. Nephron 11:101, 1973.
4. Huttunen NP: Congenital nephrotic syndrome of Finnish type: Study of 75 patients. Arch Dis Child 41:344, 1976.
5. Kestila M, Mannikko M, Holmberg C, et al: Mapping of the locus for congenital nephrotic syndrome of the Finnish type (CNF) on chromosome 19q. Am J Hum Gen 54:757, 1994.
6. Mahan JD, Mauer SM, Sibley RK, et al: Congenital nephrotic syndrome. Evolution of medical management and results of renal transplantation. J Pediatr (Paris) 105:549, 1984.
7. Norio R: Heredity in the congenital nephrotic syndrome. Ann Paediatr Fenn (Suppl) 27:1, 1966.
8. Oliver J: Microcystic renal disease and its relation to "infantile nephrosis." Am J Dis Child 100:312, 1960.
9. Sibley RK, Mahan J, Mauer SM, et al: A clinicopathologic study of forty-eight infants with nephrotic syndrome. Kidney Int 27:544, 1985.

THIN BASEMENT MEMBRANE DISEASE/BENIGN FAMILIAL HEMATURIA

It is now more appropriate to utilize the term *thin basement membrane disease* rather than benign familial hematuria, since there appears to be an increased frequency of associated glomerular diseases than previously appreciated. This lesion is a recently described disease in which there is thinning of the glomerular basement membranes. The presence of a renal disease is signaled by the presence of persistent hematuria, which may be either macroscopic or microscopic or may consist of intermittent periods of gross and microscopic hematuria. It was once thought to have a completely benign course, but it has now been shown to be associated with some other renal disease. The most recent morphometric studies of renal biopsies suggest that this lesion is very likely to be seriously underdiagnosed. This lesion has also been found in association with other diseases such as IgA nephropathy. In such cases the diagnosis relies entirely on electron microscopic findings.

Patient Presentation and Pathogenesis

In a large retrospective study of 1250 renal biopsies from adults in one American center, 54 were found to have diffuse or segmental thin glomerular basement membrane (GBM) occupying more than 50% of the filtration surface. Thirteen (24%) were normal by light microscopy, 22% had mesangial proliferative glomerulonephritis, and 18% had either IgA nephropathy or focal glomerulosclerosis. Most patients with normal histology had a benign clinical presentation, whereas those with glomerular lesions often presented with nephrotic range proteinuria, hypertension, and evidence of renal insufficiency. Evaluation of urine samples from relatives revealed that 78% had hematuria, whereas this was the case in only 62% of relatives from patients with other diseases, and in none from healthy controls.

These data compare favorably with another study of Scandinavian patients who had persistent hematuria but without azotemia, in which 17 of 54 patients (31%) had thin basement membranes. This frequency was approximately the same as in IgA nephropathy. In this recently published study, the measured glomerular basement membrane thickness in normal persons was 361 ± 69 nm and in those with thin basement membranes was 191 ± 28 nm. In agreement with others, these researchers found that patients with this lesion have persistent microscopic hematuria, and only 1 of 18 had macroscopic hematuria. A feature previously noted in Holland and thought to predict a poor outcome was that 6 of 17 patients had more than 500 mg of urine protein per 24 hours, and an additional 5 patients had 180 to 500 mg of urine protein per 24 hours. These data suggest that the presence of proteinuria, at least in this population in the

Netherlands, was not predictive of the underlying lesion. The researchers noted that 6 of 17 patients had a family history of microscopic hematuria. The mean duration of follow-up was 50 months.

The mode of inheritance is autosomal dominant, for the most part. In the American study, examination of the urine from families of patients with thin basement membrane disease revealed that 92% had at least one first-degree relative with hematuria, and 47% of family members were affected. However, in some kindreds the mode seems to be autosomal recessive inheritance. It has recently been found that some kindreds have a genetic defect in type IV (basement membrane) collagen, in the α4 chain. Thus, thin basement membrane disease joins other related genetically based basement membrane diseases.

Histology

Light Microscopy

The typical finding in the uncomplicated patient is that the biopsy material is essentially completely normal by light microscopy. A few erythrocytes may be seen within tubule lumina. The only other changes are those consistent with the patient's age.

Immunofluorescence Microscopy

Most investigators report that no immune reactants are present, but, as noted earlier, in the Netherlands study 7 of 18 patients with thin basement membranes had diffuse mesangial staining for C3.

The Goodpasture antigen appears to be present in these biopsy specimens. In addition, there is a report that the α-1 and α-2 type IV collagen chains are present in the normal distribution. The other type IV collagen α-chains have not been examined.

Of course, those with other glomerular diseases will have the findings associated with the this process.

Electron Microscopy

The thickness of the glomerular basement membranes in normal subjects has been well studied by the Minnesota and Netherlands groups, who are in agreement that it is 354 ± 55 nm. Patients in the group with thin basement membranes were very distinct from the normal subjects and from patients with various diseases, measuring 191 ± 28 nm (Fig. 7–4). There was no overlap between the latter and either of the former groups. It should be emphasized, however, that the width of the glomerular basement membranes in children

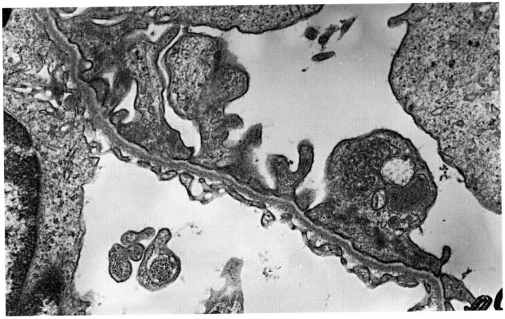

Figure 7–4. Thin basement membrane disease benign/familial hematuria. The peripheral glomerular basement membranes are uniformly thinned. The pedicels of the epithelial cells are focally spread. (Electron micrograph, ×7800.)

slowly increases as a function of age. Thus, caution must be used to match the biopsy specimen in question very carefully to the appropriate controls. In addition, the thinning of the basement membranes is more often segmental than diffuse in this disease. This is also the case in patients with associated disease.

Other lesions described in these patients, including mesangial thickening and deposits, are related to the associated diseases.

Prognosis

Most reports state that the prognosis is excellent in patients without associated diseases. This opinion is consistent with the finding that patients with glomerular basement membranes of 206 to 301 nm may have hypertension and azotemia, if there is an associated disease. Since the thickness of the glomerular basement membranes had not previously been well characterized, and the association of this syndrome with other renal diseases was not previously appreciated, some of the older reports may have to be re-evaluated.

SELECTED READINGS

1. Cosio FG, Falkenhain ME, Sedmak DD: Association of thin glomerular basement membrane with other glomerulopathies. Kidney Int 46:471, 1994.
2. Dische FE, Anerson VER, Keane SJ, et al: Incidence of thin membrane nephropathy: Morphometric investigation of a population sample. J Clin Pathol 43:457, 1990.
3. Fujigaki Y, Mitsumasa N, Kobayashi S, et al: Alterations of glomerular basement membrane relevant to hematuria. Virchow's Arch [A] 413:159, 1988.
4. Greenspan DS, Byers MG, Eddly RL, et al: Human collagen gene COL5A1 maps to the q34.2-q34.3 region of chromosome q, near the locus for nail-patella syndrome. Genomics 12:836, 1992.
5. Gubler MC, Levy M, Naizot C, et al: Glomerular basement membrane changes in hereditary glomerular disease. Renal Physiol 3:405, 1980.
6. Piel CF, Biava CG, Goodman JR: Glomerular basement membrane attenuation in familial nephritis and "benign" hematuria. J Pediatr 101:358, 1982.
7. Tiebosch T, Van Breda Vriesman P, Mooy J, et al: Thin-basement-membrane nephropathy in adults with persistent hematuria. N Engl J Med 320:14, 1989.
8. Lemmink HH, Nillesen WN, Mochizuki T, et al: Benign familial hematuria due to mutation of type IV collagen α4 gene. J Clin Invest 98:1114, 1996.

ALPORT SYNDROME

Alport syndrome was first recognized in 1902 and then fully described in 1927 as a clinical syndrome consisting of a hereditary form of progressive renal disease associated with high-frequency deafness. The syndrome was found to affect males more severely than females. The first family described had deaf members without renal disease, and although the males died of renal disease, the females did not. This syndrome is not geographically restricted, and the gene frequency estimates range from 1:5000 to 1:10,000 in the United States.

Pathogenesis

As more studies have been performed, it has become clear that the mode of inheritance is heterogeneous, with the X-linked forms representing 85 to 90% of cases, and 10 to 15% being either autosomal dominant or recessive. The genetic defect in the most common form was initially linked to Xq22, and then ascribed to the α-5 chain of type IV (basement membrane) collagen when it was mapped to that region. Finally, when the α-5 collagen chain was sequenced, it was shown that a number of the families with Alport syndrome had mutations of this gene. The number of α-5 chain mutations reported in the literature has continued to increase. In addition, it is now clear that the autosomal forms are due to mutations in either the α-3 or α-4 chain of type IV collagen.

Before the biochemical nature of the defect was known, it had been known that the glomerular basement membranes of certain kindreds lacked an epitope recognized by Goodpasture serum. This was found to localize to the noncollagenous domain of the amino terminal end of the type IV collagen molecules of the glomerular basement membranes, and now is known to be restricted to the α-5 type IV collagen chain in most cases. An interesting but unexplained finding is that the amyloid P component of the glomerular basement membranes is also missing in these patients.

Patient Presentation

The first indication of the renal aspects of this syndrome is microscopic hematuria. It may be apparent at birth and is most often apparent before school age. The hematuria may on occasion be macroscopic in males, especially after an upper respiratory infection, but microscopic hematuria is continuous. Females seldom have continuous microscopic hematuria, and some carriers never have red blood cells in their urine. Proteinuria, often absent during the first few years, slowly increases in amount in males. When renal failure and hypertension are present, the nephrotic syndrome may also be manifest, and this feature indicates the likelihood of progressive renal disease. Because females seldom develop renal failure, it is not surprising that they seldom have proteinuria.

The most common extrarenal lesion is a progressive cochlear defect that is apparent in boys by age 15. Some families without a hearing defect have been described. In affected females, the hearing defect is usually not as severe as in males, except in those women who are destined to develop severe renal lesions. Ocular defects may afflict 15 to 30% of patients, with anterior lenticonus being the most common form. Other defects have also been reported, but their frequency is low.

Histology

Light Microscopy

The morphology by light microscopy depends entirely on the stage of the disease at which the biopsy is performed. Early, the only recognizable light microscopic lesion is a slight, irregular increase in the amount of extracellular matrix in the mesangium and Bowman's capsule. Later, the glomerular changes become slightly more diffuse and evident. At this stage, the principal lesion may appear to be in the interstitium, which may be quite prominently fibrotic and contain foam cells (Fig. 7–5). This observation led previous investigators to the conclusion that foam cells in a fibrotic interstitium were the hallmarks of this disease. Not until much later was it shown that interstitial foam cells could be found in many proteinuric states and thus were not a useful diagnostic indicator for hereditary nephritides.

The glomerular changes at late stages consist of a marked increase in all aspects of the basement membranes and mesangium, ultimately resulting in complete sclerosis. The interstitial lesions progress, and tubular atrophy appears.

Immunofluorescence Microscopy

No immune reactants are found at early stages. As sclerosis appears, IgM and complement components (especially C3) may be noted. The most striking finding is that antibodies to the α-3, 4, and 5 chains of type IV collagen do not bind to the peripheral basement membrane. Types V and VI collagen appear, and anti-GBM antisera, or Goodpasture syndrome sera, most often do not bind to the glomerular basement membranes.

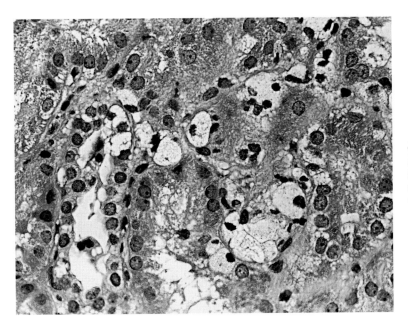

Figure 7–5. Alport syndrome. There is a mild, generalized increase in the amount of interstitial connective tissue. Foam cells are also found within the interstitium. (H&E, ×300.)

Electron Microscopy

The earliest recognizable lesions can be seen only at electron microscopic level. They consist of focal or diffuse splitting of the lamina densa. The individual laminae are thinner than the normal lamina densa. Thus, the peripheral glomerular basement membrane is multilaminated, and the individual laminae are quite irregular in contour, continuity, and thickness (Fig. 7–6). The clear areas between the laminae are of variable width and are filled with a granular, mottled material. This material has been thought to represent fragments of cell processes. These changes are irregularly distributed within and between glomerular loops, but all glomeruli are affected. The lamina densa alterations in affected females are much less severe and often consist of segmental thinning and irregularity in thickness. The basement membranes of Bowman's capsule and the tubules often show similar lesions.

Prognosis

As noted earlier, the lesions appear in boys before the age of 10 years. If signs of renal disease are not present by this time, it is quite unlikely that the patient will be affected. Affected males practically always progress to renal failure. There are kindreds in which renal failure occurs in the third decade and others in which it presents at a much later time. Females seldom have significant evidence of renal functional impairment. However, a certain number of women develop renal failure, and this outcome is most often signaled by severe basement membrane changes and proteinuria.

AUTOSOMAL RECESSIVE ALPORT SYNDROME

Four kindreds have been recently described in which an autosomal recessive pattern was

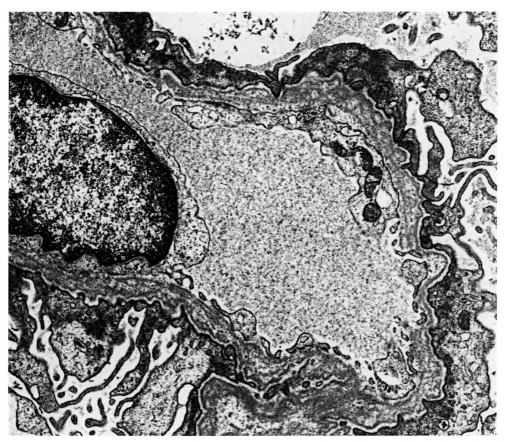

Figure 7–6. Alport syndrome. The glomerular basement membranes show diffuse multilamination and podocyte effacement. (Electron micrograph, ×4000.)

proved. All patients developed end-stage renal disease between 11 and 16 years of age. The defect was identified in the COL4A4 gene in two families and in the COL4A3 gene in another. The immunohistochemical findings were similar to those in the glomeruli of X-linked Alport syndrome patients in two families, and in one family no differences from control kidneys were found. In the latter patient the genetic defect was found to reside in the COL4A4 gene.

SELECTED READINGS

1. Alport SC: Hereditary familial congenital hemorrhagic nephritis. Br Med J 1:50, 1927.
2. Bodziak KA, Hammond WS, Molitoris BA: Inherited diseases of the glomerular basement membrane. Am J Kidney Dis 23:605, 1994.
3. Ding J, Kashtan CE, Fan WW, et al: A monoclonal antibody marker for Alport syndrome identifies the Alport antigen as the α-5 chain of type IV collagen. Kidney Int 46:1504, 1994.
4. Gubler M-C, Knebelmann B, Beziau A, et al: Autosomal recessive Alport syndrome: Immunohistochemical study of type IV collagen chain distribution. Kidney Int 47:1142, 1995.
5. Habib R, Gubler MC, Hinglais N, et al: Alport's syndrome: Experience at Hospital Necker. Kidney Int 21:S20, 1982.
6. Hostikka SL, Eddy RL, Byers MG, et al: Identification of a distinct type IV collagen α-chain with restricted kidney distribution and assignment of its gene to the locus of X chromosome-linked Alport syndrome. Proc Natl Acad Sci USA 87:1606, 1990.
7. Savage COS, Pusey CD, Kershaw MJ, et al: The Goodpasture antigen in Alport's syndrome: Studies with a monoclonal antibody. Kidney Int 30:100, 1986.
8. Spear GS, Slusser RJ: Alport's syndrome. Emphasizing electron microscopic studies of the glomerulus. Am J Pathol 69:213, 1972.

NAIL-PATELLA SYNDROME

The nail-patella syndrome has been recognized as an entity since the end of the 19th century, but not until the early 1970s was the presence of a renal lesion clearly documented. It has an autosomal dominant mode of inheritance, and the gene frequency in the population is approximately 2 per 100,000. There is a strong linkage to a locus, 9q34, containing the ABO blood group and adenylate kinase genes on chromosome 9. The multiple associated skeletal abnormalities include absence or subluxation of the patella, deformation or luxation of the radial head, iliac spurs, and fingernail dysplasia.

Pathogenesis

Essentially nothing is known about the genesis of the renal lesion in this rare condition. The fact that a disproportionate number of other congenital malformations of the skeleton and urinary tract are concomitant suggests that the lesion is generalized, but there are few studies of the extrarenal abnormalities. Recently it has been suggested that the COL5A1 gene may be involved, since this gene has been linked to the 9q34.2-9q34.3 region of chromosome 9, and the nail-patella locus has been localized to 9q34. However, no abnormalities in the COL5A1 gene have been identified.

Patient Presentation

The presence of renal disease can be the first sign of the syndrome, although kidney involvement has been found in from 30 to 60% of cases in different series. Hematuria and proteinuria are present in less than 50%, and the nephrotic syndrome is exceptional. The diagnosis is most often made in the second or third decade.

Histology

Light Microscopy

The renal tissue most often appears normal at early stages of the disease. As the disease progresses, glomerulosclerosis appears. The sclerosis is in the form of diffuse, regular thickening of the basement membranes and mesangial sclerosis. The extraglomerular connective tissue components are also affected, resulting in interstitial fibrosis and tubular basement membrane thickening.

Immunofluorescence Microscopy

No deposits are seen, because there is no evidence of an immune pathogenesis. The trapping of complement components and immunoglobulins in areas of sclerosis is observed in late lesions.

Electron Microscopy

The lesions can be appreciated only at the ultrastructural level. They consist of multiple

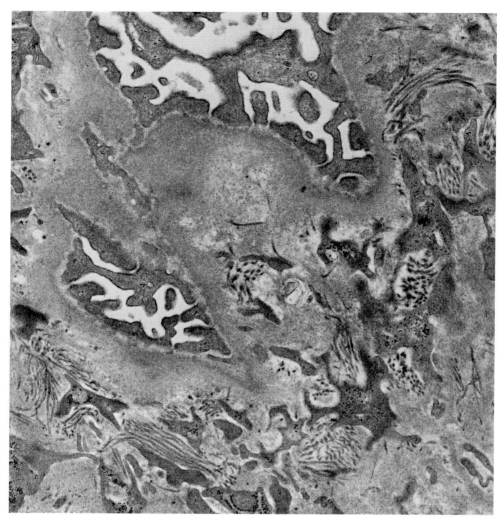

Figure 7–7. Nail-patella syndrome. Multiple banded fibrils are found within the mesangial matrix and the substance of the peripheral glomerular basement membranes. (Electron micrograph, phosphotungstic acid stain, ×6300.) (Courtesy of Dr. M.-C. Gubler.)

lucent areas within basement membranes, which contain debris and regularly banded fibrils (Fig. 7–7). The fibrils resemble interstitial collagen and are best seen after phosphotungstic acid staining. They are not seen in all lacunae and may be present in patients without proteinuria. Although most glomeruli are affected, the distribution of the lesions between individual loops or glomeruli may be very irregular.

Prognosis

In a report of 104 patients it was found that 29 progressed to renal failure. The mean age at end-stage renal failure was 33 years. Thus,

the prognosis in this syndrome may not be as benign as previously thought. It is interesting that, in transplanted patients, the basement membrane lesions do not recur; however, some of the skeletal lesions and the dystrophic nails have been reported to revert toward normal.

SELECTED READINGS

1. Ben-Bassat M, Cohen L, Rosenfeld J: The glomerular basement membrane in the nail-patella syndrome. Arch Pathol 92:350, 1971.
2. Bennett WM, Musgrave JE, Campbell RA, et al: The nephropathy of the nail-patella syndrome: Clinicopathologic analysis of 11 kindreds. Am J Med 54:304, 1973.
3. Hawkins CF, Smith OE: Renal dysplasia in a family

with multiple hereditary abnormalities, including iliac horns. Lancet 1:803, 1950.
4. Hoyer JR, Michael AF, Vernier RL: Renal disease in nail-patella syndrome: Clinical and morphologic studies. Kidney Int 2:231, 1972.
5. Looji BJ, TeSlaa RL, Hogewind BL, et al: Genetic counseling in hereditary osteo-onychodysplasis (HOOD, nail-patella syndrome) with nephropathy. J Med Genet 25:682, 1988.
6. Schleutermann DA, Bias WB, Murdoch JL, et al: Linkage of the loci for the nail-patella syndrome and adenylate kinase. Am J Hum Genet 21:606, 1969.

COLLAGEN TYPE III GLOMERULOPATHY

This is a new type of glomerulopathy seen in children presenting with early and progressive glomerular disease and hypertension. It is associated with the deposition of type III collagen in the mesangium. Until the collagen in the mesangium was typed, this lesion was referred to as primary glomerular fibrosis or collagenofibrotic glomerulopathy.

Pathogenesis

The inheritance pattern of this defect suggests that it is a genetic disease with an autosomal recessive inheritance in children. In contrast, the disease has a sporadic appearance in adults. The nature of the defect is unclear. In a study of Japanese adults, there was a tenfold increase in the circulating levels of procollagen type III propeptides. This finding has not been evaluated in other series. The increased incidence of the hemolytic-uremic syndrome in the patients and their relatives suggests that type III collagen may have something to do with this disorder.

Patient Presentation

In a study of 10 children, the most common presenting renal symptoms were proteinuria, sometimes with the nephrotic syndrome, and hematuria. Hypertension was present at onset in one half the children.

Histology

Light Microscopy

In children, the lesions are characterized by marked glomerular enlargement with both mesangial expansion and a thickened peripheral basement membrane due to the presence of poorly stained material (Fig. 7–8). Silver or PAS stains may show double contours, mimick-

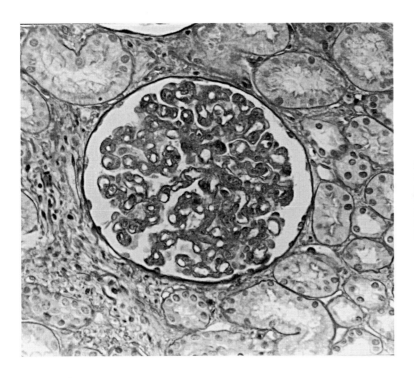

Figure 7–8. Collagen type III glomerulopathy. Diffuse, irregular thickening and duplication of the glomerular basement membrane. Vascular spaces are reduced. The mesangial spaces are mildly enlarged. (PAS, ×400.) (Courtesy of Dr. M.-C. Gubler.)

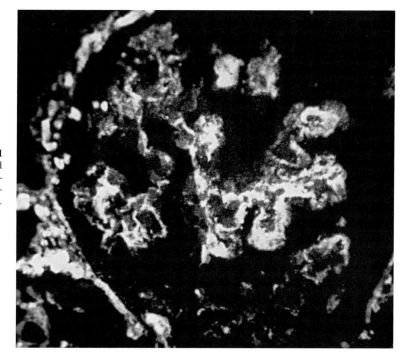

Figure 7–9. Collagen type III glomerulopathy. Mesangial and parietal deposits of type III collagen. (Immunofluorescence micrograph, ×500.) (Courtesy of Dr. M.-C. Gubler.)

ing thrombotic microangiopathy. Cell proliferation is not present. In adults, the lesions in the mesangium are more marked, sometimes becoming nodular, suggesting diabetic nephropathy, light chain systemic disease, or amyloidosis.

Immunofluorescence Microscopy

The most obvious finding is the presence of marked staining of the mesangium using antibodies to type III collagen (Fig. 7–9). This was associated with increased staining with

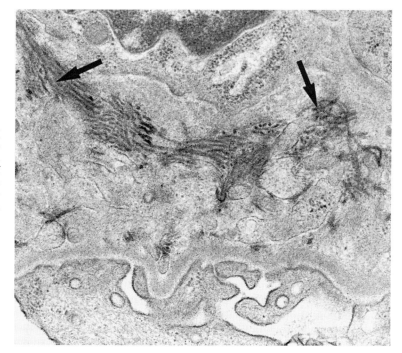

Figure 7–10. Collagen type III glomerulopathy. There is an accumulation of fibrillar collagen *(arrows)* on the inner aspects of the enlarged and irregular basement membrane. (Electron micrograph, phosphotungstic acid stain, ×30,000). (Courtesy of Dr. M.-C. Gubler.)

type IV collagen antibodies, specifically α-1 type IV collagen. The other type IV collagen α-chains were normal. Fibronectin and types V and VI collagen were found in the peripheral basement membrane—an unusual finding since they are normally restricted to the mesangium. In addition, laminin was found in a double-contour distribution in the peripheral glomerular basement membrane.

Electron Microscopy

The mesangial regions were variably, but often massively, expanded by abnormal extracellular material. This material has a clear, heterogeneous, mottled appearance. Fibrils can be seen on phosphotungstic acid (PTA) or tannic acid stains as typical collagen fibrils with the typical periodicity of 60 nm (Fig. 7–10). The peripheral basement membranes are duplicated. Between the lamellae are cell processes and cell debris. The endothelial cells have thickened cytoplasm and surface villi, giving an appearance of being activated. The pedicels of the podocytes are spread (effaced), particularly in areas with parietal lesions.

Prognosis

The renal disease progressed to end stage in 5 years in nearly one half the children. In adults, the course seems to be more benign, with renal function remaining relatively stable or slowly decreasing.

SELECTED READINGS

1. Gubler MC, Dommergues JP, Foulard M, et al: Collagen type III glomerulopathy: A new type of hereditary nephropathy. Pediatr Nephrol 7:354, 1993.
2. Ikeda K, Yokohama H, Tomosugi N, et al: Primary glomerular fibrosis: A new nephropathy caused by diffuse intraglomerular increase in a typical type III collagen fiber. Clin Nephrol 33:155, 1990.
3. Imbasciati E, Gherardi G, Morozumi K, et al: Collagen type III glomerulopathy: A new idiopathic glomerular disease. Am J Nephrol 11:422, 1991.

SICKLE CELL DISEASE

Renal disease may afflict patients with sickle cell disease (hemoglobin SS or SA). In most patients with sickle cell anemia, the renal abnormalities are not severe enough to warrant a renal biopsy. A concentrating defect is the most commonly reported lesion. However, proteinuria and the nephrotic syndrome have been described. In these cases, the underlying renal lesion is focal and segmental glomerulosclerosis or membranoproliferative glomerulonephritis. Renal lesions are seen most frequently in patients with hemoglobin SS and in children. The number of patients developing decreased renal function varies with the hemoglobin abnormality (4.2% in SS and 2.4% in SC).

Pathogenesis

It has been generally assumed that patients with sickle cell anemia have an increased glomerular hydrostatic pressure and glomerular blood flow. The current paradigm to explain the pathogenesis of progressive glomerular lesions predicts the type of glomerulosclerotic lesion in these patients. However, this hypothesis does not explain the presence of glomerular lesions of similar intensity in patients both with and without proteinuria.

The discovery of iron deposits in the mesangium of some patients suggests that the chronic anemia state also contributes to the mesangial lesions. The means by which the iron arrives in the mesangium and its relation to the glomerulosclerosis are not clear. The exact relationship between the genetic defect and the occurrence of the glomerular lesion is not known, and the small number of cases makes further study difficult.

Patient Presentation

Although sickle cell trait has been described as a potential cause of renal disease, the presence of renal lesions has mainly been restricted to autopsy studies. Thus, significant proteinuria or the nephrotic syndrome with hematuria is encountered only in sickle cell anemia. Few detailed studies of renal function have been performed, but they reveal an increase in glomerular filtration rate and renal plasma flow.

Histology

Light Microscopy

The glomeruli often appear to be distended with erythrocytes, some of which may be ab-

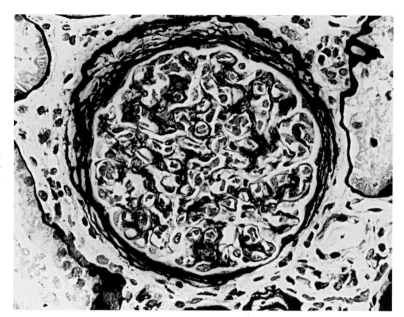

Figure 7–11. Sickle cell disease. There is segmental hypercellularity and sclerosis. The loops are distended with red blood cells. (H&E, ×250.)

normal in shape (Fig. 7–11). Some have described the glomeruli as large, but morphometric data do not exist. Deposits of iron may be revealed in glomerular and tubular cells by special stains.

Several varieties of glomerular disease have been reported, and they all share the features of mesangial sclerosis and/or hypercellularity (Fig. 7–11). The mesangium may be irregularly affected with areas of focal sclerosis. Hyalin is not detected. The glomeruli may be irregularly affected, with some being normal and some completely obsolescent (so-called global sclerosis).

The peripheral glomerular basement membranes often appear thick and wrinkled. When the glomerular basement membrane changes are marked and the mesangium is severely affected, the term *membranoproliferative glomerulonephritis* has been applied. However, the lesions are much more sclerotic than proliferative, thus the descriptor *glomerulosclerosis* seems more appropriate.

Patients with sickle cell disease may be affected by other renal diseases, but the hemoglobinopathy seems to add little to those processes.

Immunofluorescence Microscopy

There are no deposits of immune reactants due to the sickle cell disease.

Electron Microscopy

The mesangial matrix is focally increased in amount, and the glomerular basement membranes are irregularly thickened, duplicated, and wrinkled. Occasional intracellular membrane-bounded vesicles are seen to contain a granular electron-dense substance thought to represent iron-containing materials. The pedicels are irregularly effaced near areas of sclerosis.

Prognosis

Few long-term studies have been performed, but those available suggest that the prognosis in patients with glomerulosclerosis is one of slow, inexorable progression. However, this conclusion is far from established.

SELECTED READINGS

1. Buckalew VM Jr: The kidney in sickle cell disease. Kidney Int 11:11, 1978.
2. de Jong PE, Van Es LWS: Sickle cell nephropathy: New insights into its pathophysiology. Kidney Int 27:711, 1985.
3. Powars DR, Elliott-Mills DD, Chan L, et al: Chronic renal failure in sickle cell disease: Risk factors, clinical course, and mortality. Ann Intern Med 115:614, 1991.
4. Schlitt LE, Keitel HG: Renal manifestations of sickle cell disease: A review. Am J Med Sci 239:773, 1960.
5. Tejani A, Phadke K, Adamson O, et al: Renal lesions

in sickle cell nephropathy in children. Nephron 39:352, 1985.

GLOMERULOPATHY ASSOCIATED WITH FIBRONECTIN DEPOSITS

Six families have been described who have fibronectin deposits in their renal biopsy samples. The patients come to the attention of physicians at various ages but most commonly in adolescence. They have proteinuria, hematuria, and slowly decreasing renal function. Both sexes are affected, and the disease appears to have an autosomal dominant pattern of inheritance.

Light Microscopy

The glomeruli are enlarged, and there are extensive subendothelial and mesangial deposits. The glomeruli may have a lobular appearance, and the overall impression is that of membranoproliferative glomerulonephritis (MPGN) type I.

Immunofluorescence Microscopy

The major findings are the presence of large deposits of fibronectin in the mesangium in the subendothelial and mesangial regions. Laminin and types IV, III, and I collagen were not present in the deposits and did not appear in abnormal amounts or distribution. Immunoglobulins and complement components are not present in most biopsy specimens.

Electron Microscopy

Homogeneous granular deposits are present in the mesangium and subendothelial spaces. There is an admixture of fibrils in most cases, but their identification may often require considerable searching. The fibrils have a diameter of 14 to 16 nm. The mesangial matrix is not increased in amount, but the overall mesangial space is markedly enlarged by the deposits. The lamina densa appears normal.

Prognosis

Hypertension and progressive deterioration of renal function over a period of 10 to 15 years has been reported in the cohorts examined. In one transplanted patient, the deposits reappeared in the transplant, but three others appear to have normal renal function for up to 13 years after transplantation.

SELECTED READINGS

1. Buergin M, Hoffman E, Reutter FW, et al: Familial glomerulopathy with giant fibrillar deposits. Virchows Arch [A] 388:313, 1980.
2. Strom EH, Banfi G, Krapf R, et al: Glomerulopathy associated with predominant fibronectin deposits: A newly recognized hereditary disease. Kidney Int 48:163, 1995.
3. Tuttle SE, Sharma HM, Bay W, et al: A unique familial lobular glomerulopathy. Arch Pathol Lab Med 111:726, 1987.

8

GLOMERULAR DISEASES ASSOCIATED WITH SPECIFIC METABOLIC DISEASES

DIABETIC NEPHROPATHY (KIDNEY DISEASE OF DIABETES MELLITUS)

Diabetes mellitus is a common metabolic disorder characterized by a deficiency of insulin secretion or action resulting in hyperglycemia. Since the discovery of insulin and its availability as a therapeutic measure, the renal complications of diabetes have predominated as the chief causes of morbidity and mortality in this disease. They are the most common cause of end-stage renal disease (ESRD) in the United States and in many other developed countries. The incidence and prevalence of ESRD due to insulin-dependent diabetes mellitus (IDDM) vary among racial groups, being more common in whites than in blacks, Asian-Americans, Hispanics, or native Americans. The converse is true for end-stage renal disease due to non–insulin-dependent diabetes mellitus (NIDDM). It appears that the nephropathy is directly related to diabetes, since the rates appear to be directly related to the incidence and prevalence of IDDM or NIDDM in many different parts of the world.

The factor or factors that initiate the kidney disease in diabetics and that determine its subsequent rate of progression to end-stage kidney failure are unknown, but the levels of glycemia and hypertension play important roles. The role of close metabolic control in IDDM patients has been a subject of considerable controversy. Many previous studies had too few patients and often drew opposite conclusions about the effect of close metabolic control. Recently, the importance of keeping the blood glucose as close to normal as possible has been clearly documented in a prospective, long-term clinical trial of the effects of normal versus close control of glycemia with insulin, the Diabetes Control and Complications Study. Four points emerged in the group in whom blood glucose was strictly controlled, often with an insulin pump: (1) intensive therapy reduced the risk for development of sustained microalbuminuria (either at the level of 28 or 70 µg/min) or clinical albuminuria (more than 208 µg/min) by 51% and 67%, respectively; (2) there was an increase in the point prevalence of an elevated albumin excretion rate in both treatment groups, but the increase was more rapid and greater in magnitude in the conventional therapy group; (3) an analysis of the rate of change in the albumin excretion rate revealed that most of the benefits of intensive therapy were realized within the first year, and the long-term slopes of the intensive and conventional treatment groups did not differ from one another. It is important to note that many participants showed an increase in the albumin excretion rate—43% of the intensive treatment group and 45% of the conventional treatment group; and (4) a large group of patients in both treatment groups showed positive rates of progression: 43% in the intensive treatment group, and 45% in the conventional treatment group. Thus, despite the best possible control of glycemia, nearly one half of the diabetics showed progressive renal disease.

Renal disease is a major complication of diabetes, causing renal failure in approximately 20 to 30% of patients with IDDM. Diabetic nephropathy is also an important complication in NIDDM. Although its exact frequency has not been determined, most now consider that diabetic nephropathy is as common in NIDDM as in IDDM. It is responsible for about 10% of the deaths in NIDDM.

Several forms of renal disease may complicate diabetes. The most common is diabetic glomerulosclerosis, often associated with Kimmelstiel-Wilson nodules. The term *glomerulosclerosis* is used in the classic context, i.e., an overall increase in extracellular matrix in both the mesangial and peripheral basement membrane regions. Some would restrict this term to an increase in abnormal types of matrix, but we prefer the more general usage. Whether or not diabetic persons are more likely to develop renal infections than nondiabetics is currently controversial.

Pathogenesis

The first description of diabetic glomerulosclerosis was by Kimmelstiel and Wilson, in 1936. Since that time, many investigators have attempted to determine the pathogenesis of these alterations. Hyperglycemia and hypertension have both been implicated.

Recently many proteins have been shown to be nonenzymatically glycosylated in the presence of elevated glucose concentrations, at levels similar to the plasma levels found in diabetic patients. The presence of increased levels of glycosylated proteins is best measured by assessing the glycosylation of hemoglobin A1c. Glycosylation of glomerular basement membrane proteins might alter glomerular permeability, allowing the passage of high-molecular-weight substances such as albumin and immunoglobulins into the urine. Because less than one half of patients develop renal disease despite the fact that essentially all have plasma glucose levels high enough to result in nonenzymatic glycosylation, the contribution of this process to the development of nephropathy remains unclear. The clinical trials mentioned in the introduction clearly show that the control of blood sugar reduces the risk of an elevated albumin excretion rate, but reduction in risk is approximately 50%. Thus, it would appear that hyperglycemia, and perhaps an elevation in the glycosylation of proteins, is a

necessary but not sufficient stimulus. Hyperglycemia may play a role by its action on growth factors. In this regard, TGF-β1 has been most often incriminated.

Another factor that may play a role in the pathogenesis of diabetic nephropathy is systemic and microvascular hypertension. Both IDDM and NIDDM patients often have an increased glomerular filtration rate at the onset of their disease. Changes in glomerular hemodynamics, in particular elevations of intraglomerular pressure, lead to glomerulosclerosis in animals, but this outcome has not yet been clearly demonstrated in humans. The Pima Indians, a population in which nearly half the adult population develops NIDDM, has been studied biannually for over 30 years. A recent study shows that the glomerular filtration rate is elevated when glucose intolerance is first demonstrable, in all subjects. However, since nephropathy develops in somewhat less than one half, the role that increased glomerular perfusion might play in the pathogenesis of diabetic nephropathy in NIDDM patients remains somewhat unclear.

The direct role that an elevated blood pressure might play is also unclear. Nonetheless, the use of angiotensin-converting enzyme inhibitors has been shown to induce a 50% reduction in the rate at which renal disease progresses in IDDM patients. This effect appeared to be independent of the effect of these agents on systemic blood pressure, suggesting that there was some direct renoprotective effect.

There is considerable morphometric evidence of nephron hypertrophy in IDDM. Glomerular hypertrophy is present at early stages, including an increase in the mean volume of glomeruli and total mesangial volume. Mesangial expansion is inversely correlated with the total vascular area available as a filtering surface area. This may account, in part, for the decrease in renal function found in late nephropathy. In addition, hypertrophy may accentuate changes in intraglomerular pressure. There is controversy about whether glomerular hypertrophy is present in NIDDM nephropathy. Most studies of NIDDM nephropathy show that hypertrophy is not present.

The development of glomerulosclerosis in IDDM seems to depend on the overall duration of the disease, with the incidence of renal lesions continuing to increase for the first 20 years of diabetes mellitus. After that time, there is no further increase, likely because all those at risk, because of a genetic propensity, have developed nephropathy.

The development of sclerosing lesions is also related to the age of onset, especially in NIDDM. In this population, in which the onset of diabetes typically occurs at a late age, the renal lesions appear to develop at a much more accelerated rate. This accounts for the fact that the average time from the onset of diabetes to the appearance of renal dysfunction is estimated to be approximately 10 to 15 years—that is, nearly one decade shorter than in IDDM.

Patient Presentation

Renal insufficiency most often becomes evident 15 to 20 years after the onset of IDDM and after 10 to 15 years in NIDDM.

Early in the course of IDDM, the glomerular filtration rate may be elevated, renal size is usually increased, and there is exercise-induced or resting microalbuminuria (urinary albumin excretion of greater than 100 mg/day). The presence of microalbuminuria is the best predictor of the subsequent development of proteinuria and renal disease. The onset of diabetic nephropathy is suspected by the appearance of clinical proteinuria or microalbuminuria (urinary albumin excretion of greater than 300 mg/day). However, proteinuria is a marker of renal disease, not a predictor. In other words, significant renal disease may be present in the absence of proteinuria, and microalbuminuria may be present in the absence of renal disease. It is relatively unusual for patients to present with hypertension and proteinuria in the nephrotic range. The urinary sediment is inactive, although hematuria may be present.

Diabetic patients may also have nondiabetic renal disease, alone or in addition to diabetic glomerulosclerosis. This finding has been reported to occur in as many as one third of diabetic patients undergoing renal biopsy, especially in NIDDM patients. The presence of another renal disease should be suspected when the clinical and laboratory findings differ from those expected in a diabetic patient with nephropathy.

Histology

Patients with IDDM most often have a pure diabetic nephropathy lesion and have enlarged glomeruli. In contrast, in NIDDM the nephropathy is more likely to be the result of another type of glomerulopathy (one third of patients) or hypertension (one third of patients), or to be complicated by these two factors. The heterogeneity of the lesions in NIDDM patients may explain the controversy about the presence of glomerular hypertrophy in this group. The following description will consider only the classic diabetic nephropathy lesions, which do not appear to differ between biopsy material from NIDDM and IDDM patients.

Light Microscopy

The glomerular lesions are quite complex and consist of two general types: nodular and diffuse. It is not clear whether these two forms represent a continuum or whether they are two separate categories of renal disease. In any case, hypertrophy of the nephron is the earliest alteration in IDDM. The enlargement may not be obvious in the presence of renal insufficiency, although hypertrophy may still be evident in isolated, less affected glomeruli.

The characteristic glomerular alterations in the diffuse lesion include uniform thickening of glomerular basement membranes, hyalinosis, diffuse mesangial sclerosis, and an increased number of mesangial cells (Figs. 8–1, 8–2, 8–3). Hyalinosis, also referred to as an "exudative" lesion, represents an accumula-

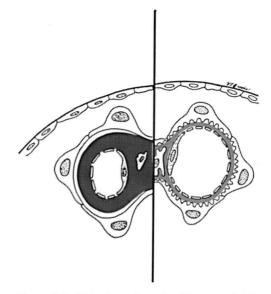

Figure 8–1. Diabetic nephropathy. Diagram of diffuse glomerular basement membrane thickening and mesangial sclerosis.

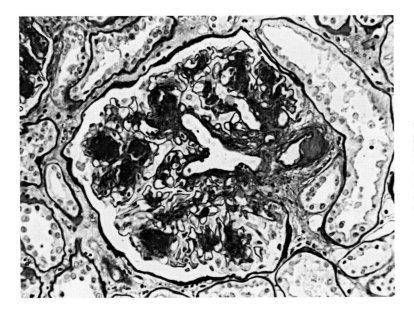

Figure 8–2. Diabetic nephropathy. There is diffuse, mild mesangial hypercellularity and mesangial sclerosis. The basement membranes of the glomerulus, Bowman's capsule, and the tubules are thickened. A large arteriolar hyalin deposit is noted at the hilum. (Periodic acid–Schiff, ×300.)

tion of plasma proteins in the subendothelial space (Fig. 8–4). The hyalin material may eventually fill the lumen. It stains bright pink with periodic acid–Schiff (PAS) stain and may contain lipid droplets or foam cells (see Figure 8–4). This is not a specific finding because similar lesions may be seen in many glomerular diseases. Their pathogenesis is not understood.

The lesion considered to be diagnostic of diabetic renal disease is the Kimmelstiel-Wilson nodule (Figs. 8–3, 8–5). These structures were first described by Kimmelstiel and Wilson in 1936. The nodules are roughly spherical in shape, appearing as large aggregates of extracellular matrix that contain a number of mesangial cells. It is to be noted that many cases lack K-W nodules and, in others they are pres-

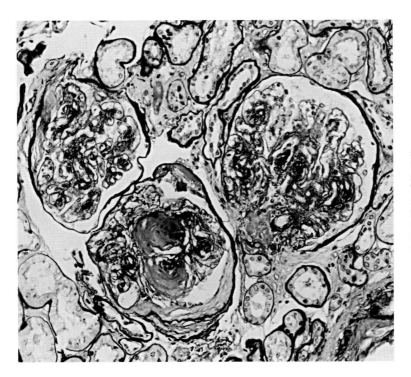

Figure 8–3. Diabetic nephropathy. In one glomerulus there are two large nodules. The two others show diffuse mesangial sclerosis. The Bowman's capsules of two glomeruli are thickened and multilaminated. There is moderate interstitial fibrosis and irregular tubular basement membrane thickening. (PAS, ×100.)

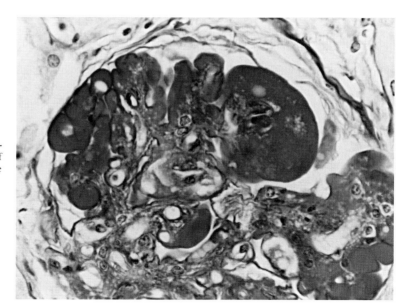

Figure 8–4. Diabetic nephropathy. Large, intraluminal masses of hyalin and capsular droplets are seen. (PAS, ×500.)

ent in a small number of the glomeruli. Among the cells in the nodules, some investigators have found an increased number of macrophages in the relatively early stages of the nodular lesions. The nodules are spread throughout the peripheral part of the glomeruli. They are seldom seen near the hilum or in the central part of the glomerulus. This pattern has been called a "horseshoe" distribution. They most commonly appear as mesangial nodules consisting of an increase in the amount of matrix. When mesangial cell proliferation is present, the cells are arranged

in a concentric pattern. The nodules stain with both PAS and silver stains. Some nodules have a distinctly laminated appearance, giving rise to the postulate that the nodules represent healed microaneurysms. The nodules in light- and heavy-chain systemic disease (see Chapter 9) can be distinguished from those in diabetes by the fact that they are quite uniform in size and distribution, whereas in diabetes they are irregular in size and have the characteristic horseshoe distribution.

The formation of enlarged peripheral vascular loops, the so-called microaneurysms (Figs.

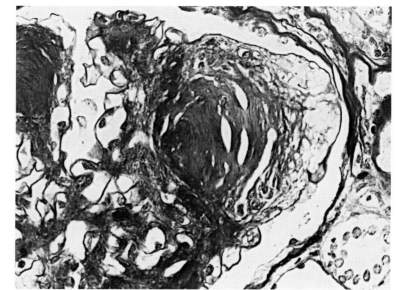

Figure 8–5. Diabetic nephropathy. The nodules have a laminated substructure. (PAS, ×500.)

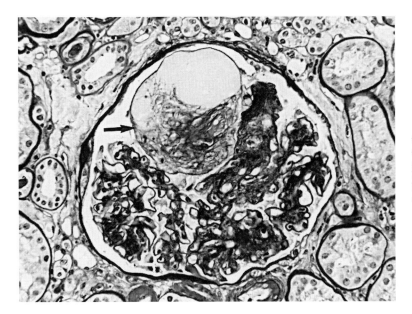

Figure 8–6. Diabetic nephropathy. There is an area of mesangiolysis *(arrow)*. Elsewhere the mesangial regions are expanded, and both the glomerular and tubular basement membranes are thickened. (PAS, ×300.)

8–6, 8–7), is thought to result from a process of mesangiolysis in which the areas of the mesangium that anchor and segregate the peripheral vascular loops are lost. This process may be seen in a variety of glomerular diseases. As these changes progress, glomerular obsolescence ensues. Although some glomeruli simply demonstrate wrinkling and collapse because of the vascular disease, other obsolescent glomeruli are normal or enlarged as a result of the sclerotic process. These large, obsolescent glomeruli may be a helpful feature in distinguishing the end-stage kidney caused by diabetes mellitus from that of other diseases in which there is progressive atrophy resulting in small, obsolescent glomeruli.

Another lesion described by Kimmelstiel and Wilson is the capsular drop or fibrin cap

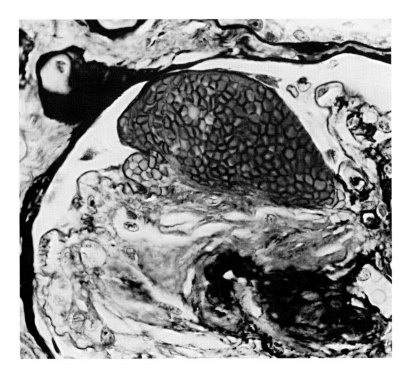

Figure 8–7. Diabetic nephropathy. A large aneurysm, filled with red blood cells, lies peripheral to the nodule. The glomerular loops are compressed to the periphery of these large sclerotic nodules. The glomerulus is markedly increased in overall size. (Periodic acid–silver methenamine, ×630.)

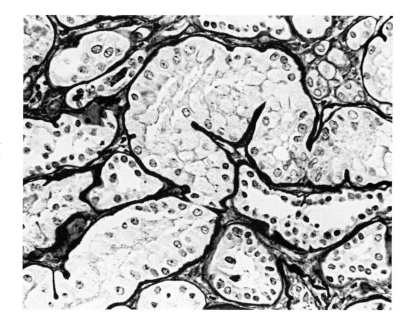

Figure 8–8. Diabetic nephropathy. The tubular basement membranes are thickened, especially in the areas of interstitial fibrosis. (Jones methenamine silver, ×300.)

(see Figure 8–4). It consists of a mass of hyalin lying within the substance of the basement membrane of Bowman's capsule. This lesion is not seen in other types of renal diseases and thus has the same specificity for diabetic glomerular disease as the Kimmelstiel-Wilson nodule.

The glomerular alterations are accompanied by tubular lesions with marked thickening of tubular basement membranes and interstitial fibrosis (Figs. 8–8, 8–9). The tubular basement membranes are often massively thickened, reduplicated, and considerably wrinkled. Tubular atrophy may also be con-

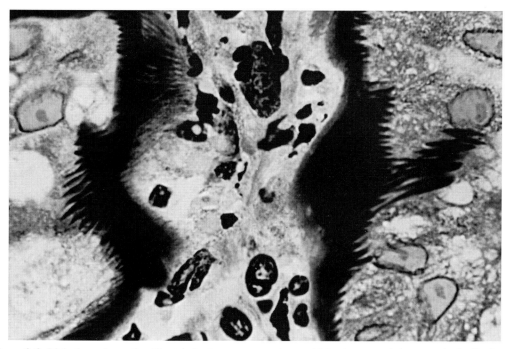

Figure 8–9. Diabetic nephropathy. The tubular basement membrane thickening extends between the basilar interdigitations of the epithelial cells, resulting in a comblike appearance. (PASM, ×1200.)

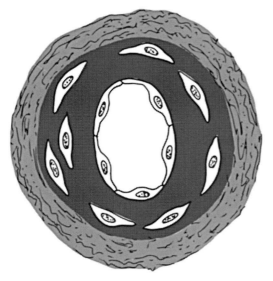

Figure 8–10. Diabetic nephropathy. Diagram of an artery with a diffuse increase in extracellular matrix of the wall.

spicuous. Inflammatory infiltrates are also to be found.

The juxtaglomerular apparatus has been noted to be very prominent in IDDM biopsy samples, and the changes are directly related to the duration of the diabetes. The initial finding is often hypercellularity. This is temporally followed by an increase in the amount of extracellular matrix. As the sclerosis increases, the cellularity is noted to decrease.

Because diabetes mellitus is often accompanied by severe atherosclerosis, large arteries often show advanced degrees of intimal thickening and internal elastic lamina reduplication.

Hyalin arteriosclerosis is identical in appearance to that which occurs in patients with hypertension (Figs. 8–10, 8–11, 8–12). However, in diabetic patients it may be present in both afferent and efferent arterioles, in which case it is considered to be pathognomonic for diabetes mellitus. In some cases, the efferent arterioles are more affected than the efferent arterioles. The deposits may invade the whole wall with concomitant cellular atrophy and reduction of the vascular lumina (Figs. 8–11, 8–12). Furthermore, the presence of numerous arterioles with hyalin deposits, particularly in young patients, should suggest the diagnosis of diabetes mellitus.

Immunofluorescence Microscopy

Antibodies to the type IV collagen α-chains reveal that the thickened peripheral basement membrane contains α-3 and α-4 type IV collagen, whereas the thickened mesangium does not, apparently being the site of other alpha-chains, including α-1 and α-2 type IV collagen chains. Late in the course, the mesangial regions also contain types I and VI collagen, especially in the nodular regions.

Diffuse linear staining of glomerular and tubular basement membranes with antibodies to IgG and albumin may be seen. Glomerular

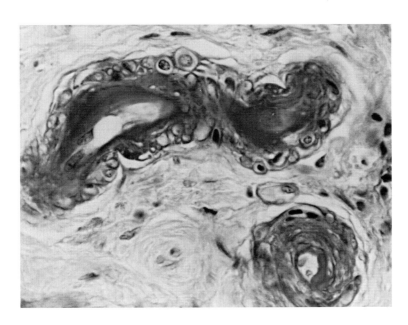

Figure 8–11. Diabetic nephropathy. The wall of one arteriole contains massive hyalin deposits. (PAS, ×400.)

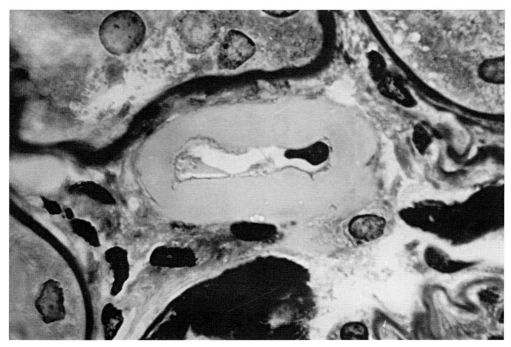

Figure 8–12. Diabetic nephropathy. The wall of this arteriole is completely replaced by a mass of hyalin material. (PASM, ×1200.)

and arteriolar deposits of hyalin contain IgM and C3 (Fig. 8–13).

Electron Microscopy

The earliest observable alteration is uniform thickening of the glomerular basement mem-branes, which may have a three- to fourfold increase, measuring as much as 1200 to 1500 nm (Fig. 8–14). The glomerular visceral epi-thelial cells may show an irregular effacement of the pedicels, although this is not a constant finding. Hyalin deposits, recognized by their subendothelial location and uniform density,

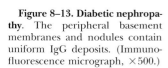

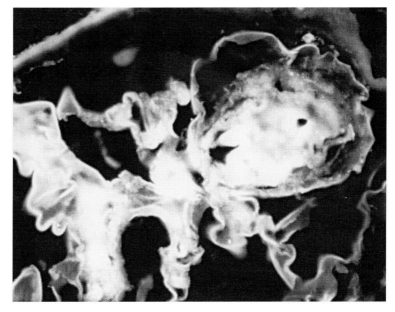

Figure 8–13. Diabetic nephropathy. The peripheral basement membranes and nodules contain uniform IgG deposits. (Immuno-fluorescence micrograph, ×500.)

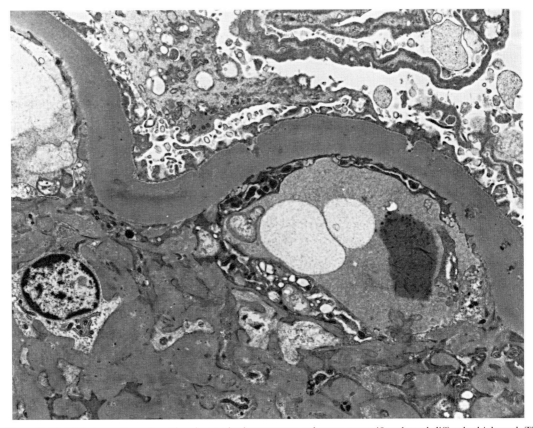

Figure 8–14. Diabetic nephropathy. The glomerular basement membranes are uniformly and diffusely thickened. The epithelial cells show microvillous transformation, and there is irregular and focal spreading of the pedicels. Marked mesangial sclerosis is also present. (Electron micrograph, ×3200.)

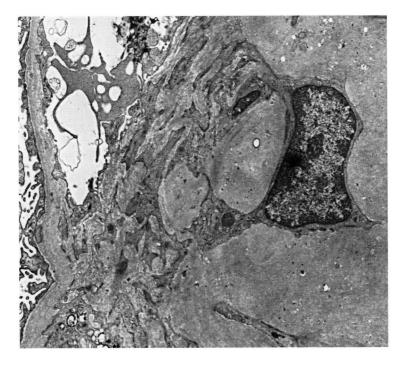

Figure 8–15. Diabetic nephropathy. The mesangial nodules consist of a large mass of homogeneous matrix. Note that the vascular spaces are relatively small. The peripheral glomerular basement membranes are irregularly thickened. (Electron micrograph, ×3000.)

may occasionally occur within the mesangium. Morphometry shows that the mesangial fraction, i.e., the volume of the whole glomerulus occupied by the mesangium, is one of the earliest changes in diabetic nephropathy. This change precedes overt glomerulosclerosis, and some have attributed a prognostic significance to this finding, believing that its presence marks those diabetics who will subsequently develop progressive renal disease. Lipids, either within macrophages or lying loose within the lesion, may also be seen. The mesangial matrix is increased in amount and may contain cell debris and microcalcifications (Fig. 8–15). Immune deposits are not identified unless another glomerular lesion is superimposed on the diabetic state. The tubular basement membranes are frequently markedly thickened and duplicated.

Prognosis

Once begun, diabetic nephropathy seems to follow an inexorably progressive course of deteriorating renal function, finally ending in renal failure requiring dialysis or kidney transplantation. As noted in the introduction, the rate of development of renal failure and death may be reduced by approximately 50% with the use of angiotensin-converting enzyme inhibitor therapy. Diabetic nephropathy has been reported to recur in transplanted kidneys at a more rapid rate than in native kidneys. Therefore, the course may be considerably shortened from the 15 to 20 years required for the evolution of the original disease. Without treatment with angiotensin-converting enzyme inhibitors and renal replacement therapy, the prognosis is grim, with mean survival time only 7 years after the onset of clinical proteinuria.

SELECTED READINGS

1. The DCCT Research Group: The effect of intensive treatment of diabetes on the development and progression of long-term complications in insulin-dependent diabetes mellitus. N Engl J Med 329:977, 1993.
2. Gambaro V, Mecca G, Remuzzi G, Bertani T: Heterogeneous nature of renal lesions in type II diabetes. J Am Soc Nephrol 3:1458, 1993.
3. Gundersen H, Osterby R: Glomerular size and structure in diabetes mellitus II. Late abnormalities. Diabetologia 13:43, 1977.
4. Kim Y, Kleppel MM, Butkowski R, et al: Differential expression of basement membrane collagen chains in diabetic nephropathy. Am J Pathol 138:413, 1991.
5. Kimmelstiel P, Wilson C: Intercapillary lesions in glomeruli of the kidney. Am J Pathol 12:83, 1936.
6. Krolewski AS, Warram JH, Christlieb AR, et al: The changing natural history of nephropathy in type I diabetes. Am J Med 78:785, 1985.
7. Kunzelman C, Pettitt D, Bennett P, et al: Incidence of nephropathy in type 2 diabetes mellitus. Am J Epidemiol 122:547, 1985.
8. Osterby R, Parving H-H, Hommel E, et al: Glomerular structure and function in diabetic nephropathy. Early to advanced stages. Diabetes 39:1057, 1990.
9. Paulsen EP, Burke BA, Vernier RL, et al: Juxtaglomerular body abnormalities in youth-onset diabetic subjects. Kidney Int 45:1132, 1994.
10. Salinas-Madrigal L, Pirani CL, Pollak VE: Glomerular and vascular "insudative" lesions of diabetic nephropathy. Electron microscopic observations. Am J Pathol 59:369, 1970.
11. Sandison A, Newbold KM, Howie AJ: Evidence for unique distribution of Kimmestiel-Wilson nodules in glomeruli. Diabetes 41:952, 1992.
12. Zatz R, Brenner BM: Pathogenesis of diabetic microangiopathy. Am J Med 80:443, 1986.

CYSTINOSIS

Cystinosis is a metabolic disorder, first described after the turn of the century. It is rare and is transmitted in an autosomal recessive manner. The gene frequency in the population is unknown, and the chromosomal localization has not been elucidated. The heterozygous carriers have no clinical symptoms but may be recognized by examination of the cystine content of their peripheral leukocytes.

There are three forms: nephropathic or infantile, intermediate or juvenile, and benign or adult. The nephropathic form is the most common and becomes manifest at birth by the presence of aminoaciduria. The juvenile form is much less common and appears after the age of 10 years, with renal failure developing in the second or third decades of life. The adult form is much milder and consists of mild elevations of cystine in various tissues, which do not lead to symptoms or signs.

The nephropathic form is associated with diffuse deposits of cystine in all organs. The deposits consist of large, intracellular accumulations of cystine crystals. The kidneys are affected early in life, and renal failure is a serious complication in this syndrome.

This stands in sharp contrast to cystinuria, in which the kidneys are the only site of increased cystine accumulation. In cystinuria, the principal defect is thought to be in the proximal tubule and is due to a defective amino acid transport process involving cystine, lysine, ornithine, and arginine. The result is that these amino acids are lost in the urine and can be found within the lumina of tubules. Cystine forms crystals and eventually renal calculi.

Pathogenesis

The defect in the juvenile form is due to a defect in carrier-mediated transport of cystine. The end result is the intracellular accumulation of cystine crystals. The entire tissue eventually becomes filled with cystine crystals within the cells. The crystals eventually reach the interstitium, where they excite an inflammatory reaction. The result is considerable distortion of the indigenous cell function, as well as of the surrounding interstitium. The eyes, kidneys, and skeleton have the most obvious lesions.

Patient Presentation

The first evidence of the infantile form may appear as polyuria and polydipsia within the first month of life. As a reflection of the proximal tubule lesions, the infants may have Fanconi's syndrome consisting of aminoaciduria, glycosuria, hyperphosphaturia, proximal renal tubular acidosis, and a concentrating defect. Affected infants develop this syndrome by approximately the sixth month of life. Thereafter, the maintenance of normal fluid and electrolyte balance, bone growth and maturation, and body growth become increasingly severe problems. Renal failure is first evident between 18 and 24 months. Renal function progressively declines and frequently reaches end stage by age 5 years, and essentially always within the first decade.

The only difference between those with the intermediate form and those with the infantile form is the rate of progression, with renal failure appearing in the mid to late teens.

Patients with benign cystinosis do not appear to have any symptoms. They are only recognized by the ophthalmologic findings.

Histology

Light Microscopy

The first renal lesions consist of the formation of lysosomal crystals in the epithelium of the glomeruli and the first part of the proximal convoluted tubule. The epithelium of this segment of the proximal tubule eventually atrophies, leading to the so-called swan neck lesion (see Figure 8–12). The visceral glomerular epithelial cells also have crystalline inclusions, and they may become multinucleated. As the disease progresses, the interstitium becomes more fibrotic, with the formation of interstitial infiltrates. Intracellular crystals with the typical rhomboid-shaped crystals are seen in many cells. Tubular atrophy, glomerular sclerosis, and nephron loss relentlessly progress. Note that the crystals are water soluble; therefore, visualization of crystals must be done in nonaqueous solvents.

Immunofluorescence Microscopy

There are no immune reactants in these biopsy specimens.

Electron Microscopy

The first lesions are those in the podocytes and the epithelium of the S1 segment of the proximal tubule. Needle-shaped crystals are found in membrane-bounded vesicles, within the first 6 months of life (Fig. 8–16). Thereafter, the podocytes may become multinucleated, and the epithelial cells of the S1 segment of the proximal tubule are replaced by a low-lying sheet of thinned cytoplasm. Tubular, glomerular, and interstitial extracellular matrix increase in concert, with mounting deposits of crystals in the kidney (Figs. 8–17, 8–18). The end result is complete nephron loss and renal atrophy.

Prognosis

An inexorable decline in renal function to end-stage renal failure by 10 years of age is the usual course in the infantile, or nephropathic, form. Those with the intermediate, or juvenile, form have the same course except that symptoms and organ failure develop in the second or third decade. The adult form is completely benign. Cysteamine has recently shown promise in preventing progression of the disease, but studies of this effect are not yet complete.

Renal transplantation has been used in many patients. The transplanted organs do not develop lysosomal deposits, but infiltrating re-

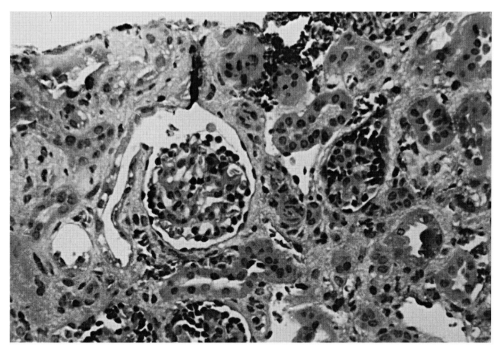

Figure 8–16. Cystinosis. The epithelium of the first portion of the proximal tubule is atrophied, resulting in the appearance of the classic "swan neck" lesion. The glomerular epithelial cells are prominent, consistent with the frequent appearance of multinucleated cells in this location by electron microscopy. (H&E, ×300.)

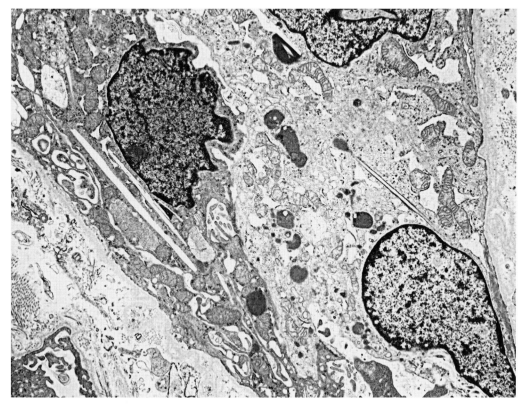

Figure 8–17. Cystinosis. Needle-shaped crystals are present in many proximal tubular epithelial cells in the region of the swan neck lesion. (Electron micrograph, ×2000.)

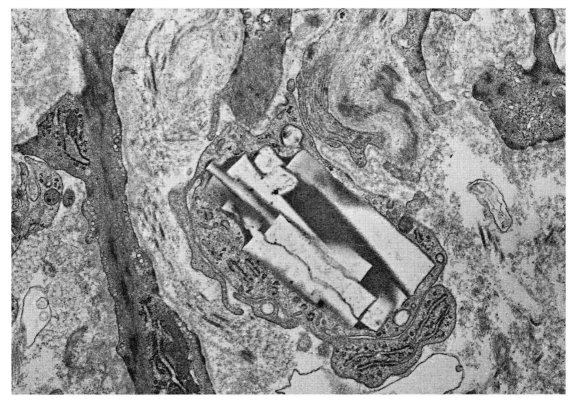

Figure 8–18. Cystinosis. Large, quadrangular crystals are present in the lysosomes of interstitial cells in the perivascular regions. (Electron micrograph, ×3000.)

cipient leukocytes contain cystine crystals, and the kidneys thus become secondarily affected.

SELECTED READINGS

1. Chesney RW: Etiology and pathogenesis of the Fanconi syndrome. Miner Electrolyte Metab 4:303, 1980.
2. Dent CE, Rose GA: Amino acid metabolism in cystinuria. Q J Med 20:205, 1951.
3. Ehrich JHH, Brodehl J, Byrd DI, et al: Renal transplantation with nephropathic cystinosis. Pediatr Nephrol 5:708, 1991.
4. Gahl EA, Schneider JA, Thoene JG, Chesney R: Course of nephropathic cystinosis after age 10 years. J Pediatr 109:605, 1986.
5. Hory B, Billerey C, Royer J, Hillier YS: Glomerular lesions in juvenile cystinoses: Report of 2 cases. Clin Nephrol 432:327, 1994.
6. Mahoney CP, Striker GE, Manning GB, et al: Renal transplantation for childhood cystinosis. N Engl J Med 283:397, 1970.
7. Schneider JA, Schulman JD: Progress in endocrinology and metabolism. Cystinosis: A review. Metabolism 26:817, 1977.
8. Schneider JA, Schulman JD: Cystinosis. In Stanbury JB, Wyngaarden JB (eds): The Metabolic Basis of Inherited Disease. New York, McGraw-Hill, 1983, pp 1844–1866.

GLYCOGENOSIS I

Glycogenosis I is characterized by the pathologic accumulation of glycogen in the kidneys, liver, and gastrointestinal tract. This disease, also known as type I glycogen storage disease or glycogenosis, is accompanied by renal dysfunction in most patients.

Pathogenesis

The disease is an autosomal recessive condition. Some patients lack glucose-6-phosphatase, and others are unable to transport glucose-6-phosphate. The result of either of these defects is the inability to transport glycogen out of the cell, resulting in its accumulation in large, intracellular vacuoles. The cause of the renal disease is the accumulation of glycogen in the various renal compartments. It is interesting that most patients have recently been shown to have significant hyperfiltration, which appears to be unrelated to hypertension, increased protein intake, or abnormal lipid levels.

Patient Presentation

Glycogenosis I is frequently manifest during childhood. The incidence of renal dysfunction in patients who survive past the age of 10 years is 70%. As in other lysosomal storage diseases, the first evidence of renal disease is the appearance of proteinuria. A few patients have the nephrotic syndrome as the presenting condition. Another small subset of patients have Fanconi's syndrome (i.e., glycosuria, aminoaciduria, and polyuria). The renal disease is one of continuous progressive loss of renal function leading to end stage.

Histology

Light Microscopy

The glomerular lesions are focal and segmental glomerulosclerosis with areas of hyalinosis. They are identical to those described in Chapter 4. These lesions progressively involve more glomeruli, and eventually they all are obsolescent.

The tubular epithelium contains large, intracellular, PAS-positive inclusions that become progressively larger.

The interstitium is initially increased in amount and contains an inflammatory cell infiltrate in the periglomerular regions. As the glomerular lesions progress, the interstitial changes become more generalized.

There are no lesions in the vasculature.

Immunofluorescence Microscopy

There are no deposits of immune reactants except for those nonspecifically trapped within sclerotic areas.

Electron Microscopy

No additional findings are revealed by electron microscopy. The mesangial matrix is irregularly increased in amount. No deposits are seen. The glomerular basement membranes may be wrinkled and thickened near the zones of marked mesangial sclerosis but are otherwise unremarkable. Large amounts of glycogen are present in the tubular epithelium, especially in the proximal tubules.

Prognosis

Most patients develop proteinuria during the second to third decade of life. Renal failure eventually ensues.

SELECTED READING

1. Chen Y, Coleman RA, Scheinman JI, et al: Renal disease in Type I glycogen storage disease. N Engl J Med 318:7, 1988.

FABRY'S DISEASE

Fabry's disease represents a deficiency of the enzyme alpha-galactosidase A. This enzyme is found in lysosomes throughout the body; therefore, the manifestations of the disease occur throughout each organ system. The result of the enzyme defect is the accumulation of the glycosphingolipid galactosylceramide. Fabry's disease is an X-linked disorder that is characteristically encountered in hemizygous males.

Pathogenesis

The X-linked defective gene is located on the long arm of the X chromosome, and it has been linked to Xq22. Although there are intra- and interfamilial variations, the gene has high penetrance. Hemizygous males are severely affected and have nearly a complete lack of the enzyme α-galactosidase A. This defect leads to accumulation of neutral glycosphingolipids with terminal α-galactosyl moieties. Curiously, females are less affected clinically. Identification of the exact biochemical defect makes it possible to diagnose the condition in utero and to identify carriers. The gene frequency has been estimated to be 1:40,000 in the United States. It is more frequently seen in whites, but it has been reported in essentially all racial groups.

Patient Presentation

The cutaneous manifestations were first recognized at the turn of the century, and the term *angiokeratoma corporis diffusum* was coined to describe the skin changes. Shortly thereafter, proteinuria and eye lesions (retinal, conjunctival, and corneal) were recognized.

The renal lesion has been the leading cause of morbidity and mortality in Fabry's disease. It most often presents as mild, asymptomatic proteinuria during early adulthood. The urine also contains oval fat bodies and occasionally a few red blood cells. Renal function gradually deteriorates during a period of 10 to 20 years, with most patients developing renal failure before the age of 50 years.

Signs and symptoms related to involvement of other organs, especially the autonomic nervous system, may develop at nearly the same time as those due to renal involvement.

Histology

Light Microscopy

The glomerular visceral epithelial cells are prominently and obviously affected. Their cytoplasm is filled with tiny, clear vacuoles that give the glomeruli a honeycomb appearance (Figs. 8–19, 8–20). The endothelial and mesangial cells are not as conspicuously affected; therefore, it may be difficult to appreciate cytoplasmic vacuoles in these cells by light microscopy.

The mesangial matrix and the peripheral glomerular basement membranes are not altered in the early stages of the disease. However, as the process evolves, diffuse mesangial sclerosis with segmental or complete sclerosis develops.

The tubules are much less affected, and the epithelial cell cytoplasm contains only a few inclusions for the most part (Fig. 8–19).

The blood vessels are often very involved, with the endothelium containing a large number of lysosomes. Hyalin deposits are commonly seen in the media as the lesion advances.

Immunofluorescence Microscopy

There are no deposits of immune reactants.

Electron Microscopy

Multiple lysosomal inclusions are seen in all renal cells (Fig. 8–21). The inclusions vary in size, shape, and intracellular location. They have been variously called myelin figures, lamellated structures, osmiophilic inclusions, zebra bodies, and so on. They may have an onion skin configuration with an array of concentric layers of electron-dense material, or the layers may consist of parallel arrays (Fig. 8–22). At high magnification, there are alternating layers of dense and light material with a periodicity ranging from 3.9 to 9.8 nm.

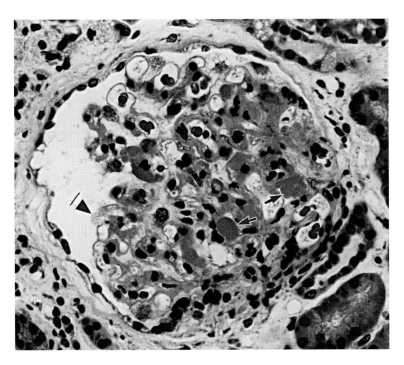

Figure 8–19. Fabry's disease. The podocytes are vacuolated *(arrowhead)*, giving the glomerulus a honeycomb appearance. There is a considerable amount of "hyalin" material *(arrows)* protruding into and compromising the vascular lumen. One of the tubules contains clear vacuoles (top left). (H&E, ×400.)

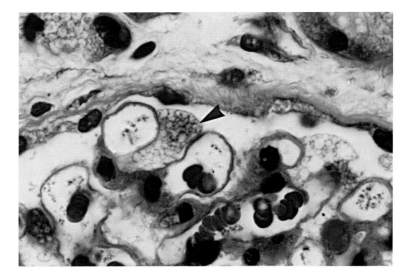

Figure 8–20. Fabry's disease. Higher magnification, showing the foamy nature of the podocyte cytoplasm *(arrowhead)*. Foam cells can also be seen in the interstitium. (H&E, ×1000.)

This configuration is considered characteristic of glycolipids.

The glomeruli are conspicuously involved, and all cells may contain large inclusions that may seriously distort the architecture of the glomerulus. Endothelial and mesangial cells contain fewer inclusions than do epithelial cells. The extracellular matrix is initially normal; however, as the disease progresses, the mesangial matrix increases in amount and the peripheral basement membranes become wrinkled and thickened.

Tubular cells also contain inclusions, in rough proportion to that appreciated by light microscopy. The distal tubules are more severely affected than the proximal tubules.

The interstitium may also contain cells filled with inclusions. The peritubular capillaries

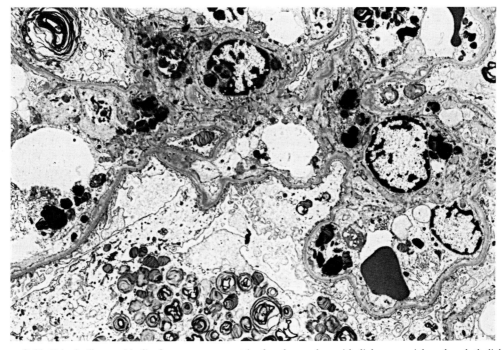

Figure 8–21. Fabry's disease. Myelin figures are present in the glomerular epithelial, mesangial, and endothelial cells. (Electron micrograph, ×2000.)

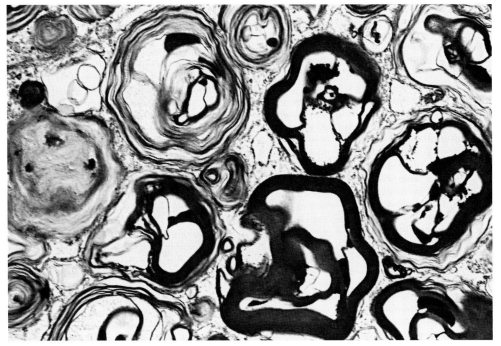

Figure 8–22. Fabry's disease. The structure of the myelin figures at high power is revealed to be multilaminated, containing rings of dark and light material. (Electron micrograph, ×10,000.)

and the arterial tree contain inclusions in the endothelial cells. The medial cells are less often involved.

Prognosis

The patients have been maintained by both dialysis and transplantation. Patients may have an increased incidence of serious infections, but this is not well established.

SELECTED READINGS

1. Brady TO, Gal AE, Bradley RM, et al: Enzymatic defect in Fabry's disease: Ceramidetrihexosidase deficiency. N Engl J Med 276:1163, 1965.
2. Desnick RJ, Bishop RJ: Fabry's disease: α-Galactosidase deficiency; Schindler disease: α-N-acetylgalactosaminidase deficiency. *In* Scriver CR, Beaudet DT, Sly WS, Valle D (eds): The Metabolic Basis of Inherited Disease. New York, McGraw-Hill, 1989, p 1751.
3. Donati DR, Novario R, Gastaldi L: Natural history and treatment of uremia secondary to Fabry's disease: European experience. Nephron 46:353, 1987.
4. Gubler MC, Lenoir G, Grunfeld JP, et al: Early renal changes in hemizygous and heterozygous patients with Fabry's disease. Kidney Int 13:223, 1978.
5. Kornreich R, Bishop DF, Desnick RJ: α-Galactosidase gene A rearrangements causing Fabry disease. J Biol Chem 265:9319, 1990.
6. Ramos EL: Recurrent disease in the renal allograft. J Am Soc Nephrol 2:109, 1991.

LECITHIN-CHOLESTEROL ACYLTRANSFERASE DEFICIENCY DISEASE

Deficiency of lecithin-cholesterol acyltransferase (LCAT) is a rare genetic disorder resulting in the accumulation of free cholesterol in many tissues. In the kidneys, these deposits are associated with progressive organ failure. The renal lesions are relatively characteristic, but the diagnosis is made on other grounds.

Pathogenesis

This deficiency was first described in Norway. It affects both sexes equally and has an autosomal recessive inheritance pattern. The relationship between the biochemical defect and the development of the renal lesions is unknown.

Patient Presentation

The characteristic features include corneal opacities, anemia, increased plasma levels of lipids and cholesterol, and undetectable levels of esterified cholesterol and LCAT. Proteinuria is a common early finding, signaling the presence of significant glomerular injury. The nephrotic syndrome may occur, but the most common finding is a progressive decline in renal function that becomes evident during the second decade of life. Hypertension occurs as a complicating factor in the renal disease and promotes the rapid loss of renal function.

Histology

Light Microscopy

The glomeruli are the principal site of the lesions in the initial phases of the disease. They have a honeycomb appearance because of the fact that the lipid accumulations are dissolved during the preparation of the tissue for sectioning (Fig. 8–23). Lipids are found in the cytoplasm of the endothelial and mesangial cells and in the glomerular basement membranes and the mesangial matrix. Silver stains reveal a mottling of the glomerular basement membranes and mesangial spaces. The vascular lumina contain large, eosinophilic coagula of material containing lipids. Later in the disease, progressive sclerosis occurs, leading to a pattern indistinguishable from the lesion of focal glomerulosclerosis. The glomeruli eventually become totally obsolescent as the sclerosis proceeds. Modest mesangial pro-

liferation has been reported. The lipids are only faintly oil-red-O-positive.

The distinction between LCAT deficiency and Fabry's disease at the light microscopic level can be based on the location of the lipid-laden lysosomes. In Fabry's disease, the visceral epithelial cells are prominently affected, whereas in LCAT deficiency, the endothelial and mesangial cells are most involved. The interstitium and the tubules also contain lipid, although the lesions are not so marked as those in the glomeruli and occur at a later time in the course of the disease.

The other condition that has similar histologic findings by light microscopy is Alagille's syndrome (a condition associated with congenital biliary atresia).

The arteries and arterioles show an atherosclerotic process that is much more advanced than would be expected for the age of the affected population.

Immunofluorescence Microscopy

The areas of focal glomerulosclerosis contain coarse, segmental deposits of IgM and C3. This pattern is consistent with that seen in other patients with focal glomerulosclerosis. Granular mesangial deposits of apolipoprotein B in the mesangium and along the glomerular basement membranes have been seen in these patients. Again, this is not a unique finding, because it has been described in membranous glomerulonephritis.

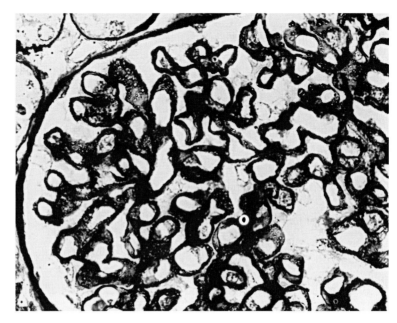

Figure 8–23. Lecithin-cholesterol acyltransferase (LCAT) deficiency. The glomerular endothelial and mesangial cells are extensively vacuolated. The glomerular basement membranes have a "honeycomb" appearance. (Jones methenamine silver, ×500.)

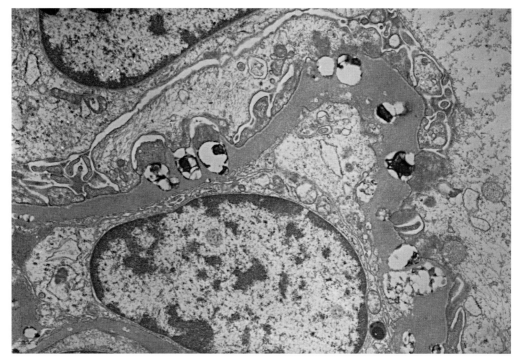

Figure 8–24. LCAT deficiency. The extensive sclerosis involving the mesangium and the peripheral glomerular basement membranes is evident. The multiple vacuoles within the mesangial cells and the glomerular basement membrane contain electron-dense and lucent lipid-laden material. (Electron micrograph, ×6000.)

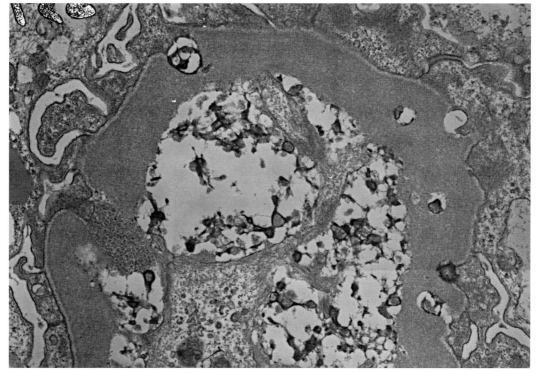

Figure 8–25. LCAT deficiency. Lipid-laden droplets lie within the substance of the glomerular basement membrane. (Electron micrograph, ×9000.)

Electron Microscopy

The glomerular basement membrane and mesangial matrix contain large lacunae filled with electron-dense, often lamellated material (Figs. 8–24, 8–25). Similar material is found in the lysosomes of endothelial and mesangial cells. It is also found in the subepithelial and subendothelial spaces. The mesangial matrix is increased in amount and contains many profiles of hyalin.

Foam cells may fill the glomerular vascular lumen. Like the endothelial and mesangial cells, the lysosomes of these cells contain electron-dense material that may have a lamellated material with a serpentine, cross-striated substructure. Comparable lesions are seen in patients with congenital biliary atresia (Alagille's disease).

The mesangial matrix and peripheral glomerular basement membranes increase in width and substance as the disease progresses.

Prognosis

The course of the renal disease is one of slow, inexorable deterioration in function to end stage. Unfortunately for these patients, the renal disease rapidly recurs in renal transplants.

SELECTED READINGS

1. Chevet D, Ramee MP, Thomas R, et al: Hereditary lecithin cholesterol acyltransferase deficiency: Report of a new family with two afflicted sisters. Kidney Int 10:185, 1976.
2. Gjone E, Norum KR: Familial serum cholesterol ester deficiency. Clinical study of a patient with a new syndrome. Acta Med Scand 183:107, 1968.
3. Magil A, Chase W, Frohlich J: Unusual renal biopsy findings in a patient with familial lecithin-cholesterol acyltransferase deficiency. Hum Pathol 13:283, 1982.
4. Norum KR, Gjone E: Familial plasma lecithin-cholesterol acyltransferase deficiency: Biochemical study of a new inborn error of metabolism. Scand J Clin Lab Invest 20:231, 1967.
5. Utermann G, Menzel HJ, Dieker P, et al: Lecithin-cholesterol-acyltransferase deficiency: Autosomal recessive transmission in a large kindred. Clin Genet 19:448, 1981.

LIPOPROTEIN GLOMERULOPATHY

This rare disease has been recently described in Japanese patients, with one case found in a Chinese man. It is characterized by prominent lipoprotein thrombi in glomeruli. First described in 1987, an additional eight cases have been described.

Pathogenesis

There are high serum levels of serum apolipoprotein E and hyperlipoproteinemia. The disease has essentially been restricted to Japanese patients, but it has recently been reported in a Chinese male. A familial pattern was documented in two families. The lipid profiles are similar to those of patients with type III hyperlipoproteinemia, with increased plasma levels of cholesterol and triglyceride and very-low-density lipoprotein enriched in apolipoprotein E. Patients with this syndrome differ from type III hyperlipoproteinemia patients in that they do not develop cutaneous or cardiovascular lesions. The defect is unknown, but it may be related to defective lipoprotein receptors.

Patient Presentation

The patients usually present with the nephrotic syndrome, hypertension, and hyperlipoproteinemia. The age at onset ranges from 8 to 46 years and the male-to-female ratio in the largest series was 5:2.

Histology

Light Microscopy

The glomeruli are enlarged and contain dilated vascular spaces filled with foamy, faintly eosinophilic material. The peripheral basement membranes are double contoured. The mesangial matrix is moderately increased. The tubules and interstitium are normal in appearance. The blood vessels are normal; specifically, there are no foam cells or eosinophilic thrombi in the lumina. The material in the glomerular vascular spaces stains positive for fat in frozen sections.

Immunofluorescence Microscopy

There is 0-trace staining for IgG, IgA, IgM, C3, C1q, and fibrin. There is bright staining of the lipid material in the vascular spaces for apo E and apo B, but not for apo A-I and apo A-II.

Electron Microscopy

The glomerular vascular loops are filled with finely vacuolated, concentrically layered material that sometimes contains platelets and fibrin strands. Similar material is seen in the subendothelial spaces in some vascular loops and occasionally in the mesangial spaces. The endothelial cells are swollen, and there is effacement of the epithelial cell pedicels. There is increased mesangial cellularity and extracellular matrix.

Prognosis

There is progressive deterioration of renal function, with end-stage renal disease being seen in the majority of patients.

SELECTED READINGS

1. Faraggiana T, Churg J: Renal lipidoses: A review. Hum Pathol 18:661, 1987.
2. Oikawa S, Suzuki N, Sakuma E, et al: Abnormal lipoprotein and alipoprotein pattern in lipoprotein glomerulopathy. Am J Kidney Dis 18:553, 1991.
3. Zhang P, Matalon R, Kaplan L, et al: Lipoprotein glomerulopathy: First report in a Chinese male. Am J Kidney Dis 24:942, 1994.

9

RENAL DISEASES ASSOCIATED WITH LYMPHOPLASMACYTIC DISORDERS

MULTIPLE MYELOMA

Multiple myeloma is characterized by the proliferation of a malignant clone of plasma cells that produces a monoclonal immuno-globulin and/or light chain (the so-called M component). There is a slight male predominance, and the incidence is 3:100,000 persons in the 50- to 70-year age group.

One of the most prominent features of this disease is the frequent occurrence of renal failure. This complication appears in almost 50% of the patients and is a frequent cause of mortality. The renal lesion is thought to be due to the renal toxicity of the free light chains, leading to damage or dysfunction of tubular epithelial cells.

Other diseases due to the M component, light-chain deposition disease and AL amyloid, will be considered separately, although they may occur in individuals with multiple myeloma.

Pathogenesis

Although patients with renal disease due to myeloma always excrete light chains, some patients with multiple myeloma who do not have renal disease excrete equally large or greater amounts of light chains. These data and information obtained in experimental animals injected with light-chain preparations suggest that light chains are not equally cytotoxic nor the only factor leading to the renal toxicity. Nonetheless, both clinical and laboratory data indicate that free monotypic light chains possess renal tubular cell cytotoxicity. One factor may relate to their size and individual or unique composition. These properties, combined with their high concentration, may enhance their propensity to precipitate in the hypertonic, acidic milieu of the distal tubules. The resultant casts (Bence Jones casts) may obstruct the lumina and magnify the cytotoxicity. There is evidence that Tamm-Horsfall protein favors cast formation.

The renal disease in multiple myeloma may be multifactorial (Table 9–1), and cast nephropathy is not the only cause of renal failure.

Patient Presentation

Weakness, fatigue, infection, and bone pain are the most common presenting features. These all are suggestive of a malignant process replacing the normal bone marrow. Many patients have albumin and light chains in the urine at the onset. Those who have overt renal

Table 9–1. Factors Contributing to Renal Failure in Myeloma

Hypercalcemia	Dehydration
Hyperuricemia	Contrast media
Pyelonephritis	

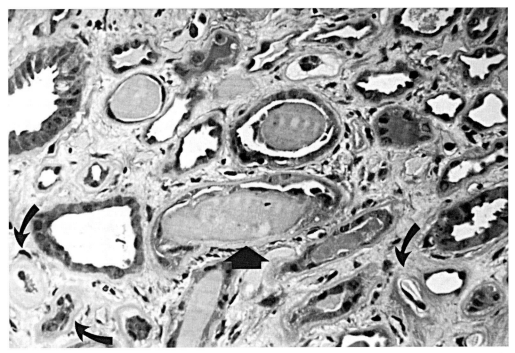

Figure 9–1. Myeloma. Most tubules contain casts similar to that noted in the center of this photomicrograph *(large arrow)*. The casts have a "hard" appearance—that is, the margins are sharp and the casts contain multiple lamellae. Many tubules are atrophied *(curved arrows)*. The interstitium is expanded and contains scattered inflammatory cells. (Hematoxylin and eosin [H&E], ×300.)

failure most often are found to have large amounts of circulating light chains, rather than intact immunoglobulins.

Histology

Light Microscopy

In contrast to the tubules, which have florid lesions, the glomeruli are usually completely normal. Glomerular lesions ranging from mild mesangial sclerosis to crescentic glomerulonephritis have been infrequently reported. These reports antedated the recognition of light-chain systemic disease as a disease entity.

The tubular lesion, light-chain cast nephropathy, consists of dilated and atrophied tubules whose lumina are filled with large and distinctive Bence Jones casts (Fig. 9–1). The casts are typical of myeloma and are characterized by an uneven size, a refractile and multilaminated appearance, and the presence of a surrounding cellular reaction that may consist of multinucleated cells (Fig. 9–2). The cellular response is composed of both tubular cells and infiltrating mononuclear cells. The casts

often appear hard and may show fracture lines. They are markedly eosinophilic, polychromatophilic, and periodic acid–Schiff (PAS) but not silver positive. They may also stain with thioflavine S and T. The periphery of the casts may be of a darker color than the center. The casts rarely exhibit the histochemical characteristics of amyloid, and when present, the "amyloid casts" are not associated with systemic amyloidosis.

Tubular epithelial cell changes are marked in the regions of the casts, the most common lesions being atrophy and/or degeneration. However, acute tubular lesions may also be found in the absence of myeloma casts. Elsewhere, the tubular cells contain lysosomes filled with proteins and other substances. The presence of crystals in the proximal tubular epithelial cells is considered characteristic of the existence of Fanconi's syndrome. The crystals are dark, elongated, PAS-positive, intracytoplasmic structures.

Interstitial changes parallel the tubular lesions in severity. Interstitial fibrosis is the predominant change in areas of tubular atrophy (Fig. 9–3). Infiltrates of malignant plasma cells are found in approximately 10% of patients.

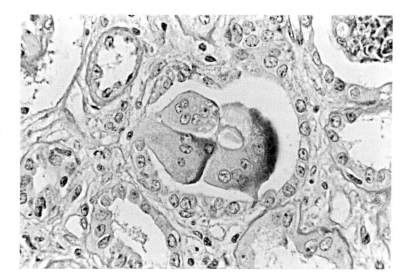

Figure 9–2. Myeloma. The characteristic tubular change is the presence of multinucleated epithelial cells surrounding the hard, waxy casts. (H&E, ×400.)

Calcium deposits, related to hypercalcemia, are generally found along tubular basement membranes, but they may also be seen within casts and areas of interstitial fibrosis by von Kossa's stains.

Acute inflammation may be present.

There are no vessel lesions apart from those expected within this age group of patients.

Immunofluorescence Microscopy

The glomeruli are negative, unless the patient has either amyloidosis or light-chain systemic disease.

The casts contain a single dominant light chain (kappa or lambda), Tamm-Horsfall protein, albumin, and occasionally fibrinogen (Fig. 9–4). The staining pattern is unusual in that the central regions may be translucent, and the periphery is brightly stained. Casts containing only the monoclonal M component are thought to be recently formed, whereas those with multiple other serum components are thought to be older, and the heterogeneity is assumed to arise from trapping materials during a period of time.

The tubular basement membranes and the tubular cell cytoplasm are generally free of immunoglobulins.

Electron Microscopy

There are few reports of the electron microscopic appearance of glomeruli in these biopsy

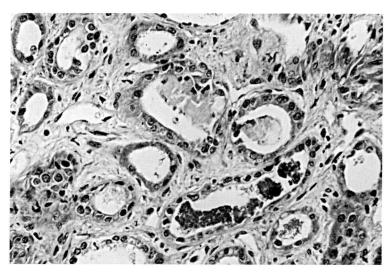

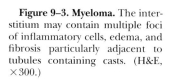

Figure 9–3. Myeloma. The interstitium may contain multiple foci of inflammatory cells, edema, and fibrosis particularly adjacent to tubules containing casts. (H&E, ×300.)

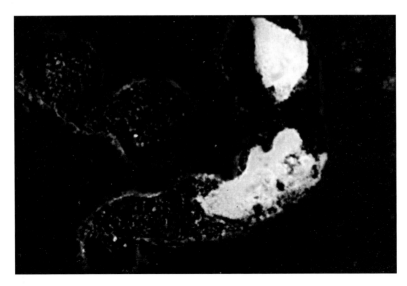

Figure 9–4. Myeloma. Immuno-fluorescence micrograph demonstrating IgA in myeloma casts. (×400.)

specimens, presumably because of the paucity of findings.

There is considerable heterogeneity in the appearance of the casts. Some contain fibrillar material, resembling Tamm-Horsfall protein, and others contain homogeneous, dense material. Others contain fibrils in parallel arrays, but they lack the periodicity characteristic of amyloid.

Crystals of various sizes are a frequent finding. They may have a fibrillar or lattice-like substructure, and the surrounding multinucleated giant cells may contain similar structures. The multinucleated giant cells resemble macrophages. The tubular cells may also contain crystals.

Prognosis

Renal disease is a frequent complication, occurring in 30% of patients at presentation and in almost 50% at some time in the course of the disease. Although acute renal failure may be present (seen in 10% of patients at presentation), the usual course is a slowly progressive decline in renal function. Amyloidosis is found at autopsy in 10% of all patients with multiple myeloma, but it may be encountered in as many as 40% of patients with IgD myeloma.

The presence of renal failure portends a poor prognosis. It was thought to be irreversible, but the development of new therapeutic strategies has altered this pessimistic viewpoint.

SELECTED READINGS

1. Cohen AH, Border WA: Myeloma kidney; An immuno-morphogenetic study of renal biopsies. Lab Invest 42:248, 1980.
2. Factor SM, Winn RM, Biempica L: The histiocytic origin of the multinucleated giant cells in myeloma kidney. Hum Pathol 9:114, 1978.
3. Levi DF, Williams RC, Lindstrom FD: Immunofluorescent studies of the myeloma kidney with special reference to light chain disease. Am J Med 44:922, 1968.
4. Meyrier A, Simon P, Mignon F, et al: Rapidly progressive ("crescentic") glomerulonephritis and monoclonal gammopathies. Nephron 38:156, 1984.
5. Pirani CL, Silva F, D'Agati V, et al: Renal lesions in plasma cell dyscrasias: Ultrastructural observations. Am J Kidney Dis 10:208, 1987.
6. Striker L, Preud'homme JL, d'Amico G, et al: Dysproteinemias and paraproteinemias. In Tisher C, Brenner B (eds): Renal Pathology. Philadelphia, JB Lippincott, 1996.

LIGHT-CHAIN AND HEAVY-CHAIN SYSTEMIC DISEASE

Among the renal consequences of the presence of the M component (abnormal immunoglobulins) is the development of light-chain systemic (or deposition) disease. This disease was recognized as a distinct clinical entity in 1976. More recently, a few cases of heavy-chain disease have also been described that share the same appearance, pathogenesis, and prognosis. Light-chain systemic disease shares several features with AL amyloidosis in that it is associated with an extracellular accumulation of immunoglobulin light chains. However, the deposits in light-chain systemic disease have a granular ultrastructure, rather than the fibril-lar/beta-pleated sheet structure, which is characteristic of amyloid. Therefore, the deposits in light-chain systemic disease do not have staining patterns similar to those of amyloid.

The majority of patients with light-chain systemic disease have a malignant lymphoplasmacytic proliferative lesion, usually myeloma. However, in one third of the patients, this association was not present.

Although the light-chain deposits may be widespread, the kidney is the most frequently involved organ, and renal involvement may dominate the clinical condition. The morphologic features of light-chain systemic disease may be recognized by light microscopy; however, the diagnosis can be made with certainty only by immunofluorescence microscopy, using antisera to kappa and lambda chains. In heavy-chain disease, antisera to gamma chains will provide the correct diagnosis.

It seems likely that this disease is the cause of a previously perplexing observation of a nodular sclerosing glomerular disease, resembling diabetic nephropathy, in patients who did not have diabetes mellitus. These reports antedated the commercial availability of antisera to light chains and did not include a long-term follow-up of the patients.

Pathogenesis

The inappropriate release of large quantities of immunoglobulin light or heavy chains, either as single entities or as a part of intact immunoglobulin molecules, leads to the development of immunoglobulin deposit systemic disease. It is likely that all patients with light-chain systemic disease have circulating light chains, although the plasma levels might be low or undetectable (possibly as a result of rapid tissue deposition, low levels of synthesis, or accelerated rates of degradation).

Attempts to study the pathogenesis of this disease have focused on two avenues, the cause of the deposition and the structure of the deposits. Some studies of the light chains have demonstrated a structural abnormality. This observation may explain, in part, both the tendency of these molecules to localize to basement membranes and the absence of the formation of beta-pleated sheets. The molecular or configurational alterations in light chains that favor deposition in basement membranes remain completely unknown.

The composition of the deposits in AL amyloid and light-chain systemic disease differ; those in the former contain mostly lambda light chains, whereas kappa chains predominate in light-chain systemic disease.

Although the emphasis has been on the differences between amyloidosis and light-chain systemic disease, both diseases may be found in the same patient, although this is certainly rare. It is not known whether the presence of both diseases in these patients reflects differences in processing the light chains at different body sites or whether they have two diseases.

Recently a small number of patients with heavy-chain disease have been reported. They have the same symptoms.

Patient Presentation

The patients are typically men over the age of 55 years (male:female ratio is 4:1). Nonselective proteinuria, often in the nephrotic range, and renal failure are frequent at presentation. A patient with multiple myeloma who has the nephrotic syndrome should be suspected of having either light-chain systemic disease or amyloidosis.

Although the renal disease dominates the presentation, deposits in the liver, heart, and brain may produce symptoms and signs.

The diagnosis rests on the histology at the immunofluorescence microscopic level, especially in patients who do not have overt myeloma.

Histology

Light Microscopy

The glomeruli are large, and the vascular spaces are markedly diminished in size. The characteristic glomerular lesions, mesangial nodules, are present in more than half the patients (Fig. 9–5). The nodules are eosinophilic and PAS positive and do not stain with silver impregnation techniques or Congo red. Almost all glomeruli contain nodules which, in contrast to those in diabetes mellitus, do not vary in size between and within glomeruli. The peripheral vascular lumina are always decreased in size. The glomerular basement membranes appear to be "stiff" and slightly thickened. The basement membranes of Bowman's capsule may be thickened and infil-

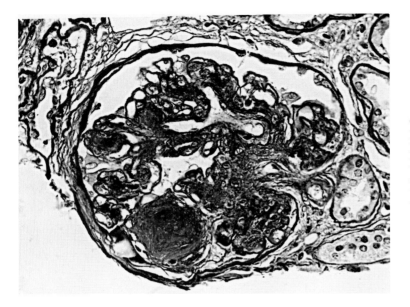

Figure 9–5. Light-chain systemic disease. The large nodules are periodic acid–Schiff (PAS) positive. They displace the glomerular lumen to the periphery. In contrast to the glomerular basement membranes in diabetes mellitus, those in LCSD are not markedly thickened. (PAS, ×400.)

trated with material similar in composition to the mesangial nodules.

Table 9–2 summarizes the differences between the glomerular nodules, basement membranes, and arterioles in diabetes mellitus and light-chain systemic disease.

The nodules are present in approximately 60% of the patients. In the other 40%, the glomerular changes vary from essentially no lesions to mild mesangial sclerosis and hypercellularity (Fig. 9–6) and/or glomerular basement membrane changes (rigidity, eosinophilia). The lesions must be differentiated from type 2 membranoproliferative glomerulonephritis. In the latter, the peripheral glomerular basement membrane ribbon-like deposits are brightly refractile, and the mesangial proliferation is more pronounced. This differentiation must be carried to the immunofluorescence microscopic level for an accurate interpretation.

Occasional patients with crescentic glomerulonephritis have been reported.

Deposits of a refractile, PAS-positive material in a ribbon-like distribution along the outer aspects of the tubular basement membranes are a uniform finding. The amount of deposits may vary, but they are predominantly found in the basement membranes of Henle's loops and distal and collecting tubules. The deposits thicken the basement membranes, resulting in the presence of homogeneous, wrinkle-free outlines that may be as thick as those in diabetic patients.

The epithelial cells are flattened and often atrophied. We found occasional Bence Jones casts in 8 of 17 patients. The casts were not numerous, and the surrounding cellular reaction was scanty in these patients, in contrast to those in multiple myeloma.

There are no specific interstitial lesions, although interstitial deposits similar to those found in basement membranes have been described.

The basement membranes in the vascular walls contain the same type of deposits as described previously.

Table 9–2. Comparison of the Lesions in Diabetes Mellitus and Light-Chain Systemic Disease

	Diabetes	Light-Chain Systemic Disease
Nodules		
Argyrophilia	Strongly positive	Negative
Size	Variable	Uniform
Number	Variable	Uniform
Glomerular basement membranes	Thickened, aneurysms	Mild thickening
Arterioles		
Efferent arteriolar sclerosis	Present	Absent
Capsular drops	Present	Absent

Immunofluorescence Microscopy

This diagnosis cannot be made without using antibodies to immunoglobulin light

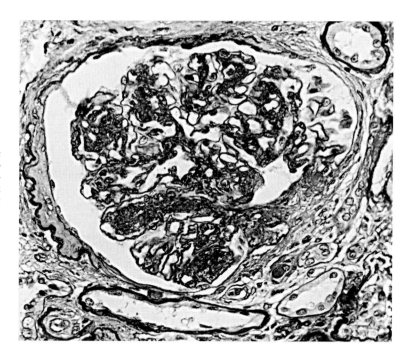

Figure 9–6. Light-chain systemic disease. There is marked mesangial sclerosis and diffuse thickening of the tubular basement membranes. (Periodic acid–silver methenamine [PASM], ×400.)

chains. Kappa chains are found in most patients, but lambda chains as the principal light chains have also been reported in a few cases. Heavy chains are of the gamma type.

The abnormal chains may be found both along the peripheral glomerular basement membranes and in the nodules (Fig. 9–7). Granular C3 deposits have also been found in the mesangium of such patients. Patients who do not have mesangial nodules may have no glomerular deposits.

In contrast, peritubular deposits are always present, and the diagnosis is most often made by the finding of brightly staining deposits in this region (Fig. 9–8). The distal parts of the nephron are most frequently involved, but the proximal tubular basement membranes may also be affected. The peritubular deposits stain more intensely than do those in the glomeruli. They are distributed in a smooth, linear pattern even if they appear to be sparse and irregular by PAS stains. The rare instances in which

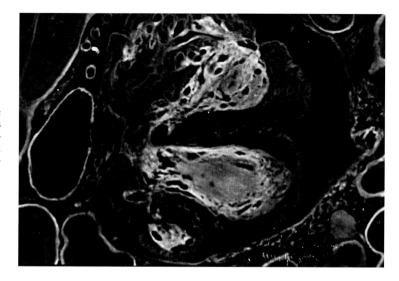

Figure 9–7. Light-chain systemic disease. The glomerular nodules and basement membranes are diffusely positive for kappa light chains. (Immunofluorescence micrograph, ×400.)

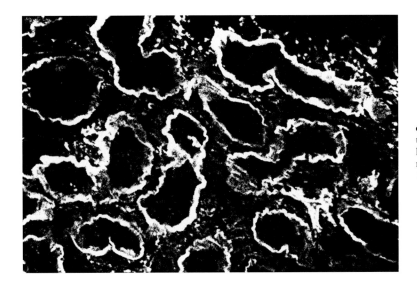

Figure 9–8. Light-chain systemic disease. There are diffuse, linear tubular basement membrane kappa light-chain deposits. (Immunofluorescence micrograph, ×250.)

monotypic heavy chains have been detected has been termed *monoclonal immunoglobulin deposition disease.*

Deposits may be present along capillary and arterial basement membranes.

Electron Microscopy

The glomerular lesions consist of deposits of a nonfibrillar, electron-dense material in both the mesangial nodules and along the glomerular basement membranes. The deposits are finely granular and generally lie in the lamina rara interna, separated from the endothelial cells by electron-dense, fluffy material (Fig. 9–9). They rarely are seen within the lamina densa, although the exact limits between the two elements may be difficult to discern. No substructure is seen in most biopsy samples, although fibrils of varying types have occasionally been reported. The cellular changes in the glomerulus consist of effacement of some pedicels, patchy mesangial encroachment on the vascular spaces, and an increase in the number of cells in the mesangium.

Like the immunofluorescence microscopic findings, the electron microscopic changes in the tubular compartment are diagnostic. Finely granular deposits are present along the interface of the tubular basement membranes and the interstitium of almost all tubules (Fig. 9–10). They may be quite large, but a substructure is not present. The adjacent tubular cells

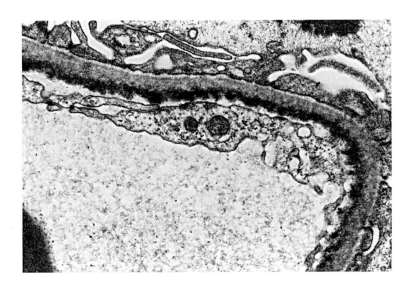

Figure 9–9. Light-chain systemic disease. Finely granular deposit along the inner aspects of the glomerular basement membranes. (Electron micrograph, ×10,000.)

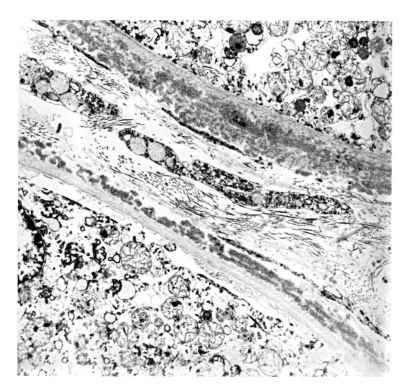

Figure 9–10. Light-chain systemic disease. Finely granular deposits at the interface of the tubular basement membranes and the interstitium. (Electron micrograph, ×10,000.)

contain many lysosomes and sometimes crystalline inclusions.

Prognosis

Although it has been speculated that some patients who have mild mesangial changes may subsequently develop more diffuse lesions and even nodular glomerulosclerosis, this transition has been documented only in rare patients. The rarity of light-chain systemic disease makes it difficult to determine its normal pattern of evolution. Some patients have a fulminant course with multiorgan involvement, whereas others may develop renal failure and remain quite well-managed on dialytic therapy without other sequelae. The survival appears to parallel that of patients with multiple myeloma with renal failure. Some patients with light-chain systemic disease do not manifest signs of multiple myeloma for months or even years.

Chemotherapy is indicated in patients in whom multiple myeloma is diagnosed. It is less well established whether the indications are the same in the absence of overt myeloma, although some patients are reported to have shown a decrease or stabilization of the amount of deposits after therapy.

SELECTED READINGS

1. Aucouturier P, Khamlichi AA, Touchard G, et al: Brief report: Heavy chain deposition disease. N Engl J Med 329:1389, 1993.
2. Gallo GR, Feiner HD, Katz LA, et al: Nodular glomerulopathy associated with nonamyloidotic kappa light chain deposits and excess immunoglobulin light chain synthesis. Am J Pathol 99:621, 1980.
3. Ganeval D, Mignon F, Preud'homme JL, et al: Visceral deposition of monoclonal light chains and immunoglobulins: A study of renal and immunopathologic abnormalities. *In* Grunfeld JP, Maxwell MH (eds): Advances in Nephrology. Chicago, Year Book Medical Publishers, 1982, pp 25–63.
4. Hofmann-Guilaine C, Nochy D, Jacquot C, et al: Association of light chain deposition disease (LCDD) and amyloidosis. One case. Pathol Res Pract 180:214, 1985.
5. Preud'homme JL, Aucouturier P, Touchard G, et al: Monoclonal immunoglobulin deposition (Randall type). Relationship with structural abnormalities of immunoglobulin disease. Kidney Int 46:965, 1994.
6. Preud'homme JL, Morel-Maroger L, Brouet JC, et al: Synthesis of abnormal immunoglobulins in lymphoplasmacytic disorders with visceral light chain deposition. Am J Med 69:703, 1980.
7. Randall RE, Williamson WC Jr, Mullinax F, et al: Manifestations of systemic light chain deposition. Am J Med 60:293, 1976.
8. Sanders PW, Herreras GA, Kirk KA, et al: Spectrum of glomerular and tubulointerstitial renal lesions associated with monotypical immunoglobulin light chain deposition. Lab Invest 64:527, 1991.
9. Silva FG, Meyrier A, Morel-Maroger L, et al: Proliferative glomerulonephropathy in multiple myeloma. J Pathol 130:229, 1980.

AMYLOIDOSIS

The term *amyloidosis* refers to accumulations of amorphous, homogeneous-appearing extracellular deposits with a fibrillar structure at the ultrastructural level and a characteristic beta-pleated sheet structure by x-ray diffraction. The beta-pleated sheet structure lends the characteristic tinctorial and optical properties evident by Congo red staining. More importantly, this configuration leads to the resistance of this material to proteolytic digestion. As a consequence, amyloid accumulates and progressively impairs the function of the kidneys. The amyloid substances are derived from various precursors, and it has been well established that the accumulation of amyloid fibrils may complicate the course of various diseases. The current classification system for amyloidosis is based on the protein composition of amyloid fibrils in different disease states (Table 9–3).

Other precursors of the amyloid fibrils have been described. These include beta$_2$-microglobulin, hormones, and albumin, but they have not been described in the kidneys.

Pathogenesis

Each of the several varieties of amyloidosis has a separate origin, biochemical composition of the fibrils, and pathogenesis. Despite this heterogeneity, the histologic and electron microscopic patterns are indistinguishable. The two species of amyloid (i.e., AA and AL) that affect the kidney may thus reflect many different diseases.

AL Amyloidosis

AL amyloid components are composed of light chains, usually lambda chains. Patients who have AL amyloidosis either have myeloma or synthesize monoclonal light chains and may be considered as having a plasma cell dyscrasia.

AL amyloidosis complicates the course of approximately 10% of cases of multiple myeloma. It is most frequent in patients with IgD myeloma, followed by those with light-chain myeloma. The other patients with AL amyloidosis are considered to have primary amyloidosis; nonetheless, they have a population of cells responsible for the production of monoclonal light chains. These data suggest that there may be a continuum between primary amyloidosis and myeloma.

AA Amyloidosis

Although the morphologic and ultrastructural characteristics are similar to those in patients with AL amyloidosis, the biochemical composition of the fibrils in AA amyloidosis is completely different. The origin of the deposits in AA amyloidosis is a large serum precursor, serum amyloid A protein. The serum levels of this protein are increased in chronic infectious and inflammatory diseases, in certain neoplasias, and in familial Mediterranean fever. Serum amyloid A protein is a high-density lipoprotein synthesized by the liver and belongs to the family of proteins collectively designated as acute phase reactants. The exact relationship between the elevated levels of serum amyloid A protein and the development of amyloidosis is not known, because only a small number of patients with the previously listed diseases develop amyloidosis. The amino acid structure of serum amyloid A protein varies among individuals, a fact that may partially explain the variability among patients with respect to the propensity to develop amyloidosis. It has also been suggested that individuals who develop amyloidosis have an impaired ability to degrade serum amyloid protein.

All amyloid deposits, without regard to the nature of the precursor protein, contain a glycoprotein that has been given the designation of the P component. This component repre-

Table 9–3. Classification of Amyloid Fibrils

Clinical Classification	Fibril Type	Precursor
Myeloma-associated	AL	Immunoglobulin light chain (mostly lambda)
Primary amyloidosis	AL	Immunoglobulin light chain (mostly lambda)
Secondary amyloidosis	AA	Serum amyloid A
Familial amyloidosis	AA	
Familial Mediterranean fever	AA	Serum amyloid A

sents as much as 10 to 15% of the total fibril weight. The P component is identical to a serum protein called serum amyloid P component. The biologic function of the P component is unknown, but it has also been identified in normal glomerular basement membranes.

Patient Presentation

Although the nature of the fibrils and the inciting causes of AA and AL amyloidosis are quite different among patients, the renal findings are comparable. Massive proteinuria, often associated with the nephrotic syndrome, is the most common presentation in these patients. Hematuria is most often absent, and hypertension is found only in advanced cases. Enlargement of the kidneys is a characteristic finding and reflects infiltration of the renal parenchyma by the amyloid deposits. Renal function, often normal at onset, rapidly deteriorates to end-stage renal failure in the majority of the patients. Glycosuria and other signs of tubular dysfunction are often found.

AA amyloidosis often affects younger patients. In developing countries, chronic infections such as tuberculosis and leprosy are the major underlying diseases. Elsewhere, the most commonly associated diseases include rheumatoid arthritis, chronic inflammatory diseases, and cancer. Adenocarcinoma of the kidney is the most common carcinoma associated with the development of AA amyloidosis. Drug abuse, especially when associated with subcutaneous injections, is also commonly as-

sociated with the development of AA amyloid. Finally, patients with familial amyloidosis and most of those with familial Mediterranean fever have deposits consisting of AA amyloid fibrils. AA amyloid is rarely found as an isolated event.

By contrast, AL amyloid occurs as part of a plasma cell dyscrasia or as a primary process. Ninety per cent of patients with AL amyloid have an M component in the plasma or the urine. There is a clear male predominance, and the median age at diagnosis is 65 years. AL amyloidosis is characterized by peripheral neuropathy, congestive heart failure, and hypotension. The median survival is very poor, being approximately 1 year.

Newer therapeutic avenues, including the use of colchicine in AA amyloid and melphalan in the AL type, may delay the deterioration of renal function. Thus it is useful to determine the composition of the deposits.

Histology

Light Microscopy

Amyloidosis is characterized by the extracellular deposition of an amorphous, weakly eosinophilic material (Figs. 9–11, 9–12). The deposits may be present in glomeruli, tubular basement membranes, interstitium, and blood vessels. Large deposits are easily recognizable, but small deposits, especially when localized to the mesangial areas, may easily be overlooked. Special attention should be paid to biopsies of nephrotic patients who are older than 50 years

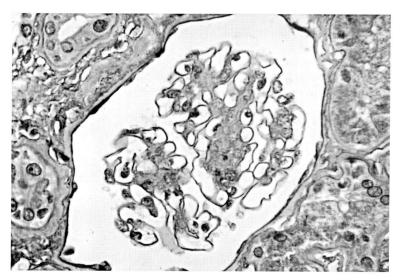

Figure 9–11. Amyloid. A glomerulus that contains irregular, nodular masses of homogeneous, poorly staining material. This material is largely restricted to the mesangium. (PASM, ×250.)

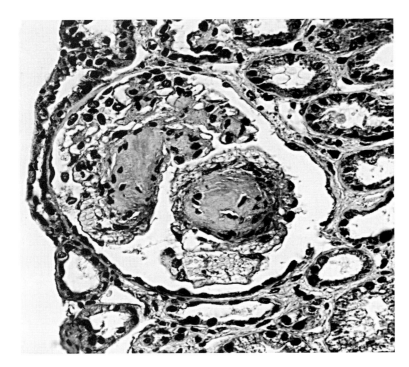

Figure 9–12. Amyloid. Large nodules displace the nuclei at the periphery. The center of the nodules is amorphous and has a "glassy" appearance. (Masson's trichrome, ×250.)

and who have minimal lesions or a mild increase in the mesangial extracellular matrix material. In these cases, thick sections (8 μm at a minimum) should be stained with Congo red or crystal violet. The metachromasia following crystal violet staining is most easily detectable on cryostat sections from frozen tissue.

The glomerular mesangium is invaded by the extracellular material that presents a smooth, homogeneous appearance. This histologic feature is often referred to as hyalin. Apart from the acidophilia, amyloid is very weakly stained pale pink by PAS and is not stained by silver impregnation (Fig. 9–11). As a rule, no glomerular cell proliferation is associated with the presence of amyloid deposits. There is a decrease in the number of nuclei. Congo red staining reveals orange to rose deposits that show a characteristic apple-green birefringence when examined with polarizing light. This staining pattern is considered the most reliable diagnostic criterion for the presence of amyloid fibrils at the light microscopic level. The deposits stain with thioflavine T by fluorescence microscopy, but this feature is not specific for amyloid fibrils. Although the amyloid deposits are initially localized to the mesangial spaces, as they increase in amount the peripheral glomerular basement membrane becomes progressively invaded. As an

end result, there is a gradual loss in the patency of the glomerular vascular loops. In some cases, the mesangial deposits form nodular masses, but, unlike those seen in diabetes, the nodules are acellular (Figs. 9–13, 9–14).

The differentiation of an advanced amyloidotic lesion from that of light-chain systemic deposit disease may be difficult, but the pale, glassy appearance of amyloid deposits and their typical Congo red fluorescence pattern allow their differentiation.

At early stages, the amyloid deposits are restricted to the vascular pole and exist in a segmental and focal distribution. As the peripheral vascular loops become involved, the deposits are first observed in the paramesangial and subendothelial regions. As the amount of deposit increases further, subepithelial deposits are observed, and these are often associated with conspicuous subepithelial glomerular basement membrane abnormalities consisting of irregular, spikelike projections (Fig. 9–14). These spikes are large and usually irregular in distribution. Thus they should not be confused with the subepithelial spikes present in membranous glomerulonephritis. Although an uncommon finding, multinucleated cells may be found surrounding the periphery of the amyloid deposits. The giant cells are assumed to be derived from macrophages. Cellular crescents occur in some

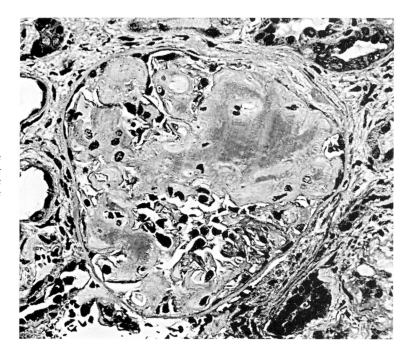

Figure 9–13. Amyloid. These large amyloid masses have replaced most of the tuft. Note the quasi-absence of cells within the amyloid material. (H&E, ×400.)

advanced cases, but in the great majority of cases the glomeruli are striking by their hypocellularity. Even when completely invaded by amyloid deposits and completely obsolescent, the glomeruli remain large. In late cases, the deposits may lose some of the histochemical properties of amyloid.

Tubular basement membranes often con-

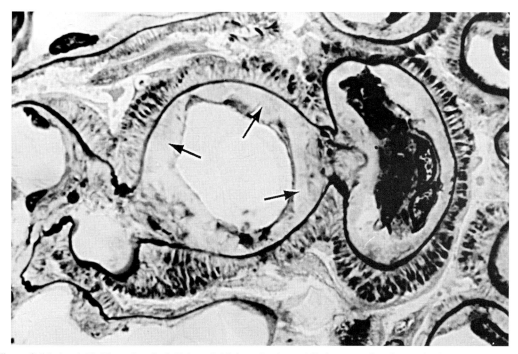

Figure 9–14. Amyloid. The subendothelial amyloid deposits *(arrows)* lie between the glomerular basement membrane and a thin layer of endothelial cytoplasm. The subepithelial amyloid deposits are interspersed with spikelike projections of basement membrane. (PASM, ×1200.)

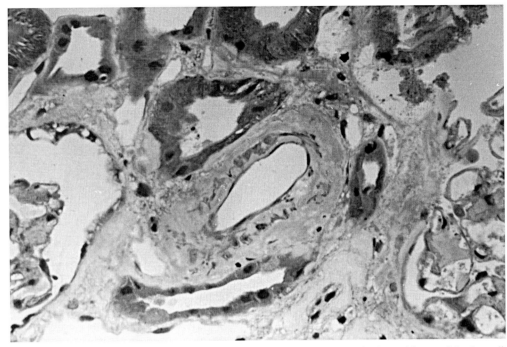

Figure 9–15. Amyloid. Homogeneous, eosinophilic amyloid deposits lie within the interstitium and in the wall of an artery. The arterial smooth muscle cells are displaced and distorted by the deposits. (H&E, ×600.)

tain amyloid deposits recognizable as ribbon-like, bright refractile deposits. These are preferentially localized to the basement membranes of distal tubules. Epithelial cells often show atrophy and/or hyalin droplets. Bence Jones casts have been described in patients with amyloidosis, but they are very rare in our experience. However, large, proteinaceous casts are extremely common and often numer-

ous. Amyloid plaques may be found in the interstitial tissue, especially in the medulla.

The interstitium often contains a disseminated lymphocytic and plasmacytic infiltrate in patients with advanced disease.

Amyloid deposits may be found in each of the layers of the arterial and arteriolar walls (Figs. 9–15, 9–16). As in other structures, the deposits are acellular and irregularly invade

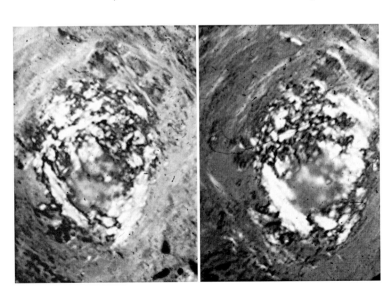

Figure 9–16. Amyloid. The amyloid deposits in this artery, stained with Congo red, show the characteristic apple-green birefringence with polarized light (compare left vs. right). (×300.)

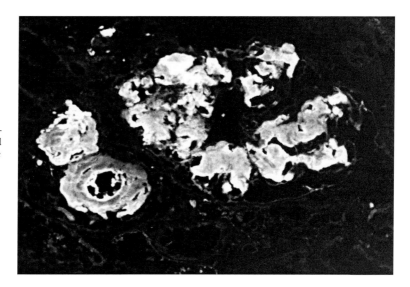

Figure 9–17. Amyloid. The glomeruli contain large AA amyloid deposits. (Immunofluorescence micrograph, ×250.)

and displace the native extracellular matrix. In patients with minimal or no proteinuria, the arteries may be the only element of the renal parenchyma containing amyloid deposits.

The differentiation between AL and AA amyloid at the light microscopic level may also be possible using the differential sensitivity of the fibrils to trypsin digestion. When slides are prestained with Congo red, they are subjected to trypsin digestion. Only AA amyloid deposits are degraded, when assessed for the loss of apple-green birefringence.

Immunofluorescence Microscopy

It has been suggested that amyloid deposits nonspecifically trap serum component, including immunoglobulins, complement, and fibrinogen. Although this may be true, it should not lead to confusion, because commercially available antibodies to AA allow the differentiation of amyloid and immunoglobulin deposits (Fig. 9–17).

Conversely, in AL amyloid the deposits react only with the antibody directed against the light chain (usually lambda chains) composing the fibrils (Fig. 9–18). Therefore, immunofluorescence microscopy may be used to categorize the type of amyloid in the deposits. In addition, immunoperoxidase methods yield good results on paraffin-fixed material. The deposits do not contain serum amyloid A protein.

Electron Microscopy

The use of electron microscopy is critical to confirm the presence of amyloid fibrils, especially when the deposits are small. The ultrastructural features allow one to make the diagnosis of amyloidosis, but they do not allow differentiation between the different types of fibril composition. Their identical morphologic appearance provides the best justification for their aggregation under the generic descriptor of amyloidosis.

Amyloid deposits consist of fibrils with a regular nonbranching topography (Fig. 9–19). They vary in width from 8 to 10 nm and in length from 330 nm to several micrometers. They exist in disorderly arrays, appearing like straws in a haystack. Individual fibrils may show a beaded substructure with a 5-nm periodicity. The deposits exist as compact aggregates when they are adjacent to the cell profiles but appear more loosely arranged when they are at a distance. The fibrils are extracellular and initially invade the mesangial matrix. The cell limits, which are often imprecise, may give the impression that the fibrils are present in the cytoplasm of mesangial cells. It seems likely that the cells in the mesangium, which have been said to contain fibrils in certain rare occasions, are bone marrow–derived macrophages. In the early stages, the extracellular matrix adjacent to the deposits remains normal, but with time it becomes distorted and increased in amount. The fibrils may extend through the basement membrane, and the basement membrane itself may undergo marked alteration. The endothelial cells lose their fenestrae in the areas adjacent to the deposits. When podocytes are in contact with the deposits, the pedicels may show spreading.

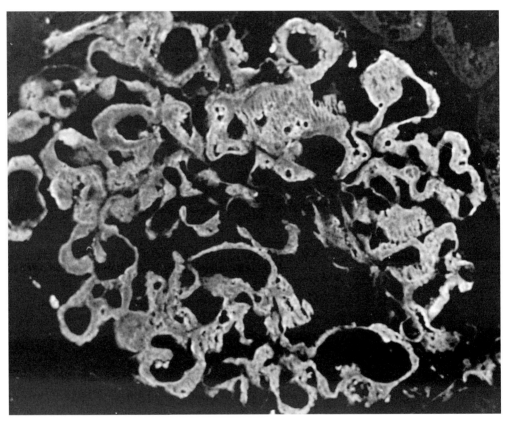

Figure 9–18. Amyloid. The subendothelial and mesangial deposits are strongly positive for lambda light chains. (Immunofluorescence micrograph, ×400.)

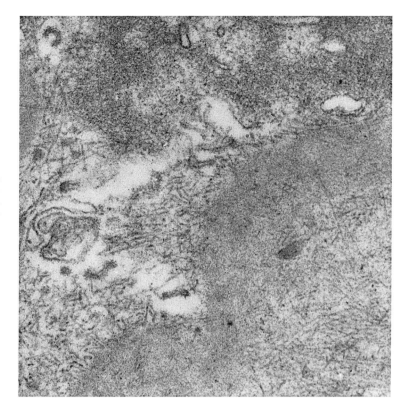

Figure 9–19. Amyloid. The appearance of amyloid fibrils is one of a tangled mass of straight, non-branched fibrils that are randomly arrayed. (Electron micrograph, ×10,000.)

In addition, a new layer of basement membrane may appear between the epithelial cells and the fibrils, appearing to encircle the cells.

Deposits in the other renal basement membranes share the same ultrastructural features as those in the glomeruli.

Prognosis

Patients who do not have treatable underlying causes of amyloidosis have a poor prognosis. Patients with AL amyloid, especially those with an overt myeloma, have a much more rapidly progressive course than those with AA amyloid. Patients with AA amyloid on the basis of an underlying chronic inflammatory or infectious process may show arrest or regression of the deposits if the underlying process has resolved.

New forms of therapy show promise for the resolution of deposits, but the evidence is too fragmentary to make generalizations at this point. One patient has been recently reported who had amyloid deposits secondary to chronic drug abuse, and in whom proteinuria markedly diminished when drug abuse was stopped. The amount of renal deposits did not appear to diminish, however.

Finally, amyloid deposits have been shown to recur in renal transplants if the underlying condition has not resolved before placement of the graft.

SELECTED READINGS

1. Crowley S, Feinfeld DA, Janis R: Resolution of nephrotic syndrome and lack of progression of heroin-associated renal amyloidosis. Am J Kidney Dis 13:333, 1989.
2. Dikman SH, Churg J, Kahn T: Morphologic and clinical correlates in renal amyloidosis. Hum Pathol 12:160, 1981.
3. Gallo GR, Feiner HD, Chuba JV, et al: Characterization of tissue amyloid by immunofluorescence microscopy. Clin Immunol Immunopathol 39:479, 1986.
4. Glenner GG: Amyloid deposits and amyloidosis. The beta-fibrilloses. N Engl J Med 302:1283, 1980.
5. Isobe T, Osserman EF: Patterns of amyloidosis and their association with plasma-cell dyscrasia, monoclonal immunoglobulins and Bence Jones proteins. N Engl J Med 290:473, 1974.
6. Nolting SF, Campbell WG: Subepithelial argyrophilic spicular structures in renal amyloidosis: An aid in diagnosis. Hum Pathol 12:724, 1981.
7. Wright JR, Calkins E, Humphrey RL: Potassium permanganate reaction in amyloidosis. Lab Invest 36:274, 1977.

MIXED CRYOGLOBULINEMIA

Glomerular lesions have been a recognized occurrence in mixed cryoglobulinemia for more than 20 years. It is still debated whether or not this disease is a plasma cell dyscrasia. *Cryoglobulin* is the generic term given to immunoglobulins that precipitate on cooling and resolubilize on warming. The cryoglobulins most often associated with renal disease contain at least two different immunoglobulins and are called mixed cryoglobulins.

A syndrome consisting of purpura, weakness, arthralgias, and (frequently) glomerular disease was first described in the mid-1960s. This multisystem involvement is characteristic of the acute disease.

Cryoglobulins may be present in a number of diseases, but the term *mixed essential cryoglobulinemia* is restricted to those patients with the characteristic clinical symptoms and cryoglobulins of the IgM anti-IgG type. There is disagreement about the number of patients who develop renal disease—between 20 and 55%—often several years after the onset.

The disease is common; several hundred cases have been reported. There are wide, unexplained variations in the incidence of the disease among different geographic regions. It occurs only in adults, and there is a slight female predominance. Many of the reported cases are in northern Italy.

Pathogenesis

The glomerular lesions are thought to be due to the localization of the immunoglobulin aggregates to the glomeruli. The complexes fix complement and serve as chemoattractants for macrophages. The released products from these processes have been implicated in the proliferation of resident glomerular cells. This simplistic explanation does not account for the fact that only one third of the patients with cryoglobulinemia develop a renal lesion, that the glomerular lesions are so diverse, and that there are wide regional and geographic variations.

It is clear that the presence of IgM rheumatoid factor is important in the development of the renal lesion. It is often an IgM kappa monoclonal response against polyclonal IgG. It is not known whether the IgG is directed against a single antigen or whether it is a collection of immunoglobulins. Some researchers have suggested that the IgG is directed against hepatitis C antigens, but this remains as a speculation.

The mechanism of the cryoprecipitation is also unknown, but the cryoglobulin concentration in the circulation does not appear to be directly related to the presence, absence, or intensity of the underlying glomerular lesion.

It has been suggested that the IgM is an anti-idiotypic anti-IgG antibody. The single most well-established fact is that when the cryoglobulins are composed of a single type of immunoglobulin (known as type II), they are not usually associated with a glomerular lesion.

Patient Presentation

The signs and symptoms vary widely. The acute nephritic syndrome is present in 20 to 30% of patients and is characterized by hematuria, heavy proteinuria, hypertension, and the sudden onset of renal failure. Renal involvement may not be obvious. Oliguric acute renal failure may occur in 5%.

The majority of patients with mixed cryoglobulinemia have a more indolent and protracted renal course, presenting with proteinuria, hypertension, and hematuria. The renal disease most often appears several years after the onset of the extrarenal systemic signs and symptoms. Most patients have depressed serum complement component levels.

Histology

Light Microscopy

The glomerular lesions in patients with cryoglobulinemia are diverse, and several patterns have been recognized:

- Diffuse proliferative and exudative glomerulonephritis
- Membranoproliferative glomerulonephritis
- Focal and segmental glomerulonephritis

Any of these histologic patterns may be associated with an acute small vessel vasculitis. Although rare, this association contributes to the diagnosis of the lesion.

Exudative Glomerulonephritis. This is the characteristic lesion of the glomerulonephritis of cryoglobulinemia. The glomeruli are large, with diffuse, marked intraglomerular hypercellularity (Fig. 9–20). The intravascular cells are

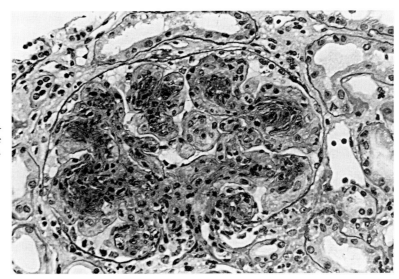

Figure 9–20. Mixed cryoglobulinemia. There is marked, diffuse intraglomerular hypercellularity. (Masson's trichrome, ×400.)

mainly macrophages, which can be recognized by a nonspecific esterase stain. Their clear cytoplasm is also useful to differentiate them from resident glomerular cells. Neutrophils are present in small numbers. The vascular loops are distended, but the glomerular basement membranes are not thickened.

The lumina may be almost obliterated by the infiltrating macrophages, proliferating resident glomerular cells, and deposition of an eosinophilic, amorphous proteinaceous mass that is often called a "thrombus." This material represents local precipitates of cryoglobulins in the vascular spaces (Fig. 9–21). There may be multiple profiles of this material within a single glomerulus, particularly if there is an associated nephritic syndrome. The presence of this material in combination with a proliferative and exudative glomerulonephritis is very suggestive of mixed cryoglobulinemia. These thrombi are not always plentiful and may be absent if the biopsy is performed at a time that the disease is relatively quiescent.

Membranoproliferative Glomerulonephritis. This is the lesion most frequently found in patients with chronic renal involvement. There is diffuse mesangial cell proliferation and infiltration with macrophages. Neutrophils are uncommon. The peripheral glomerular basement membranes are extensively dupli-

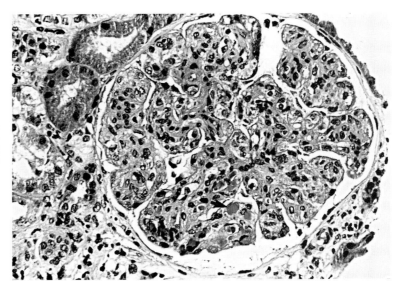

Figure 9–21. Mixed cryoglobulinemia. Multiple rounded, pale-staining "hyalin thrombi" *(arrow)* are found within the glomerular lumen. (H&E, ×300.)

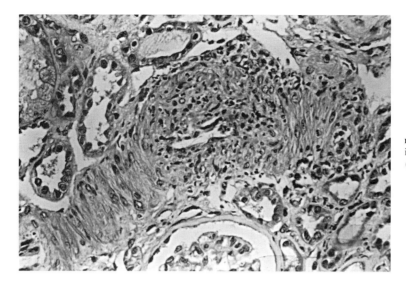

Figure 9–22. Mixed cryoglobulinemia. The arterial wall is locally infiltrated with inflammatory cells. (Masson's trichrome, ×250.)

cated, and there is diffuse mesangial sclerosis. In contrast to the acute glomerulonephritis described earlier, there are few luminal thrombi at this stage. Crescents may be seen, but they are not present in a large number of glomeruli.

A lobular pattern may be seen after treatment in patients with long-standing disease. In these instances, the macrophage infiltrate is inconspicuous, and the mesangial nodules are large and strongly PAS positive.

Focal and Segmental Proliferative Glomerulonephritis. The mesangial proliferation is fo-cal, and there often is a mixture of cellular and fibroepithelial crescents.

The tubules and interstitium do not have specific abnormalities; rather they reflect those in the glomerular compartment.

No matter what type of glomerular lesion exists, a small vessel vasculitis is quite common. This is one of the few conditions in which a small vessel vasculitis coexists with a proliferative and exudative glomerulonephritis. The lesions affect either the interlobular arteries or the afferent arteries. They vary from an

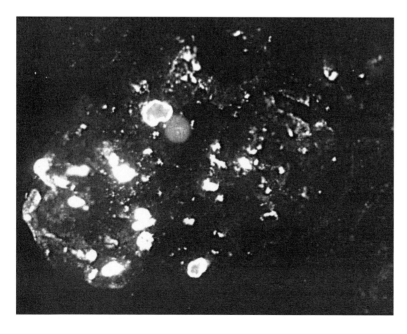

Figure 9–23. Mixed cryoglobulinemia. The hyalin thrombi contain IgM. (Immunofluorescence micrograph, ×400.)

acute necrotizing arteritis involving the whole arterial wall, including the intima and media, to various degrees of perivascular inflammatory infiltrate (Fig. 9–22). Occlusion of the small arterioles by material similar to that found within glomeruli may also occur. In our experience, the most common vascular lesion is an abundant, periadventitial infiltrate. The interlobular arteries are frequently affected. The lesions are often quite focal, so multiple sections should be obtained in the search for these lesions.

Immunofluorescence Microscopy

The glomerular deposits have the same composition as the circulating cryoglobulins. Thus deposits of IgG and IgM are present in many locations of the glomeruli. The large, intravascular thrombi contain IgG and IgM as well as complement components (Fig. 9–23). These large, intraluminal aggregates may be the only deposits found in patients with acute cryoglobulinemic glomerulonephritis, but diffuse granular deposits may also be present.

IgG, IgM, C1q, C4, and C3 are found in a peripheral glomerular basement membrane distribution in patients with membranoproliferative glomerulonephritis.

The deposits in patients with the focal lesions seen by light microscopy have the same types of immunoglobulins as in acute glomerulonephritis. However, in contrast to the focality of the lesions by light microscopy, diffuse, granular mesangial deposits are seen by immunofluorescence microscopy.

As might be expected, in patients with IgA cryoglobulinemia the glomerular deposits contain IgA.

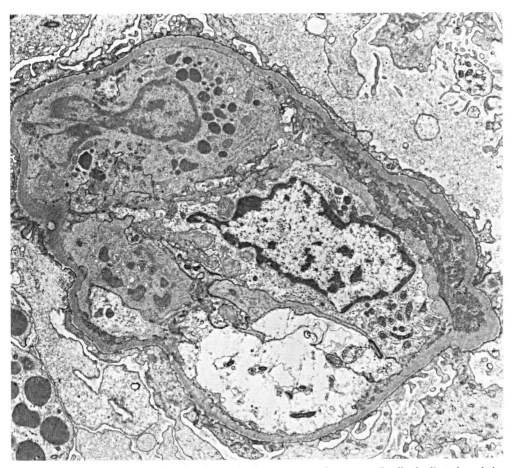

Figure 9–24. Mixed cryoglobulinemia. The glomerular basement membranes are focally duplicated, and there are subendothelial deposits. These changes, along with the infiltrate of monocytes, lead to occlusion of the glomerular loops. (×4230.) (Courtesy of Dr. G. D'Amico and the Department of Pathology, San Carlo Hospital, Milan, Italy.)

Electron Microscopy

The similarity between the substructure of the glomerular aggregates in the luminal thrombi and that of circulating cryoglobulin precipitates has been noted by many investigators. Thus, the diagnosis of cryoglobulinemia can be made by the finding of deposits with this characteristic fibrillar substructure containing annular or cylindric structures with spokes. The curved cylinders are 250 nm in width and are arranged in parallel arrays. They may show parallel cross striations. The fibrillar material is often surrounded by amorphous osmiophilic extracellular material. The deposits that represent the cryoglobulin precipitates in the glomeruli are the most characteristic finding in this glomerulonephritis.

A large number of macrophages are seen within the glomerulus, particularly in the vicinity of the fibrillar material (Fig. 9–24).

Prognosis

The lesions in the patients with acute glomerulonephritis are said to resolve without sequelae. Although probably true, this conclusion is based on the study of only a few patients. In some patients, the deposits disappear but the mesangial proliferation persists and mesangial sclerosis develops. Persistence of the glomerular disease is usually associated with the findings of either focal and segmental or membranoproliferative glomerulonephritis.

Recurrent episodes of acute nephritis have been documented. The exact course and renal prognosis are not clear from either the literature or the personal experience of those who have seen many such patients. It is most likely true that no more than 10 to 20% of the patients with mixed cryoglobulinemia develop end-stage renal disease.

Many immunosuppressive and antiviral regimens have been promulgated, but the small number of patients, coupled with the wide variety of renal manifestations, has not allowed the development of meaningful broad generalizations about therapy.

SELECTED READINGS

1. D'Amico G, Fornasieri A: Cryoglobulinemic glomerulonephritis: A membranoproliferative glomerulonephritis induced by hepatitis C virus. In-depth review. Am J Kidney Dis 25:361, 1995.
2. Feiner H, Gallo G: Ultrastructure in glomerulonephritis associated with cryoglobulinemia. Am J Pathol 88:145, 1977.
3. Ferrario F, Castiglione A, Colasanti G, et al: The detection of monocytes in human glomerulonephritis. Kidney Int 28:513, 1985.
4. Ferri C, Greaco F, Longobardo G: Antibodies to hepatitis C virus in patients with mixed cryoglobulinemia. Arthritis Rheum 34:1606, 1991.
5. Morel-Maroger L, Verroust P: Glomerular lesions in dysproteinemias. Kidney Int 5:249, 1974.
6. Sinico RA, Winearls CG, Sabadini E, et al: Identification of glomerular immune deposits in cryoglobulinemic glomerulonephritis. Kidney Int 34:109, 1988.
7. Tarantino A, Mariarosaria C, Giovanni B, et al: Long-term predictors of survival in essential mixed cryoglobulinemic glomerulonephritis. Kidney Int 47:618, 1995.
8. Verroust P, Mery JP, Morel-Maroger L, et al: Glomerular lesions in monoclonal gammopathies and mixed essential cryoglobulinemias. Adv Nephrol 1:161, 1971.

MONOCLONAL GAMMOPATHY

Monoclonal gammopathy, the presence of a peak of an electrophoretically homogeneous immunoglobulin, may occur in individuals without myeloma or Waldenström's macroglobulinemia. Other terms have been used to define this benign condition: *benign, atypical, idiopathic paraproteinemia,* and monoclonal gammopathy of undetermined significance (MGUS). This anomaly appears to be associated with glomerular disease with an increased frequency.

Pathogenesis and Patient Presentation

The pathogenesis of the glomerular lesions in this syndrome is unknown. Monoclonal gammopathy most commonly affects adults over the age of 50 years. A monoclonal cryoglobulin has been reported in several patients.

Histology

Light Microscopy

In most of the cases there is some degree of endocapillary glomerular proliferation. The proliferation may be diffuse or focal and segmental. Infiltration of the glomeruli by macrophages has been reported in patients with the acute nephritic syndrome.

Patients who also have cryoglobulinemia may show glomerular lesions resembling those with mixed cryoglobulinemia—namely, intraluminal deposits, macrophages in the glomerular loops, and occasionally membranoproliferative glomerulonephritis. Membranous glomerulonephritis and minimal change disease have also been described.

Immunofluorescence Microscopy

No clear-cut pattern has emerged from the various case reports of this syndrome. A relationship between the circulating pathologic immunoglobulin and the glomerular deposits can be confirmed only when they have the same composition. This has been the case in a few patients who had an IgG monoclonal gammopathy and cryoprecipitates in the glomeruli containing IgG (type I cryoglobulins).

Electron Microscopy

The absence of large series and the lack of documented cases make it difficult to describe the renal lesions accurately. Intracellular crystals and fibrillar deposits have been reported in a few patients with diffuse proliferative glomerular lesions. The fibrils form parallel bundles, are most frequently found in patients with cryoglobulinemia, have a width of 20 to 40 nm, and lack the periodicity of amyloid fibrils.

Prognosis

Too few cases have been reported to establish a prognosis for this condition.

WALDENSTRÖM'S MACROGLOBULINEMIA

This is not normally an indication for renal biopsy, since the renal signs are usually minimal. Most patients excrete determinants of mu chains in the urine. There have been reports of the following associated conditions: minimal change nephrotic syndrome, membranoproliferative glomerulonephritis type I, and amyloid disease. The most characteristic feature is the presence of large deposits in the glomerular loops, without marked proliferation (Fig. 9–25). The deposits contain exclusively IgM, which has led to the hypothesis that they are due to the local precipitation of the M component, favored by the hyperviscosity commonly present in these patients.

GLOMERULAR LESIONS IN MALIGNANCIES

Glomerular Lesions in Carcinoma

Membranous Glomerulonephritis

The most common renal lesion noted in patients with carcinoma is membranous glomerulonephritis. It accounts for more than half the glomerular lesions in carcinoma. Most investigators point out the strong relationship between membranous glomerulonephritis and carcinoma, although this link is the subject of some controversy.

The association between the nephrotic syn-

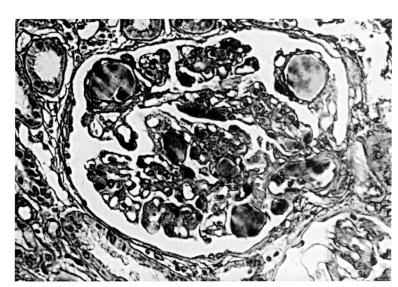

Figure 9–25. Waldenström's macroglobulinemia. There are large occlusive "thrombi" occluding many loops. (PAS, ×250.)

drome and cancer was first recognized in 1966 in a 10-year follow-up study of 101 patients in the United States. It was observed that in adults presenting with the nephrotic syndrome, neoplasia was discovered within a period of 14 months in 10.9%. Membranous glomerulonephritis was the renal lesion in nine of these ten patients. A similar incidence was found in another study of 44 British adults with membranous glomerulonephritis; 4 were found to have carcinomas. We reported that in a series of patients with membranous glomerulonephritis in France, 7 of 86 had a carcinoma. Finally, in a report on 3476 patients with proteinuria in the United Kingdom, 42 had an underlying carcinoma, and the principal histologic lesion in this group was membranous glomerulonephritis. Thus, there appears to be a privileged relationship between membranous glomerulonephritis and carcinoma in adults.

Pathogenesis

The pathogenesis is not clear. Attempts to isolate substances from the circulation are too sparse to draw general conclusions. The cancers most commonly associated with membranous glomerulonephritis are pulmonary, with bronchogenic being the predominant lesion. Other sites include the colorectal area, kidney, breast, and stomach.

Histology

The features are the same as those described in Chapter 4.

Prognosis

The prognosis is essentially determined by the underlying tumor.

Membranoproliferative Glomerulonephritis

Membranoproliferative glomerulonephritis has been most often reported in association with gastrointestinal carcinomas. However, it has also been reported that in a series of 40 patients with hypernephromas, 35% had mesangial deposits of immunoglobulins and complement. In a series of 57 patients with renal cell carcinoma, we also found mesangial changes ranging from moderate-to-severe sclerosis. A few specimens showed glomerular epithelial cell proliferation with or without synechiae and crescents.

Amyloidosis

The renal amyloid deposits in patients with carcinomas have been shown to be of the AA type in those few cases studied by modern techniques, and it seems reasonable to assume that many of the others are similar. The incidence of amyloidosis in one series of 4033 autopsies of patients with cancer was 0.4%. Only 7 of 16 affected patients had an associated carcinoma, but membranous glomerulonephritis was the most frequent renal lesion. In this and other series, the most frequent tumors associated with renal amyloidosis are hypernephromas.

Glomerular Lesions in Lymphoma

Hodgkin's Disease

Amyloidosis was the most common renal lesion before 1963, but it has largely disappeared as a complication. Currently the most frequent is minimal change. This change may antedate the diagnosis of Hodgkin's disease. Its appearance correlates with the initial onset and recurrences, and it often disappears with remissions.

Renal lesions of other types are much less frequently associated with Hodgkin's disease. They include focal sclerosis, membranous glomerulonephritis, membranoproliferative glomerulonephritis, proliferative glomerulonephritis, and crescentic glomerulonephritis with circulating antiglomerular basement membrane antibodies.

Non-Hodgkin's Lymphoma

The renal lesions are of quite diverse types, in contrast to those associated with Hodgkin's disease. In these cases, it has been difficult to implicate directly the hematologic malignancy in the pathogenesis of the renal lesion.

Glomerular Lesions in Leukemias

Chronic Lymphocytic Leukemia

Glomerular lesions are found as frequently in chronic lymphocytic leukemia as in lymphoid malignancies (Fig. 9–26). The most

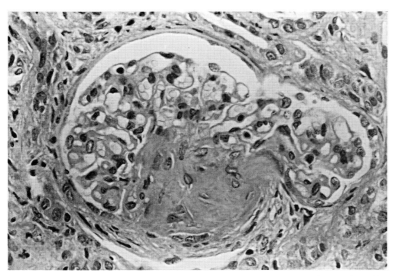

Figure 9–26. Chronic lymphocytic leukemia. Focal sclerosis affecting one half of the glomerulus. There is also interstitial fibrosis and an infiltrate of mononuclear cells. (Masson's trichrome, ×250.)

commonly reported histologic type is membranoproliferative glomerulonephritis. Monoclonal gammopathy has been found in several patients, and cryoglobulinemia was reportedly present in another series. Fibrillary or immunotactoid glomerulopathy has been reported in a few patients. Our experience is similar and suggests that in patients with chronic lymphocytic leukemia with a proliferative glomerular lesion, slightly more than half have an associated monoclonal gammopathy.

SELECTED READINGS

1. Dabbs D, Striker L, Mignon F, et al: Glomerular lesions in lymphomas and leukemia. Am J Med 80:63, 1986.
2. Davison AM: The United Kingdom Medical Research Council's glomerulonephritis registry. Contrib Nephrol 48:24, 1985.
3. Eagen JW, Lewis EJ: Glomerulopathies of neoplasia. Kidney Int 11:297, 1977.
4. Gilboa N, Durante D, Guggenheim S, et al: Immune deposit nephritis and single-component cryoglobulinemia associated with chronic lymphocytic leukemia. Nephron 24:223, 1979.
5. Lee JC, Yamaushi H, Hopper J: The association of cancer and the nephrotic syndrome. Ann Intern Med 64:41, 1966.
6. Moulin B, Ronco P, Mougenot B, et al: Glomerulonephritis in chronic lymphocytic leukemia and related B-cell lymphomas. Kidney Int 42:127, 1992.
7. Silva FG, Pirani CL, Mesa-Tejada R, et al: The kidney in plasma cell dyscrasias: A review and a clinicopathologic study of 50 patients. *In* Fenoglio C, Wolff M (eds): Progress in Surgical Pathology. New York, Masson, 1984, pp 131–176.

IMMUNOTACTOIDS AND FIBRILS IN THE GLOMERULI

The name *immunotactoid* or *fibrillary glomerulonephritis* was coined to designate a glomerular disease with fibrillar nonamyloid glomerular deposits that could be detected only by electron microscopy. Fibrillary glomerulonephritis refers to deposits composed of 16 to 24 nm fibrils, while immunotactoid glomerulonephritis refers to deposits of fibrils of 30 nm or more.

Patient Presentation

Hypertension and chronic microscopic hematuria and proteinuria are common presenting findings. The patients described so far have not had plasma cell dyscrasias. Nonamyloid fibrils have also been described in patients with other types of glomerular diseases, such as cryoglobulinemia and IgG monoclonal benign gammopathy.

Histology

Light Microscopy

The amount of mesangial matrix is increased, with various degrees of mesangial cell proliferation. Crescents are present in 30% of cases.

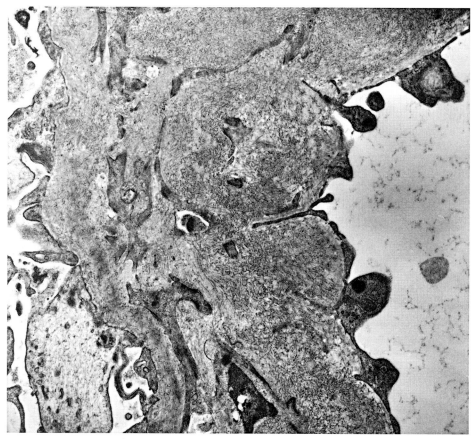

Figure 9–27. Fibrillary glomerulonephritis. Bundles of nonbranched fibrils are present in both the mesangial and subendothelial regions. (Electron micrograph, ×14,000.)

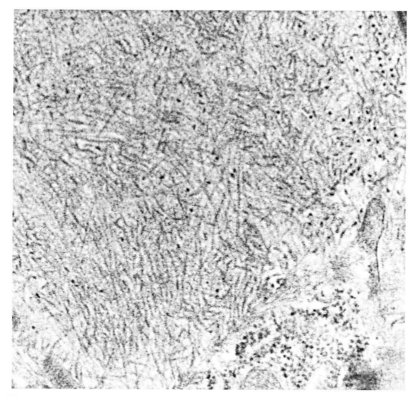

Figure 9–28. Fibrillary glomerulonephritis. At higher power, the fibrils are irregularly arranged, and no substructure is visible. (Electron micrograph, ×35,000.)

Immunofluorescence Microscopy

Irregular granular deposits of polyclonal IgG, IgM, and C3 are seen in the mesangial and subendothelial areas.

Electron Microscopy

Bundles of fibrils without a recognizable periodicity have been described in the mesangial and subendothelial areas (Fig. 9–27). The individual size of the microfibrils approximates 20 nm in fibrillary glomerulonephritis (Fig. 9–28). They are usually distributed in the same regions as the deposits seen by immunofluorescence microscopy. It has been suggested that they represent altered immunoglobulins based on immunoelectron microscopic findings.

Prognosis

Fibrillary glomerulonephritis often progresses to renal failure. There is most often no response to immunotherapy.

SELECTED READINGS

1. Alpers CE, Rennke HG, Hopper J Jr, et al: Fibrillary glomerulonephritis: An entity with unusual immunofluorescence features. Kidney Int 31:781, 1987.
2. Duffy JL, Khurana E, Susin M, et al: Fibrillary renal deposits and nephritis. Am J Pathol 113:279, 1983.
3. Hsu HC, Churg J: Glomerular microfibrils in renal disease: A comparative electron microscopic study. Kidney Int 16:497, 1979.
4. Korbet SM, Schwartz MM, Lewis EJ: The fibrillary glomerulopathies. Am J Kidney Dis 23:751, 1994.
5. Mery JP: Glomerulopathies fibrillaires. Nephrologie 14:123, 1993.

10

GLOMERULAR DISEASES ASSOCIATED WITH PREGNANCY

TOXEMIA OF PREGNANCY

Pregnancy may be associated with a number of diseases. It may, for instance, exacerbate renal diseases that existed before the pregnancy. The only syndrome that is specific for pregnancy is preeclampsia, or toxemia of pregnancy. Although the frequency of the disease is decreasing, preeclampsia still represents a common problem during the third trimester of pregnancy. This condition was clearly delineated in the 1960s with the help of detailed pathologic studies, but the use of biopsies in this setting is much more restricted now.

Many diseases that antedate a pregnancy, in particular those with a hypertensive component, may be exacerbated during the late part of pregnancy. A pathologist thus may have to recognize an underlying glomerular disorder from those abnormalities characteristic of toxemia of pregnancy.

Pathogenesis

Toxemia of pregnancy is associated with intravascular coagulation, and as in thrombotic microangiopathies, the glomerular endothelium is the principal site affected. The pathogenesis, although not completely elucidated, is presumably related to a combination of factors. Pregnancy predisposes to intravascular coagulation and to the effect of endotoxins, as shown in a number of experimental conditions. In the third trimester of pregnancy, ischemia of the uterus and placenta may trigger the release of thromboplastic substances. Finally, there may be a genetic propensity to develop preeclampsia in response to immunologic reactivity against the fetal antigens. A vasospasm of the arterioles may be the initiating factor leading to the endothelial damage sometimes referred to as endotheliosis, progressing to local thrombosis in the glomeruli.

Patient Presentation

The disease typically affects primiparas and occurs during the third term of pregnancy. Hypertension, proteinuria, and edema are characteristic. Another feature is retinal arteriolar spasm, which correlates with the severity of the glomerular lesions. Other clinical findings include a decline in glomerular filtration rate and hyperuricemia. Proteinuria is moderate, and the nephrotic syndrome, although possible, is a rare event.

Histology

Light Microscopy

The glomerular changes are diffuse and regular, consisting of enlargement and loss of the vascular spaces by an expanded mesangium and endothelial cell swelling (Figs. 10–1, 10–2). Hypercellularity is not a feature of this disease, although the glomeruli may appear to

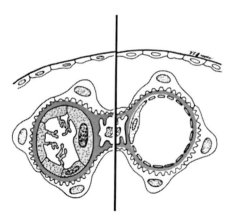

Figure 10–1. Toxemia of pregnancy. Diagram of endothelial cell swelling.

have an increased number of cells because of the cytoplasmic swelling. The glomerular basement membranes appear thickened on hematoxylin and eosin (H&E) stains, but silver stains reveal normal contours (Fig. 10–3). The subendothelium is widened and filled with a flocculent material.

Aside from endothelial swelling, the blood vessels do not show lesions.

The tubules and interstitium are generally unremarkable, unless tubular necrosis is present. Hyalin droplets may be present in tubular epithelium, and casts may be seen in the lumina if the patient has significant proteinuria.

Immunofluorescence Microscopy

There is considerable discussion about the amount and type of deposits in this syndrome. Suffice it to say that there is little evidence to implicate an immunologic component in this process at the present time. Deposits of IgG and IgM have been found along the glomerular basement membranes in approximately 10% of biopsy samples and are most frequently present in the severe forms of the disease. Fibrin may also be found in the glomeruli. As was the case with immunoglobulin deposits, fibrin is most commonly found in specimens of patients with severe lesions.

Electron Microscopy

The major changes occur on the luminal aspects of the glomerular basement membranes. The endothelial cells are swollen and vacuolated. The lamina rara interna is markedly expanded and contains flocculent mate-

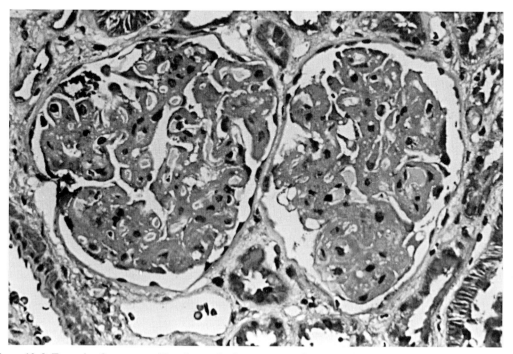

Figure 10–2. Toxemia of pregnancy. The glomerular basement membranes in all glomeruli have a thickened, refractile profile. The vascular spaces are markedly compressed. The number of intraglomerular cells is not increased. The interstitium is edematous. (H&E, ×300.)

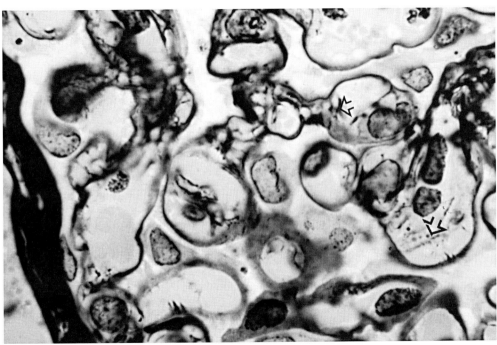

Figure 10–3. Toxemia of pregnancy. At higher power, the widened subendothelial spaces are clearly visible *(right lower arrow)*. The luminal aspect of the endothelial cell cytoplasm is widely separated from the glomerular basement membrane by deposits *(right upper arrow)*. (PASM, ×1200.)

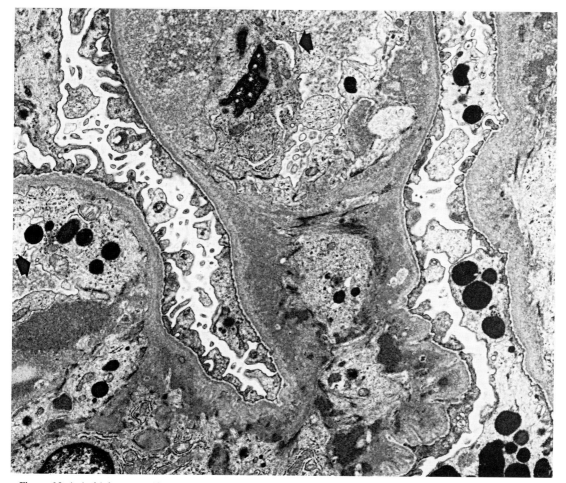

Figure 10–4. At higher magnification, the endothelial cell cytoplasmic prominence is apparent (arrowhead), and the large subendothelial deposits are easily appreciated. Large lysosomes are present in both endothelial and mesangial cells. (×4000.)

rial and electron-dense strands of material resembling basement membranes (Fig. 10–4). As noted by light microscopy, the mesangial cells also appear swollen, and the mesangial matrix is expanded and contains electron-dense material. Material resembling fibrin may be seen in the vascular spaces.

The epithelial cells may contain an increased number of lysosomes, but they are otherwise unremarkable.

Prognosis

Most investigators agree that the lesions associated with preeclampsia are completely reversible. However, few long-term studies have been performed, and renal biopsies have not been a part of the follow-up evaluation.

SELECTED READINGS

1. Kincaid-Smith P: Participation of intravascular coagulation in the pathogenesis of glomerular and vascular lesions. Kidney Int 7:242, 1975.
2. Pirani CL: Coagulation and renal disease. *In* Bertani T, Remuzzi G (eds): Glomerular Injury 300 Years after Morgagni. Milan, Italy, Wichtig Editore, 1983, pp 119–138.
3. Pollak VE, Nettles JB: The kidney in toxemia of pregnancy: A clinical and pathological study based on renal biopsies. Medicine 39:469, 1960.
4. Pollak VE, Pirani CL, Kark RM, et al: Reversible glomerular lesions in toxemia of pregnancy. Lancet 2:59, 1956.
5. Spargo B, McCartney CP, Winemiller R: Glomerular capillary endotheliosis in toxemia of pregnancy. Arch Pathol 68:593, 1959.
6. Wagoner RA, Holley KE, Johnson W: Accelerated nephrosclerosis and post-partum acute renal failure. Ann Intern Med 69:237, 1968.

11

TRANSPLANTATION

Introduced nearly 30 years ago, renal allo-transplantation is now one of the most rapidly advancing fields in clinical nephrology, in part due to the development of more efficacious and less toxic forms of immunosuppression. Over 11,000 renal transplants were performed in the United States in 1994 (of which approximately three fourths were cadaveric and one fourth living donor). One year survival rates are over 85% for cadaveric transplants and 95% for living related transplants. Immunoprophylaxis typically consists of cyclosporine, prednisone, and a third immunosuppressive agent such as imuran or mycophenolate mofetil. These drugs affect different phases of the immune response. Prednisone inhibits interleukin-1 (IL-1) production by monocyte/macrophage cells and cyclosporine inhibits interleukin-2 (and other lymphokine) synthesis by activated T-cells. This complex blocks NF-kappa B activation, a transcription factor for IL-2. Imuran and mycophenolate are inhibitors of purine synthesis and interfere with lymphocyte proliferation more distally in the immune effector response.

Despite improvements in immunosuppression, rejection continues to be the major cause of graft dysfunction. Most renal allografts suffer one or more rejection episodes. Their timely and accurate detection and treatment are clinically important for long-term graft function. Renal biopsy remains the gold standard for the diagnosis of rejection, despite the recent introduction of newer diagnostic tools such as the fine needle aspirate and radionuclide scintigraphy. Renal biopsies can be performed repeatedly, and complication rates are low because of the superficial location of the allograft in the iliac fossa.

The differential diagnosis of graft dysfunction is large; thus, renal biopsy has an indispensable diagnostic role (Table 11–1). Light microscopy and immunofluorescence microscopy are routinely performed, and electron microscopy is used when primary or de novo glomerular disease is suspected. Frozen sections are reserved for extremely urgent situations, such as suspected hyperacute rejection.

REJECTION

Allograft rejection has been divided into several major subgroups according to the time at which it occurs, the nature (humoral vs. cellular) of the immune response, and the character of the renal lesions produced.

Table 11–1. Causes of Renal Allograft Dysfunction

Rejection
  Hyperacute
  Accelerated vascular
  Acute
  Chronic
Postoperative acute tubular necrosis
Perfusion injury
Drug toxicity
  Cyclosporine
  FK-506
  OKT_3
Obstruction
Major vascular occlusion
  Renal artery
  Renal vein
Recurrent glomerular disease
De novo glomerular disease
Infections
Lymphoma (Post-transplant lymphoproliferative
  disease)

Hyperacute Rejection

Pathogenesis and Patient Presentation

Hyperacute rejection is an immediate form of graft rejection. It is generally irreversible and occurs within hours of placement of the graft. When it occurs at 24 to 48 hours, it is called *delayed hyperacute rejection.*

Hyperacute rejection is mediated by pre-formed circulating antibodies to donor endothelial cells, such as ABO blood group antigens, HLA Class I antigens, or (rarely) HLA Class II antigens. Fortunately, it affects less than 0.2% of transplants, since standard cross-match tests detect donor-specific antibody prior to transplantation. However, some antibody levels are below the detection level or are directed to vascular-endothelial antigens shared by monocytes and are not routinely screened in standard cross-match tests. Antibodies may also have been acquired in the course of previous transplantations, pregnancy, or blood transfusions. Cold agglutinin IgM antibodies have also been implicated in grafts not adequately warmed prior to reperfusion.

Graft injury is mediated by binding of antibody (usually of the IgM class) to endothelial cells of the glomeruli, interstitial capillaries, and small arteries. Complement activation causes chemotactic complement (C3 and C5a) release and neutrophil accumulation. Endothelial lysis mediated by membrane attack complexes (C5b to C9) leads to endothelial denudation and activation of the coagulation cascade, with formation of occlusive fibrin-platelet thrombi and renal infarction. If this occurs immediately, the graft may turn dusky blue and cyanotic within minutes of surgical vascularization, and sections reveal widespread vascular thrombosis. Later, hyperacute rejection may present as the sudden development of oliguric renal failure in the early postoperative period, and the kidney most often has to be removed to prevent a serum sickness–like reaction.

Histology
Light Microscopy

The earliest changes are endothelial swelling and necrosis and neutrophil margination, most evident in peritubular capillaries and glomeruli. Later, there is thrombosis of glomeruli, arterioles, and small arteries by fibrin-

platelet thrombi, which results in diffuse ischemic injury (Fig. 11–1). Even after infarction, microthrombi may still be detectable by Masson's trichrome stain, which stains fibrin red; by phosphotungstic acid hematoxylin, which stains fibrin purple; or by modified Fraser Lendrum, which stains fibrin orange. There is usually no polymorphonuclear leukocyte infiltration of the graft interstitium. Patchy tubular necrosis, present early, is rapidly followed by total infarction (Figs. 11–2, 11–3). Interstitial hemorrhage is common as the infarction progresses.

Immunofluorescence Microscopy

Since hyperacute rejection is humorally mediated, diagnosis is confirmed by the detection of linear to semilinear staining for IgM or IgG and C3 along all endothelial surfaces. Although immunoglobulins may not be detectable in many cases, especially late in the course of hyperacute rejection, IgM is more often positive than is IgG. There is strong staining for fibrin-related antigen throughout the microvasculature, and often focally in the interstitium, corresponding to areas of interstitial hemorrhage. In cases of cortical necrosis, the necrotic tissue may have yellowish autofluorescence.

Electron Microscopy

The early ultrastructural findings are endothelial swelling and necrosis accompanied by neutrophil margination, erythrocyte congestion, and fibrin-platelet thrombi. This is followed by necrosis of all the renal compartments.

Accelerated Vascular Rejection

Pathogenesis and Presentation

This form usually occurs within the first 6 weeks and has a poor prognosis, with 50 to 75% graft failure. It is thought to be primarily mediated by donor-specific HLA Class I antibodies. Since the advent of cyclosporine, it now occurs in fewer than 1% of renal allografts.

Histology
Light Microscopy

There is endothelial injury and thrombosis of glomeruli and small arteries, producing le-

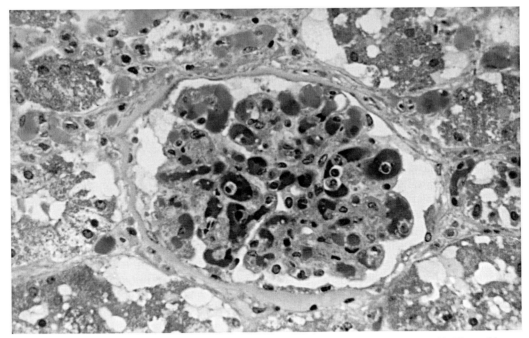

Figure 11–1. Hyperacute rejection. The glomerular spaces are filled with extensive fibrin thrombi. The architecture of the basement membrane is extensively altered, and there appears to be mesangiolysis. In addition, the surrounding tubules are necrotic. (Hematoxylin and eosin [H&E], ×300.)

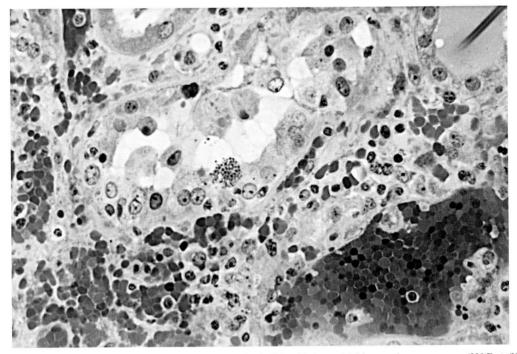

Figure 11–2. Hyperacute rejection. Tubular necrosis and tubulitis with interstitial hemorrhage are seen. (H&E, ×300.)

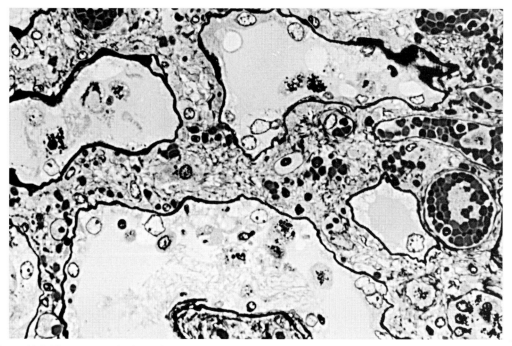

Figure 11–3. Hyperacute rejection. The interstitium is filled with edema and inflammatory cells. The tubules are nearly completely necrotic, and the epithelial cells are sloughing into the lumen. (Silver stain, ×300.)

sions similar to those described in hyperacute rejection. Glomerular endothelial necrosis may be accompanied by mesangiolysis, a dissolution of the mesangial matrix similar to that seen in other forms of thrombotic microangiopathy (Fig. 11–4). Larger arteries may display medial fibrinoid necrosis, i.e., fibrin and plasma proteins in the vessel wall and necrosis of myocytes. There may be neutrophil or lymphocytic infiltration of the media, mimick-

ing the vascular lesions in polyarteritis nodosa (Fig. 11–5). Differential diagnosis includes the hemolytic uremic syndrome due to cyclosporine toxicity.

Immunofluorescence Microscopy

There is variable glomerular and arterial endothelial staining for IgM, IgG, and C3. Heavy fibrin/fibrinogen staining is seen in the loca-

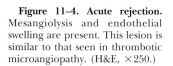

Figure 11–4. Acute rejection. Mesangiolysis and endothelial swelling are present. This lesion is similar to that seen in thrombotic microangiopathy. (H&E, ×250.)

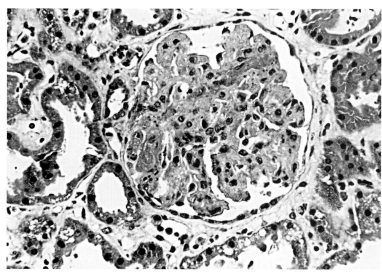

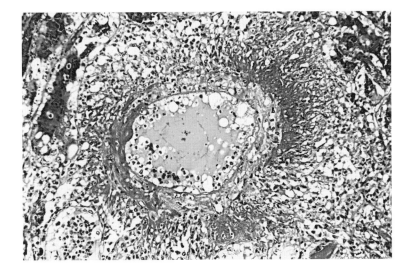

Figure 11-5. Accelerated vascular rejection. An interlobular artery showing transmural inflammation composed of lymphocytes and neutrophils. There is circumferential medial fibrinoid necrosis. The endothelium is swollen and there are subendothelial leukocytes. (H&E, ×250.)

tion of the thrombi. Vascular staining for immunoglobulin and complement and involvement of interstitial capillaries are helpful distinguishing features of accelerated vascular rejection.

Electron Microscopy

Glomeruli demonstrate narrowing of lumina due to endothelial swelling and obliteration of fenestrations as well as hypercellularity. There is focal detachment of the endothelium from the glomerular basement membrane (GBM), with deposition of fibrillar fibrin in the subendothelial space and vascular lumina plus obliteration of fenestrations. Subendothelial electron-lucent flocculent ("fluffy") material may lie in the widened lamina rara interna and likely represents partially degraded coagulation products. Arterioles and arteries are focally narrowed by endothelial swelling and denudation, with intraluminal and intimal accumulation of fibrin and electron-dense plasma proteins accompanied by myocyte necrosis.

Acute Rejection (Cellular)

Pathogenesis and Patient Presentation

This is the most common form of rejection and is primarily T-cell–mediated. Although acute cellular rejection occurs most frequently in the first 1 to 2 months, it may develop years following transplantation, especially if the level of immunosuppression has been reduced. Clinical signs include a rising serum creatinine

level and, less often, graft tenderness. Renal biopsy is generally performed after prerenal (hemodynamic) and postrenal (obstructive) causes of graft dysfunction have been ruled out. Over 90% of patients will recover graft function following therapy. The choice of therapy is dictated by the type and severity of the acute rejection. Commonly used protocols include high-dose intravenous corticosteroid therapy, polyclonal antilymphocyte sera, antithymocyte globulin, and OKT$_3$ (a non–complement-fixing mouse monoclonal antibody of the IgG$_{2\alpha}$ subclass that is specific for CD$_3$).

Histology

Light Microscopy, Tubulointerstitial Lesions

The standards for a diagnosis of acute rejection are controversial. Most agree that the hallmark of acute tubulointerstitial cellular rejection is interstitial mononuclear leukocyte infiltration and edema together with leukocyte infiltration of the tubular epithelium, a lesion called *tubulitis* (Fig. 11-6). The interstitial infiltrate is predominantly perivascular early in the rejection process but becomes more diffusely distributed and peritubular in severe rejection. Note that the diagnosis of acute rejection cannot be based solely on the finding of interstitial inflammation, since *significant interstitial infiltrates may be present in nonrejecting allografts, especially in the first month post-transplant.* Therefore, the diagnosis of acute rejection requires additional histologic features, i.e., tubulitis and/or infiltration of the vascular walls by inflammatory cells (arteritis).

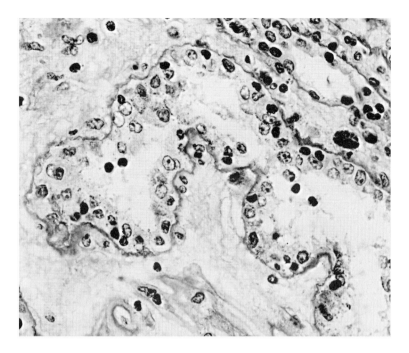

Figure 11–6. Acute rejection. Tubulointerstitial region showing infiltration of the tubular epithelial cell layer by inflammatory cells (tubulitis). There is also interstitial edema and inflammation. (Periodic acid–Schiff, ×400.)

The "BANFF working classification" requires greater than four mononuclear cells per tubular cross-section or group of ten tubular cells and interstitial inflammation involving more than 25% of the biopsy surface area to differentiate "borderline" from "grade 1" acute rejection (Table 11–2). Others feel that the diagnosis of acute rejection is more secure if tubulitis is accompanied by histologic evidence of tubular injury in the form of tubular degenerative and regenerative changes. Since the prevalence of tubulitis is an index of the magnitude of the rejection, the BANFF classification defines moderate (grade 2) acute rejection as greater than ten infiltrating leukocytes per tubular cross-section.

In severe acute rejection, cortical infarcts and interstitial hemorrhage may occur, particularly in the medulla. Both infarction and interstitial hemorrhage predict a poor prognosis, and the presence of either one warrants a diagnosis of severe acute rejection (BANFF grade 3).

The composition of the interstitial inflammatory infiltrate is mixed, consisting predominantly of T-lymphocytes, lymphoblasts, and macrophages, with a smaller number of plasma cells, granulocytes (neutrophils, eosinophils, and basophils), and NK (natural killer) cells. While CD4+ T-cells are common in early rejection, particularly in the perivascular areas, CD8+ cells usually predominate in fully developed acute rejection. Both CD4+ and CD8+ cells may infiltrate the tubular epithelium in areas of tubulitis. Tubular epithelial expression of DR antigen, IL-8, VCAM-1, and ICAM-1 are upregulated in acute cellular rejection and may be important in the media-

Table 11–2. BANFF Classification of Acute Rejection and Chronic Rejection

---

I. Acute Rejection

Grade 1 (mild acute)
1. interstitial inflammation >25% parenchyma affected
   and
2. tubulitis >4 mononuclear cells/tubular cross-section, or groups of 10 tubular cells

Grade 2 (moderate acute)
1. significant interstitial inflammation and tubulitis >10 mononuclear cells/tubular cross-section
   and/or
2. mild or moderate intimal arteritis

Grade 3 (severe acute)
1. severe intimal arteritis and/or transmural arteritis with fibrinoid change and necrosis of medial myocytes
   and/or
2. focal infarction or interstitial hemorrhage

II. Chronic Allograft Nephropathy

Grade 1. mild interstitial fibrosis and tubular atrophy
Grade 2. moderate interstitial fibrosis and tubular atrophy
Grade 3. severe interstitial fibrosis and tubular atrophy

Adapted from Solez K, Axelsen RA, Benediktsson H, et al: International standardization of nomenclature and criteria for the histologic diagnosis of renal allograft rejection: The BANFF working classification of kidney transplant pathology. Kidney Int 44:411, 1993.

tion of T-cell infiltration. T-cell recruitment and cellular cytotoxicity to tubular epithelium may be mediated by release of a host of T-cell cytokines, including interferon-gamma, tumor necrosis factor α and β, interleukins such as IL-2 and IL-6, and perforin.

Immunofluorescence Microscopy, Tubulointerstitial Lesions

The major finding is focal C3 staining of the tubular basement membranes, often in a semilinear distribution. Since deposits of immunoglobulin are not found, the C3 activation may be Ig-independent.

Electron Microscopy, Tubulointerstitial Lesions

Electron microscopy does not generally aid in the diagnosis of acute rejection.

Light Microscopy, Arterial Lesions

This lesion is generally termed *endothelialitis* or *endovasculitis*, because there is arterial sub-endothelial mononuclear leukocyte infiltration, often accompanied by intimal edema and endothelial swelling, proliferation, and degeneration (Fig. 11–7). If very severe, there may also be intimal and intraluminal deposition of fibrin. These lesions may be identified in arteries at all levels of the vascular tree but are most common in larger arteries of arcuate or interlobar caliber. Thus, endothelialitis is often missed in renal biopsies sampling only the outer cortex. Although originally thought to be humoral in nature, T-cells and monocytes and in some cases neutrophils are present. These lesions heal by the progressive appearance of intimal fibrosis. The presence of a sparse mononuclear leukocyte infiltrate within a zone of intimal fibrosis aids in detecting healing foci of endovasculitis in late lesions.

Although endovasculitis is a characteristic feature of acute rejection, it is far less commonly identified than is tubulointerstitial rejection. The BANFF schema recognizes endovasculitis as a feature of moderate or severe rejection. Its presence increases the classification to grade 2, whereas necrotizing arteritis receives a grade 3 designation.

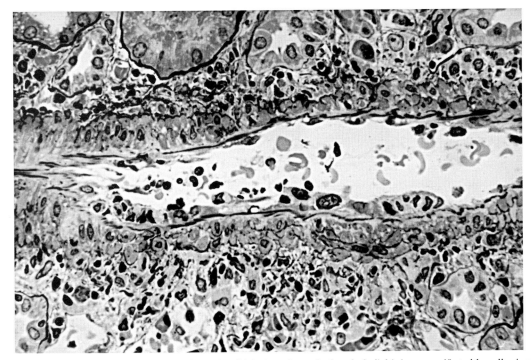

Figure 11–7. Acute rejection. A vascular lesion in which there is marked endothelial injury, manifested by adhesion of neutrophils, vacuolation and proliferation of endothelial cells, and an inflammatory cell infiltrate in the subendothelial space (so-called endothelialitis or endovasculitis). (Periodic acid–silver methenamine [PASM], ×300.)

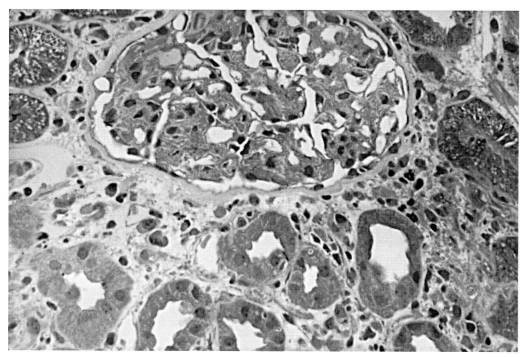

Figure 11–8. Acute rejection. The glomerulus has endothelial cell swelling, moderate hypercellularity in the mesangium, and marked reduction of the lumen. The surrounding interstitium is markedly edematous and contains many inflammatory cells. (H&E, ×250.)

Immunofluorescence Microscopy, Arterial Lesions

Fibrinogen, IgM, C3, and C1 are most commonly identified in the involved vessels. They may be present in areas of intimal edema and coagulation due to altered permeability.

Light Microscopy, Glomerular Lesions

Although glomeruli are usually unaffected in acute cellular rejection, in approximately 10% there is prominent infiltration of the glomerular tuft by mononuclear leukocytes. This process, known as *transplant glomerulitis*, is usually accompanied by other tubulointerstitial and/or vascular features of acute rejection. In the rare instances in which it is the major histologic manifestation of the acute rejection, it must be differentiated from recurrent or de novo glomerulonephritis. The distribution of lesions ranges from focal to diffuse and from segmental to global. There is swelling and hypercellularity of glomerular endothelial cells and infiltration of the glomerular capillaries by CD4+ and CD8+ T-cells and monocytes (Fig. 11–8). Mild mesangial hypercellularity and segmental double contours of the glomerular basement membrane may also be identified.

Immunofluorescence Microscopy, Glomerular Lesions

Variable staining for fibrin, immunoglobulin (IgM and/or IgG), C3, and C1 may be seen, in a semilinear subendothelial distribution.

Electron Microscopy, Glomerular Lesions

Vascular spaces are severely narrowed or occluded by endothelial swelling and hypercellularity, with loss of endothelial fenestrations. Mononuclear leukocytes are closely apposed to endothelial cells but generally do not infiltrate the mesangium. The subendothelial accumulation of electron-lucent fluffy material or fibrin is sometimes observed but electron-dense immune deposits are not seen.

Chronic Rejection

Pathogenesis and Patient Presentation

Chronic rejection is a clinical term referring to a gradual diminution in graft function developing over months to years, often accompanied by proteinuria that may reach nephrotic levels. Chronic rejection may appear after one or more clinical episodes of acute rejection,

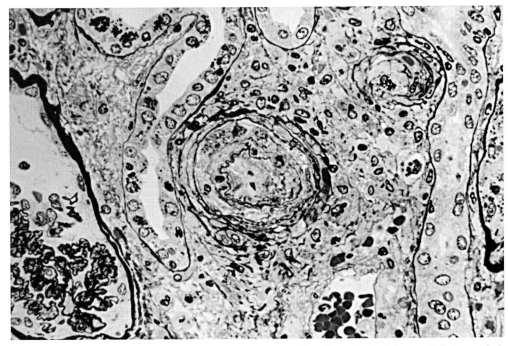

Figure 11–9. Chronic rejection. The small artery in the center has dense intimal hypercellularity, and there is endothelial hypertrophy. The vascular lumen is nearly occluded. The arteriolar lesions *(upper right quadrant)* consist mainly of endothelial cell swelling and smudging of some of the nuclei of cells within the media. (PASM, ×400.)

or it may develop without overt bouts of acute rejection. Chronic rejection remains the major cause of graft failure, with a 10-year graft survival of 40% for cadaveric grafts, 50% for parental (1 haplotype mismatch) grafts, and 70% for HLA-identical grafts. Although antirejection therapy is effective in reversing acute rejection episodes and improving 1-year graft survival, long-term graft survival has not been appreciably altered.

Histology

Light Microscopy, Vascular Lesion

A major feature of chronic rejection is progressive narrowing of medium-sized and large-caliber arteries by dense intimal fibroplasia (Fig. 11–9). Small arteries and arterioles are involved to a lesser degree. The endothelium is intact, and there is little or no leukocyte infiltration of the intima. There is abundant intimal collagen, and elastic membranes may be duplicated. Intimal foam cells are sometimes observed. After graft failure, nephrectomy specimens may show acute vascular rejection superimposed on chronic vascular changes.

Light Microscopy, Tubulointerstitial Lesions

There is extensive interstitial fibrosis and tubular atrophy, accompanied, in some patients, by tubulitis and interstitial hemorrhage as evidence of continuing rejection (Fig. 11–10). It is not often possible to determine the extent to which chronic rejection, ischemia, hypertension, and chronic cyclosporine toxicity have contributed to the tubulointerstitial scarring. For this reason, the BANFF group advocated the use of the term *chronic allograft nephropathy* rather than *chronic rejection* (Table 11–2).

Light Microscopy, Glomerular Lesions

The glomerular lesions are varied. In some specimens the lesions are ischemic, with global wrinkling, thickening and retraction of glomerular basement membrane, and contraction of the tuft, which is termed *ischemic glomerulopathy* in the BANFF classification. In other samples the remaining glomeruli are hypertrophied and have focal segmental glomerulosclerosis.

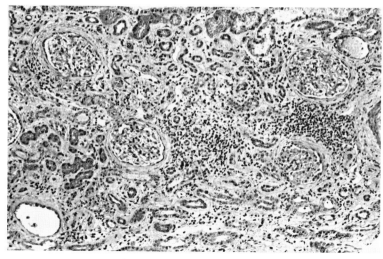

Figure 11–10. Chronic rejection. This low-power view demonstrates the dense interstitial fibrosis, loss of proximal tubules, atrophy of many remaining tubules, and irregular aggregates of mononuclear cells. Note that the glomeruli appear to be relatively unaffected. (H&E, ×80.)

Transplant Glomerulopathy

Patient Presentation and Pathogenesis

This condition is unique to renal transplant and occurs in a small number of patients, who all present with heavy proteinuria or the nephrotic syndrome. Its frequency is approximately 20% of all glomerular lesions that can be encountered in a transplant.

Histology

Light Microscopy, Glomeruli

Transplant glomerulopathy is characterized by diffuse thickening of the glomerular walls (Fig. 11–11). The presence of diffuse tramtracks on silver-stained biopsies has even led some to call this disease membranoproliferative, but the lesions are quite distinct from the usual forms of membranoproliferative glomer-

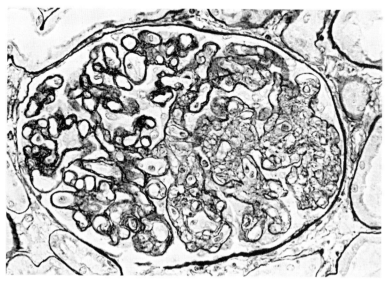

Figure 11–11. Transplant glomerulopathy. The right half of the glomerulus is involved with a process consisting of simplification of the vascular loops and duplication of the peripheral basement membranes. The mesangial spaces are enlarged and are filled with a poorly stained material. The left half of the glomerulus is less severely involved, but the underlying process is similar, i.e., thickened and duplicated peripheral basement membranes, mesangial widening, and simplification of the vascular loops. (Silver stain, ×250.)

ulonephritis. The thickening of the capillary walls is due to clear, fluffy subendothelial material located between double contours of the glomerular basement membrane. Monocytes and lymphocytes are often marginated in the glomerular capillary lumina. Endothelial cells are swollen. There is usually no marked mesangial or endocapillary proliferation, although a small increase in the number of mesangial nuclei may occur. The mesangial matrix appears swollen and contains fine fibrillar material. Some of the mesangial areas may even show overt mesangiolysis. Occasional aneurysmal dilations of the peripheral loops may be present. These lesions result in a considerable decrease in the patency of the glomerular vascular loops, reminiscent of those seen in hemolytic-uremic syndrome.

Immunofluorescence Microscopy, Glomeruli

There are small, filamentous, subendothelial deposits along the glomerular loops, which contain IgM, C3, C1, and in some cases fibrin. Staining for IgG is typically weak or absent. These features are useful to distinguish transplant glomerulopathy from recurrence of other forms of glomerulonephritis.

Electron Microscopy, Glomeruli

The major finding is the presence, between the inner aspect of the GBM and the endothelial cytoplasm, of a flocculent, electron-lucent material similar to that seen in chronic thrombotic microangiopathies (Fig. 11–12). This material may be separated from the endothelium by a thin layer of newly formed basement membrane, producing a double contour. The subendothelial zone often contains cellular debris and mesangial cell cytoplasmic elements. Foot process effacement and hypertrophy of the visceral cells are also commonly observed. The absence of electron-dense deposits is useful to differentiate transplant glomerulopathy

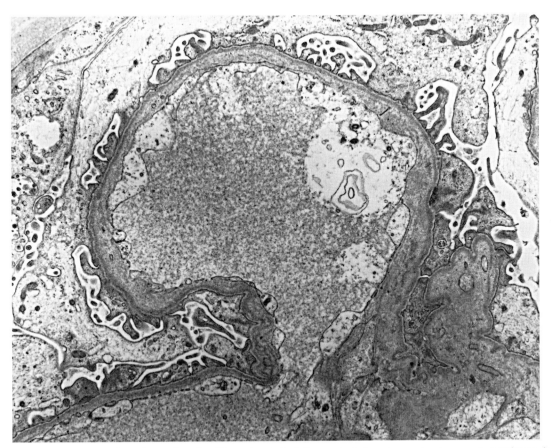

Figure 11–12. Transplant glomerulopathy. The subendothelial aspect of the glomerular basement membrane is widened, containing an electron-lucent flocculent material. There is an irregular, thin layer of basement membrane–like material adjacent to the endothelium, resulting in a double-contour configuration of the basement membrane. (Electron micrograph, ×10,100.)

from de novo or recurrent glomerulonephritis.

Prognosis

Some distinguish two phases. In the first, there are monocytes in the capillary lumina but no conspicuous subendothelial deposits. At this stage the lesions appear reversible. In the late phase as described earlier, the lesions are chronic and progress to graft loss in 60% of the cases, although the slope of deterioration varies widely between patients.

POSTOPERATIVE ACUTE TUBULAR NECROSIS

Pathogenesis and Patient Presentation

Acute tubular necrosis (ATN) is a significant cause of primary graft failure. It is most common in cadaveric grafts that have been subjected to prolonged warm or cold ischemia time, but it may also occur in living donor grafts if operative time has been protracted. It is recognized clinically in the first 1 or 2 weeks post-transplant by the presence of a persistently elevated serum creatinine level and oliguria or anuria. Differentiation from acute rejection is critical to spare the patient unnecessary antirejection therapy, especially since ATN renders the kidney particularly sensitive to cyclosporine toxicity. After 1 or more weeks on dialysis, renal function usually resumes.

Histology

Light Microscopy

The findings do not differ from ATN in other situations. The proximal tubules show a spectrum of changes, from frank coagulation necrosis with desquamation of epithelial cells to subtle tubular simplification, ectatic irregular tubular lumina, loss of the brush border, and regenerative enlarged tubular nuclei with nucleoli and increased mitotic figures. Interstitial infiltrates and tubulitis are not present.

Immunofluorescence Microscopy

No deposits are found.

Electron Microscopy

No lesions other than those related to ATN are present (see Chapter 13).

CYCLOSPORINE NEPHROTOXICITY

Pathogenesis and Patient Presentation

Cyclosporine nephrotoxicity is not limited to renal allograft recipients; it has also been found in recipients of heart, liver, and bone marrow transplants and in patients with a variety of autoimmune and inflammatory conditions. Cyclosporine toxicity may be acute or chronic and may affect all the kidney compartments (Table 11–3). Cyclosporine nephrotoxicity was found in nearly 40% of cyclosporine-treated transplant recipients with graft dysfunction in one recent series. Since it may be superimposed on acute or chronic rejection, the detection of cyclosporine toxicity may be very difficult and quite often requires careful clinical-pathologic correlations.

Functional Toxicity

Therapeutic cyclosporine doses may be associated with a reduced renal plasma flow and

Table 11–3. Renal Manifestations of Cyclosporine Nephrotoxicity

Type	Renal Biopsy Findings
1. Functional toxicity	No morphologic abnormalities
2. Prolonged acute renal failure in early postoperative period	Acute tubular necrosis
3. Acute toxicity	
Tubules	Vacuolization
	Microcalcification
	Giant mitochondria
Vascular	Microthrombosis (HUS-like syndrome)
	Endothelial and myocyte necrosis
4. Chronic toxicity	
Vascular	Hyaline arteriolopathy
Tubulointerstitial	Linear, focal fibrosis
	Diffuse interstitial fibrosis and tubular atrophy
Glomerular	Focal and segmental glomerulosclerosis

HUS, hemolytic-uremic syndrome.

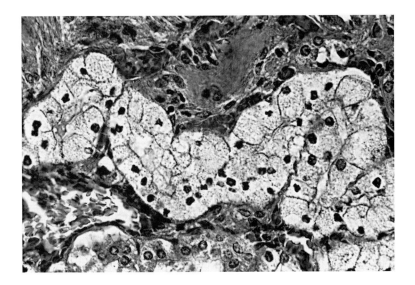

Figure 11–13. Cyclosporine, acute toxic tubular injury. A proximal tubule showing marked vacuolation of the cytoplasm. The vacuoles are of similar size (so-called isometric vacuoles). Some tubular cell nuclei appear shrunken and pyknotic. (H&E, ×400.)

glomerular filtration rate, in the absence of structural renal lesions. These functional changes are most common in the early post-transplant period, may occur at any time, and are reversible upon lowering the cyclosporine dosage.

Prolonged Post-Transplant Oligoanuria

Acute tubular necrosis renders the allograft particularly sensitive to cyclosporine toxicity, and the combination of these two conditions may cause prolonged oligoanuria. For this reason, cyclosporine is usually withheld until good allograft function has been established. The biopsy findings are those of postoperative acute tubular necrosis.

Acute Tubular Toxicity

The incidence of this reversible lesion, sometimes called *acute toxic tubulopathy*, has decreased as maintenance doses of cyclosporine have been lowered. The histologic lesion consists of a clear vacuolization of the cytoplasm of the straight segments (S_2 and S_3) of the proximal tubule. The vacuoles are of similar size (so-called isometric), contain aqueous fluid, may be very focal, and are best visualized, after formalin-fixation, with hematoxylin and eosin or trichrome stains (Fig. 11–13). Vacuolated epithelial cells may be identified in the urinary sediment. By electron microscopy, the vacuoles represent dilated smooth endoplasmic reticulum, and they are rarely accompanied by giant mitochondria in proximal tubular epithelial cells.

Other morphologic features of tubular toxicity include increased numbers of phagolysosomes, producing eosinophilic cytoplasmic inclusions visible at the light microscopic level. Increased tubular calcifications have also been described.

Acute Vascular Toxicity

The lesion, a form of acute thrombotic microangiopathy, may cause the hemolytic-uremic syndrome (see Chapter 6). Microthrombi are present in glomeruli, arterioles, and interlobular arteries. Glomeruli may show mesangiolysis, endothelial swelling and necrosis, and entrapment of distorted erythrocytes (schistocytes) in the thrombi.

This lesion is difficult to differentiate from accelerated vascular rejection. The absence of leukocyte infiltration, tubulitis, and endovasculitis and the lack of linear staining of vessel lumina with antisera to immunoglobulins (IgG or IgM) favor the diagnosis of cyclosporine toxicity. The outcome is variable; renal failure has been irreversible in most patients, but some have had complete restoration of renal function.

Chronic Toxicity

Chronic cyclosporine toxicity is a form of vascular toxicity accompanied by interstitial fibrosis, tubular atrophy, and progressive glomerulosclerosis. The afferent arterioles at the glomerular hilus, as well as the most distal portions of the interlobular arteries, are the

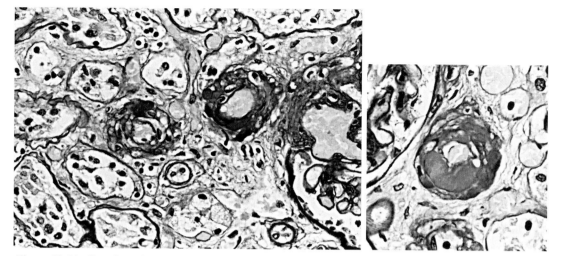

Figure 11–14. Chronic cyclosporine toxicity. The two small arteries demonstrate moderate *(right)* and severe *(left)* lesions consisting of swelling, vacuolation, and necrosis of medial smooth muscle cells as well as deposits of hyalin. The hyalin deposits are nodular *(inset)* and are often circular *(left)*. (Silver stain, ×400.)

site of the predominant lesions. There is swelling, vacuolization, and necrosis of individual medial myocytes, followed by nodular hyalinosis (Fig. 11–14). Although these lesions resemble the arteriolar hyalinosis associated with hypertension, aging, or diabetes, they differ in that the hyalin involves the media as well as the intima. Hyalin extends to the outermost boundary of the media, producing a "pearl necklace" pattern with paucicellular media. This pattern may be due to the replacement of myocytes by the hyalin. By immunofluorescence microscopy, the areas of hyalinosis stain with antisera to IgM, C3, and C1.

In severe lesions, the arteriolar lumen is narrowed or occluded by hyalinosis. It is usually associated with the development of chronic tubulointerstitial lesions. The most common pattern is linear zones of fibrosis and tubular atrophy in the distribution of medullary rays, an area of the kidney particularly vulnerable to ischemic injury (Fig. 11–15). In later lesions, there is more diffuse interstitial fibrosis and tubular atrophy. Although a modest interstitial infiltrate of mononuclear leukocytes is often present, there is no tubulitis. In some patients, nephrotic-range proteinuria develops. Renal biopsy specimens have shown residual glomeruli to be hypertrophied, with focal segmental glomerulosclerosis and hyalinosis and frequent hyperplasia of the juxtaglomerular apparatus.

The vascular lesions may be partially reversible, as assessed by one study of repeat renal

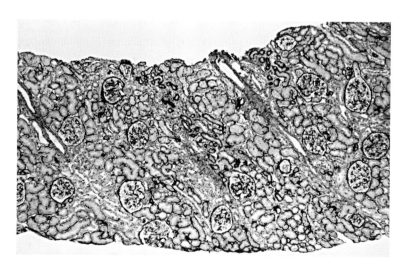

Figure 11–15. Chronic cyclosporine toxicity. This low-power view reveals linear zones of interstitial fibrosis and tubular atrophy. This distribution pattern appears to follow medullary rays. (PASM, ×40.)

biopsies 6 to 18 months after reduction of the cyclosporine dose. Whereas the arterioles underwent remodeling, with resorption of hyaline deposits, the interstitial fibrosis was a relatively irreversible lesion.

FK-506 NEPHROTOXICITY

Although clinical experience with FK-506 is more limited, FK-506 and cyclosporine may induce similar lesions. Greater experience with the drug is required to determine whether FK-506 toxicity is reversible.

OKT₃ TOXICITY

There are rare reports that high-dose OKT_3 may induce allograft thrombosis, at the level both of the glomeruli and large vessels. This effect has been postulated to be due to OKT_3-induced release of tumor necrosis factor, IL-2, and gamma-interferon, which triggers endothelial activation and increased endothelial expression of leukocyte adhesion factors and tissue factor procoagulant. In some cases, acute renal vein thrombosis following OKT_3 therapy has led to graft rupture in the early post-transplant period.

RECURRENT GLOMERULAR DISEASE

Although morphologic evidence of recurrent disease is not unusual in allograft biopsy specimens when these are studied by light microscopy, fluorescence microscopy, and electron microscopy, it is uncommon for recurrent glomerular disease to be a cause of graft failure.

Dense deposit disease (membranoproliferative glomerulonephritis type II) has the highest recurrence rate, 95 to 100%; however, less than 15% of these recurrences cause graft loss. Other glomerular diseases that frequently recur in the transplanted kidney include membranoproliferative glomerulonephritis type 1 (40 to 70%), IgA nephropathy and Henoch-Schönlein purpura nephritis (30 to 50%), focal segmental glomerulosclerosis (20 to 40%), hemolytic-uremic syndrome (10 to 30%), membranous glomerulopathy (10%), anti-GBM disease (5 to 10%), Wegener's granulomatosis (less than 10%), and lupus nephritis (less than 5%). Recurrent glomerulonephritis most often occurs within the first 6 months post-transplant. Focal segmental glomerulosclerosis with the nephrotic syndrome has been reported to recur within the first 24 hours post-transplant. In these cases, the identification of a circulating "permeability factor" may predict that subset of patients likely to develop recurrent disease.

There may be morphologic evidence of recurrent disease that does not have functional significance. For example, recurrent IgA deposits may be seen by immunofluorescence microscopy in a transplant biopsy sample as an incidental finding, without mesangial hypercellularity or hematuria.

Some systemic metabolic diseases have also been reported to recur in the transplant. These include amyloidosis, diabetes, oxalosis, and Fabry's disease. As a rule, the recurrence of systemic diseases such as diabetes or amyloidosis takes several years. Diabetic nephropathy usually does not recur before 2 to 2.5 years post-transplant. Nonetheless, this time course is much shorter than the approximately 10-year time span required for development of diabetic glomerulosclerosis in the native kidney.

DE NOVO GLOMERULONEPHRITIS

A variety of glomerular diseases may occur de novo in the allograft. The clinical onset of de novo disease is often heralded by the appearance of proteinuria, the nephrotic syndrome, an active urinary sediment, or reduced renal function. As in the case of recurrent disease, it is unusual for de novo glomerular disease to cause graft failure.

The most common glomerular disease to occur de novo in the transplant is membranous glomerulopathy. The incidence of de novo membranous glomerulopathy in large biopsy series ranges from 2 to 5%, and it would likely be higher if immunofluorescence and electron microscopy were performed on all allograft biopsies. Spikes are not always identifiable, and subepithelial deposits tend to be small (membranous stage 1 to 2).

In some cases, linear IgG deposits can be detected in the transplant in patients without overt nephritis. Linear deposits of IgG may also occur in up to 15% of transplanted Alport's disease patients, but severe crescentic glomerulonephritis leading to graft failure rarely occurs.

The most common nonspecific, and probably nonpathogenic, glomerular histologic change is a focal segmental sclerotic lesion. This lesion has been identified in 10 to 20% of allografts, as a complication of ischemia, hypertension, chronic rejection, and cyclosporine toxicity. It is rarely associated with the nephrotic syndrome, allowing it to be differentiated from recurrent or de novo focal segmental glomerulosclerosis.

INFECTIONS

A variety of pathogens may infect the transplant kidney, including bacteria, viruses, fungi, and protozoa. The most common viral pathogen, cytomegalovirus, may produce the typical intranuclear and cytoplasmic inclusions in tubular epithelium, urothelium, interstitial capillary endothelium, or glomerular endothelium. Cytomegaloviral inclusions are a frequent incidental finding in a biopsy specimen with features of acute or chronic rejection. Multinucleation may be a feature of herpesvirus infection. Adenovirus infection typically produces nuclear "smudging." In some cases, viral infection can incite an inflammatory response that mimics acute cellular rejection. The detection of viral antigen by immunoperoxidase staining may help differentiate viral infection from acute rejection.

POST-TRANSPLANT LYMPHOPROLIFERATIVE DISEASE

Lymphoma, a rare complication in the transplant kidney, may be seen with the development of transplant-related lymphomas. Most of these cases are associated with Epstein-Barr virus (EBV)-induced transformation of B-lymphocytes, producing a spectrum of histopathologic and clinical lesions ranging from polymorphic B-cell hyperplasia to overt lymphoma. When these lymphomas affect the kidney, they can usually be differentiated from the infiltrates of rejection by their monomorphic appearance, enlarged pleomorphic nuclei, nucleoli, and reactivity with B-cell markers such as L-26 (which is reactive in formalin-fixed paraffin-embedded tissue). Post-transplant lymphomas rarely manifest a T-cell phenotype.

Post-transplant lymphoproliferative disease complicates approximately 1% of renal transplant patients, whereas it has been seen in 5% of cardiac transplant recipients. These differences in incidence may be related to the different levels of immunosuppression used in these two populations. Common presentations include an acute mononucleosis–like syndrome with fever and lymphadenopathy, as well as gastrointestinal and central nervous system involvement. As many as 25% of cases may be reversible with reduction of immunosuppression and antiviral agents; others may require additional chemotherapy or radiation therapy.

SELECTED READINGS

1. Brockmeyer C, Ulbrecht M, Schendel D, et al: Distribution of cell adhesion molecules (ICAM-1, VCAM-1, ELAM-1) in renal tissue during allograft rejection. Transplantation 55:610, 1993.
2. Cameron JS: Recurrent primary disease and de novo nephritis following renal transplantation. Pediatr Nephrol 5:412, 1991.
3. Colvin RB: Renal allograft pathology. *In* Colvin RB, Bhan AK, McCluskey RT (eds): Diagnostic Immunopathology. 2nd ed. New York, Raven Press, 1995, pp 329–365.
4. D'Agati V: Morphologic features of cyclosporin nephrotoxicity. Contrib Nephrol 114:84, 1995.
5. Kiss D, Landman J, Mihatsch M, et al: Risks and benefits of graft biopsy in renal transplantation under cyclosporin-A. Clin Nephrol 38:132, 1992.
6. Mihatsch MJ, Thield G, Ryffel B: Morphologic diagnosis of cyclosporin nephrotoxicity. Semin Diagn Pathol 5:104, 1988.
7. Noronha IL, Weis H, Hartley B, et al: Expression of cytokines, growth factors and their receptors in renal allograft biopsies. Transplant Proc 25:891, 1993.
8. Solez K, Axelsen RA, Benediktsson H, et al: International standardization of nomenclature and criteria for the histologic diagnosis of renal allograft rejection: The Banff working classification of kidney transplant pathology. Kidney Int 44:411, 1993.

12

RENAL LESIONS IN HYPERTENSION

The definition of hypertension established by the World Health Organization is the presence of blood pressure exceeding 160/95 mm Hg.

Hypertension affects approximately 40 million people in the United States. However, there are large variations among different ages and races. For instance, the incidence of hypertension in blacks is very high (33%). The differences between blacks and nonblacks become even more striking if one considers that the risk of developing end-stage hypertensive renal disease is 20-fold higher in blacks than whites in the 20- to 40-year-old population. The frequency with which hypertensive patients develop renal disease is unknown but is the subject of current investigation.

Finally, renal biopsies are not a standard part of the workup of a hypertensive patient, unless there is a suspicion of associated kidney lesions, such as glomerular abnormalities or acute tubulointerstitial lesions. The renal lesions in hypertension can be categorized as shown in Table 12–1.

No cause can be discerned in 95% of hypertensive patients, leading to the diagnosis of essential or idiopathic hypertension. This condition is generally associated with a slow, progressive loss of nephrons. In 1 to 7% of patients with benign hypertension, there is a sudden and unexplained progression to the malignant phase—i.e., a sudden and severe worsening of hypertension with a diastolic blood pressure of over 120 mm Hg. The syndrome also consists of papilledema, nausea/vomiting, and convulsions progressing to hypertensive encephalopathy. Renal function rapidly deteriorates, and renal failure may appear. This rapid evolution of hypertension and the renal damage it causes, so-called malignant nephrosclerosis, often produce a clinical picture of acute renal failure. The causes of secondary hypertension include other forms of renal disease, which are reviewed in other chapters.

BENIGN NEPHROSCLEROSIS

Benign hypertension, which is associated with the changes known as benign nephrosclerosis (also known as hypertensive nephropathy), is an insidious disease usually producing no symptoms. It usually begins before the age of 50 years and is more common in women than in men and in blacks. Several mechanisms are believed to play a part in the genesis of essential hypertension. These include modi-

Table 12–1. Causes of Renal Lesions in Hypertension

Cause	% of Total
Idiopathic	
Benign nephrosclerosis	90
Malignant nephrosclerosis	5
Known Cause	5
Renal artery stenosis	
Chronic renal disease	
Fibromuscular dysplasia	
Endocrinopathies	
Atheroembolic embolism	

fications of the renin-angiotensin system, an increase in blood volume, abnormalities in mineralocorticoids, and some type of dysregulation of the autonomic nervous system. Among the genetic factors that may play a role, some investigators have incriminated an insufficient number of nephrons at birth. Angiotensinogen polymorphism may favor hypertension in whites. The term *nephrosclerosis* is used to describe the renal pathologic alterations resulting from benign hypertension. These include lesions in the arcuate and interlobular arteries and afferent arterioles. Fibrinoid necrosis characterizes malignant hypertension and is not a part of the description of nephrosclerosis. Various degrees of glomerular and tubulointerstitial damage are associated with the vascular changes. The diagnosis of nephrosclerosis should be entertained only after other parenchymal renal diseases associated with hypertension have been excluded on the renal biopsy.

Patient Presentation

In the early stages of benign nephrosclerosis, there is no apparent reduction in renal function. Examination of the urinary sediment may reveal occasional hyaline and granular casts and, rarely, red blood cells. Small amounts of protein may be present in the urine. The earliest detectable abnormality of renal function is a decrease in the renal plasma flow. A reduction in the glomerular filtration rate occurs later. Progression of the renal injury eventually results in a slowly rising serum creatinine level. The presence of proteinuria, including the nephrotic syndrome, should cause one to entertain other diagnoses. As noted in Chapter 2, elevation of the serum creatinine level may not occur until the glomerular filtration rate has fallen to less than 50% of normal and is thus not a good screening tool to evaluate renal damage.

Histology

Light Microscopy

Many glomeruli are normal, especially those at a distance from the capsule. Some show ischemic changes characterized by collapse of peripheral capillary loops, a decrease in overall size, and thickening and multilamination

of the basement membrane of Bowman's capsule. These glomeruli are often smaller than normal. These changes tend to occur in linear sclerotic zones characterized by interstitial fibrosis and tubular atrophy. The glomeruli within the fibrotic areas appear to be clustered together because of the tubular atrophy. Periodic acid–Schiff (PAS) or silver stains demonstrate the "wrinkling" of the glomerular basement membranes, with apparent thickening and decrease in glomerular size (Figs. 12–1, 12–2). When this change is severe, the vascular spaces are decreased (Fig. 12–3). These changes are most evident near the mesangial regions and progressively involve the rest of the tuft. There is a progressive disappearance of nuclei as the tuft shrinks and becomes obsolescent. Bowman's space fills with extracellular matrix, best seen on trichrome stain. The degree of glomerulosclerosis correlates with the severity of generalized atherosclerosis and with increased intrarenal vascular disease. Depending on the age, or the etiology of the lesions, there may be hyperplasia of the juxtaglomerular apparatus, sometimes associated with connective tissue deposition.

Tubular atrophy characterized by atrophy of epithelial cells and wrinkled and thickened basement membranes occurs both near affected glomeruli (Fig. 12–4) and in areas near normal-appearing glomeruli. These data have

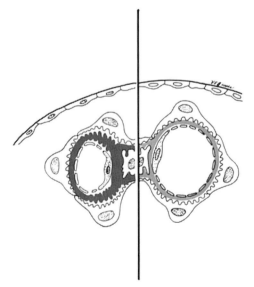

Figure 12–1. Benign nephrosclerosis. Diagram of an ischemic glomerulus. The major change is wrinkling and thickening of the glomerular basement membranes, particularly near the mesangium.

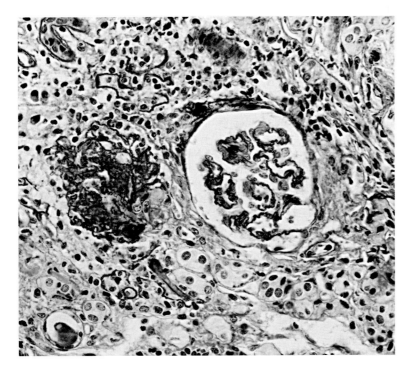

Figure 12–2. Benign nephrosclerosis. The basement membranes of the glomeruli are wrinkled. One is nearly obsolescent. The basement membrane of Bowman's capsule is thickened and multilaminated. (Periodic acid–silver methenamine [PASM], ×100.)

been taken as evidence that the tubules have an increased susceptibility to ischemia.

Interstitial fibrosis is present in a patchy distribution and is frequently accompanied by an inflammatory infiltrate composed of small lymphocytes. The fibrosis surrounds atrophic tubules, which often contain hyaline casts. The areas of atrophied tubules filled with casts resemble thyroid tissue, and the process has been known as pseudothyroid change. The zones of atrophy vary in size, depending on the number of nephrons supplied by the af-

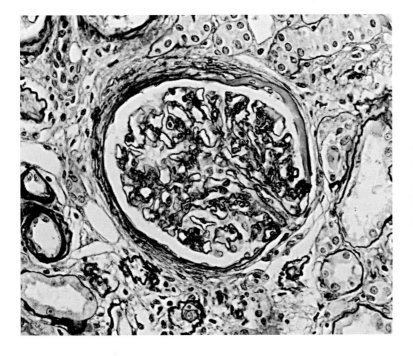

Figure 12–3. Benign nephrosclerosis. Ischemic glomerulus surrounded by a multilaminated Bowman's capsular basement membrane. The tubular basement membranes are thickened around the atrophic tubules. (Periodic acid–Schiff [PAS], ×200.)

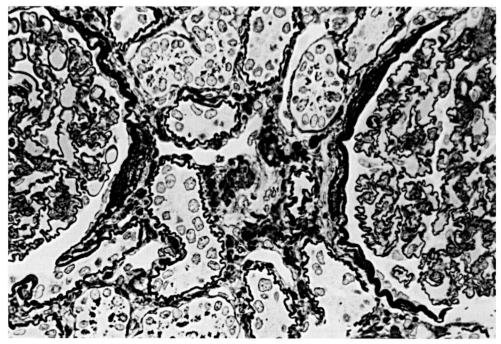

Figure 12–4. Benign nephrosclerosis. Areas of tubular atrophy and interstitial fibrosis *(center)* alternate with less affected zones. The tubular basement membranes are thickened around the atrophic tubules. (PASM, ×400.)

fected vessel, and alternate with areas of hypertrophied tubules. This irregularity in the distribution of tubulointerstitial lesions is characteristic of chronic ischemic lesions.

Abnormalities affect all of the vessels. The interlobular arteries show intimal thickening with consequent reduction of the lumina (Figs. 12–5, 12–6). The intimal thickening is frequently accompanied by multilayering (so-called reduplication) of the internal elastic lamina. Whereas the media may appear normal, there is often an increase in its thickness,

due to proliferation of the smooth muscle cells. The arterioles and small arteries develop arteriosclerosis, characterized by the accumulation of a homogeneous, eosinophilic hyaline material within the vessel wall, often associated with loss of smooth muscle cells (Fig. 12–7). The hyalin contains multiple plasma components, suggesting an abnormality in the permeability of the vascular wall, which may have resulted from damage. Hyalin arteriosclerosis also results in narrowing of the lumina.

Immunofluorescence Microscopy

The changes by immunofluorescence microscopy include staining of the hyalin deposits by C3 and very commonly IgM in the glomeruli and the arterioles. This pattern is nonspecific and may be seen in conditions associated with hyaline deposits and/or sclerosis. C1q often codistributes with C3.

Electron Microscopy

Electron microscopic examination confirms collapse of the capillary loops, with extensive wrinkling and thickening of glomerular basement membranes. The wrinkling is most marked near the mesangial regions, often giv-

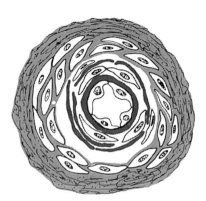

Figure 12–5. Arteriolosclerosis. Diagram of a small artery with multilayering of the internal elastic lamina and its associated connective tissue.

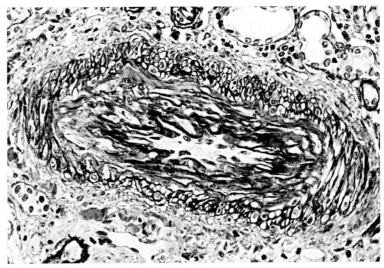

Figure 12–6. Arteriosclerosis. The multiple lamellae (duplication) in the subintima are visible in this silver-stained preparation. The endothelium is prominent. (PASM, ×300.)

ing the false impression of mesangial sclerosis. The glomerulus has a relatively hypocellular appearance.

Hyalin arteriolosclerosis is manifested by the appearance of homogeneous acellular material within the arterial wall, often replacing smooth muscle cells (Fig. 12–8).

Prognosis

The Framingham study has shown that both stroke and cardiovascular disease are more common in patients with hypertension. Recent studies indicate that treatment of patients with even very mild elevations of blood pressure

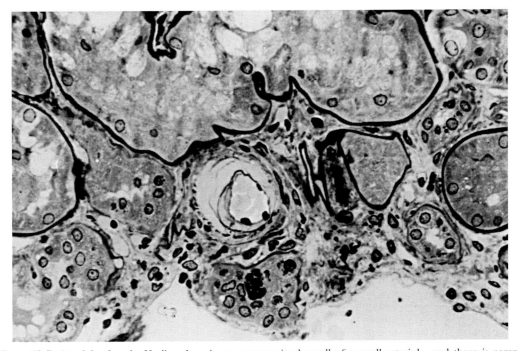

Figure 12–7. Arteriolosclerosis. Hyaline deposits are present in the wall of a small arteriole, and there is complete atrophy of the smooth muscle cells in the media. (PASM, ×400.)

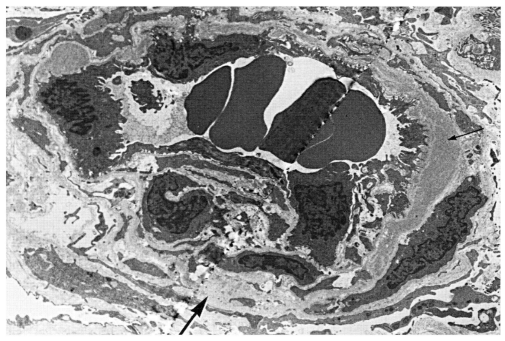

Figure 12–8. Arteriolosclerosis. The areas between the intima and the surrounding smooth muscle layer contain irregular, large deposits of hyalin *(arrows)*. The smooth muscle cells are absent in the regions of the hyalin deposits. (Electron micrograph, ×1000.)

results in decreased morbidity and mortality from stroke and cardiovascular diseases. A recent evaluation of a large study of patients with mild-to-moderate hypertension shows that hypertension is a risk factor for renal disease.

MALIGNANT NEPHROSCLEROSIS

Malignant hypertension most often occurs in patients who have a previous history of poorly controlled benign essential hypertension. This complication occurs in 1 to 7% of patients with essential hypertension. Malignant hypertension is defined as a diastolic blood pressure that is persistently greater than 120 mm Hg and eye changes consisting of papilledema with retinal hemorrhages and exudates. Males are affected more frequently than females, and the highest frequency is in blacks. Malignant nephrosclerosis may also be seen in various other diseases that affect the kidneys.

Few of these patients are subjected to renal biopsy, since the risks of bleeding are very high due to the hypertension and frequent association of coagulation abnormalities.

Patient Presentation

The presenting symptoms include headache, dizziness, weight loss, and difficulties with vision. The documentation of an extreme elevation of blood pressure, in combination with the typical funduscopic alterations, confirms the diagnosis. Examination of the urine reveals either gross or microscopic hematuria and proteinuria, which may attain nephrotic levels. The peripheral blood smear may contain the findings of microangiopathic hemolytic anemia, including fragmented red blood cells and a reduction in platelets. Renal function may appear to be normal at the onset, but it rapidly declines.

Histology

Light Microscopy

The changes of malignant nephrosclerosis are frequently superimposed on those of preexisting nephrosclerosis. A discussion of the latter changes is found in the preceding section.

The glomerular lesions are characterized by

ischemic alterations, hemorrhage, thrombosis, and fibrinoid necrosis. Some glomeruli are small, with wrinkled and thickened glomerular basement membranes and an apparent decrease in the number of cells, whereas others are unaffected (Fig. 12–9). The most striking alteration is segmental fibrinoid necrosis, affecting 5 to 20% of glomeruli. This lesion often predominates in the vicinity of the vascular pole and may be in continuity with a necrotic or thrombosed afferent arteriole. Necrosis, most easily identified using the PAS-methenamine silver stain, is recognized as a mass of fibrinoid material that has an intense pink color and is admixed with red blood cells. Destruction of the glomerular basement membrane as well as loss of definition of the glomerular architecture may also be present. Cellular crescents are sometimes observed, in association with areas of necrosis.

Rarely, small infarcts may occur as a result of arterial occlusion. Interstitial edema is commonly present.

The most characteristic vascular change is fibrinoid necrosis involving the small interlobular arteries and the arterioles (Fig. 12–10). As in the glomeruli, necrosis is recognized by the presence of a bright pink–staining, granular material within the wall of the vessel, the loss of nuclei, and thrombi in the lumina (Fig. 12–11). Fibrin may be detected by special stains. Fragmented red blood cells are often present in the thrombi. Arteries of all sizes show intimal narrowing of three distinct patterns. The first is the so-called onionskin change, which consists of concentric layers of proliferating intimal cells (Fig. 12–12). The second change, often referred to as mucinous degeneration in older texts, is characterized by the presence of a loose material in the intima that is stainable with Alcian blue (Fig. 12–13). There is an associated multilayering of basement membrane material in the subintimal space. The third, fibrous intimal thickening, is typical of the changes in benign nephrosclerosis, although the extent of luminal narrowing may be more severe in malignant hypertension. This consists of multiple layers of basement membrane and collagen, with considerable narrowing of the vascular lumina and the disappearance of smooth muscle cells in the media.

Immunofluorescence Microscopy

Large amounts of fibrinogen are always found in areas of fibrinoid necrosis in glomeruli and blood vessels.

Electron Microscopy

The glomeruli show severe wrinkling and thickening of glomerular basement membranes. In addition, there is subendothelial widening, often containing a granular or flocculent material. Fibrin tactoids may on occasion be found in this space. Loss of the normal architecture of the basement membranes and mesangial matrix may be seen in areas of large fibrin deposits. Platelets and fragmented red blood cells are frequently present. Endothelial cells show swelling and disruption and occa-

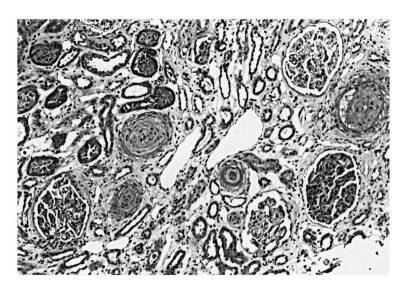

Figure 12–9. Malignant nephrosclerosis. The glomeruli are severely ischemic, with loss of the lumina. There is interstitial edema, tubular atrophy, and complete occlusion of blood vessels. (Masson's trichrome, ×80.)

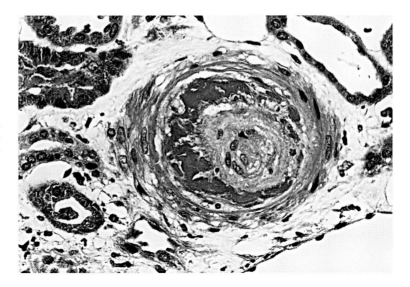

Figure 12–10. Malignant nephrosclerosis. The small arteriole is thrombosed, and there is necrosis of the wall near the thrombus. (Masson's trichrome, ×400.)

sionally may be atrophied. Epithelial cells manifest focal effacement but are otherwise unremarkable.

The vessels show endothelial swelling and multilamination of the basement membranes. The cells in the intimal onionskin lesions represent modified smooth muscle cells. The lucent areas contain extracellular matrix. The cells and the extracellular matrix of the media may be disrupted in the areas of fibrinoid necrosis.

Prognosis

Before the development of effective antihypertensive agents, 90% of patients with malignant hypertension died within 1 year after the diagnosis was established. The most common cause of death was acute renal failure. This grim outlook has dramatically changed, since pharmaceutical agents are now available to control the blood pressure in most patients. Patient survival at 5 years is now 90%, and

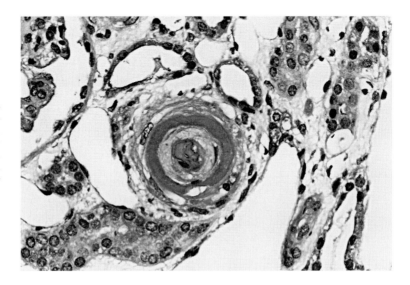

Figure 12–11. Malignant nephrosclerosis. This arteriole has a circumferential deposit of fibrin in the region of the smooth muscle layer. The intima is edematous, and the lumen is filled with a thrombus. (Hematoxylin and eosin [H&E], ×400.)

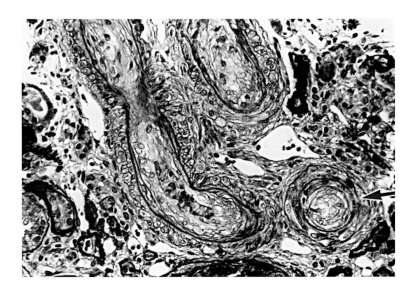

Figure 12–12. Malignant nephrosclerosis. There is onion-skin proliferation in one small arteriole *(arrow)*. The intima of the other two shows mucoid degeneration. (PAS, ×250.)

Figure 12–13. Malignant nephrosclerosis. Thrombosis and intimal proliferation of two interlobular arteries. In one the thrombus contains fibrin and cellular debris. (PAS, ×400.)

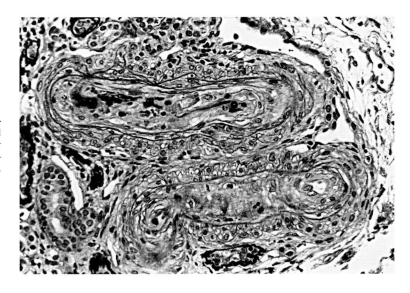

renal function remains adequate in 40% at this time.

RENAL ARTERY STENOSIS

Patient Presentation

An underlying cause of hypertension may be defined in 10% of patients. Certain features suggest a particular etiology. For instance, renal artery stenosis secondary to arteriosclerosis is the most common lesion in young white patients who develop the sudden onset of malignant hypertension or an unexpected acceleration of benign hypertension. Renal artery dysplasia is most common in young women.

Histology

Light Microscopy

The glomeruli distal to the stenotic vessel remain relatively well preserved, whereas the tubules are atrophic. As a result, the glomeruli appear to be closer together than normal. The contralateral kidney may show changes of benign or malignant hypertension, depending on the blood pressure and the state of its corresponding artery.

The blood vessels in the kidneys distal to the stenotic renal artery are likely to show minor changes, unless there had been pre-existing hypertension.

Prognosis

The course and prognosis depend on the nature of the lesion causing the hypertension, its response to treatment, and the amount and degree of renal disease induced by the hypertension.

RENAL ATHEROEMBOLIC DISEASE

Embolization of material from aortic atherosclerotic plaques can cause acute renal failure, if the embolization is massive. The more common presentation is a slowly progressive loss in renal function. Showers of plaque emboli may occur without a precipitating event but more commonly appear as a complication of an intra-arterial procedure such as angiography or vascular surgery. Coexistent hypertension is also a precipitating factor.

Patient Presentation

Atheromatous emboli to the kidneys occur most frequently in elderly patients and in-

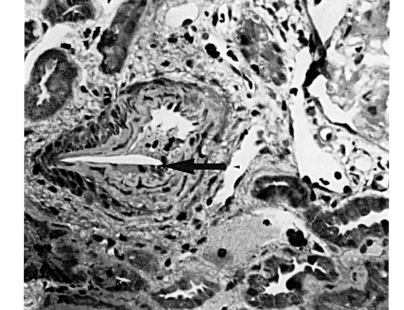

Figure 12–14. Atheroembolic disease. An elongated, pointed crystalline structure *(arrow)* and amorphous material surrounding it partially occlude the lumen of this small artery. (H&E, ×300.)

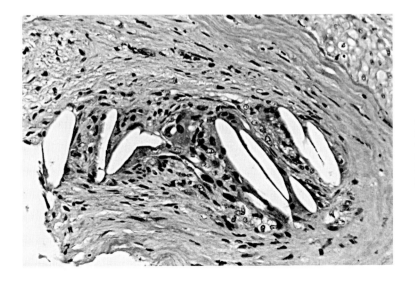

Figure 12–15. Atheroembolic disease. This large artery has a large mass of material occluding the lumen. The luminal material contains needle-shaped crystals surrounded by multinucleated cells and amorphous debris. (H&E, ×300.)

crease in incidence with age. This diagnosis should be entertained in any elderly patients with acute renal failure of unknown origin, especially in the presence of advanced atherosclerosis.

Renal involvement is signaled by the onset of acute renal failure, often accompanied by hypertension, which may be difficult to control. When this syndrome follows angiographic procedures, it is necessary to determine whether the renal lesion is due to contrast medium nephrotoxicity or embolization. In the former, renal failure occurs immediately and resolves within 2 weeks. However, renal failure associated with emboli may occur as late as 2 to 6 weeks after the embolic event.

The symptoms and signs may mimic a systemic illness such as vasculitis and hypocomplementemia may occur. Peripheral eosinophilia ranging between 6 and 18% may be noted.

Histology

Light Microscopy

Needle-shaped crystals, together with other amorphous eosinophilic material, may be seen in the thrombosed blood vessels (Fig. 12–14). At later times, the embolic material is incorporated into concentric layers of proliferating cells in the subendothelium. The crystals may be associated with giant cells, giving the appearance of a granuloma (Fig. 12–15).

These lesions have an irregular distribution. The emboli may lodge in the glomerulus. The most common glomerular change is ischemia with wrinkling and thickening of the glomerular basement membranes. Tubular, interstitial, and vascular changes reflect the pre-existing vascular disease. Those changes due to the embolic process vary from mild ischemia to foci of necrosis, depending on the severity of the vascular occlusion secondary to the embolization.

Prognosis

The course depends on the severity and distribution of the emboli. There is no effective therapy.

SELECTED READINGS

1. Genest J, Kuchel O, Hamet P, et al (eds): Hypertension. 2nd ed. New York, McGraw-Hill, 1983.
2. Heptinstall RH: Renal biopsies in hypertension. Br Heart J 16:133, 1954.
3. Hsu H, Churg J: The ultrastructure of mucoid "onionskin" intimal lesions in malignant nephrosclerosis. Am J Pathol 99:67, 1980.
4. Kincaid-Smith P, McMichael J, Murphy EA: The clinical course and pathology of hypertension with papilloedema (malignant hypertension). Q J Med 27:117, 1958.
5. Klag MJ, Whelton PK, Randall BL, et al: Blood pressure and end-stage renal disease in men. N Engl J Med 334:13, 1996.
6. McManus JFA, Lupton CH Jr: Ischemic obsolescence of renal glomeruli. The natural history of the lesions and their relation to hypertension. Lab Invest 9:413, 1960.
7. Nagle RB, Kohnen PW, Bulger RE, et al: Ultrastructure of human renal obsolescent glomeruli. Lab Invest 21:519, 1969.
8. Sommers SC, Relman AS, Smithwick RH: Histologic studies of kidney biopsy specimens from patients with hypertension. Am J Pathol 34:685, 1958.

13

TUBULAR AND INTERSTITIAL LESIONS

Conditions in which the initial injury is directed at the tubules are nearly always associated with changes in the interstitium because of their anatomic proximity and their functional interdependence. Similarly, interstitial changes lead to tubular changes. Nonetheless, one is often able to determine which of the two areas is the principal or initial site of involvement.

ACUTE TUBULAR NECROSIS

Acute tubular necrosis is a clinicopathologic syndrome characterized by the presence of acute renal failure clinically and histologic evidence of renal tubular cell injury. The renal failure may vary from mild, transient oliguria (or even isothenuric polyuria) to prolonged anuria. Similarly, cell injury varies from modest cell swelling to complete necrosis. This syndrome has also been called acute tubulointerstitial nephritis. Another name proposed for this syndrome is *ischemic acute tubular necrosis,* because this is the most common underlying cause. However, it seems more accurate and generic to retain the term *acute tubular necrosis,* which does not imply a specific or unique pathogenetic mechanism.

Acute tubular necrosis includes lesions that are primarily, or almost exclusively, restricted to the proximal tubules. The laboratory data and clinical history are so characteristic that renal biopsies are not often necessary to establish the diagnosis, except in very unusual cases. The utility of a renal biopsy in establishing the diagnosis is to rule out other causes of acute renal failure.

Pathogenesis

The pathogenesis of acute tubular necrosis is not understood. There are multiple causes, and both the initial injury and subsequent renal response determine the outcome. The causes of tubular necrosis are multiple (Table 13–1) and include ischemia due to hypovolemia, chemical toxins, drugs (especially antibiotics such as aminoglycosides), and the precipitation of toxic proteins in the tubules (i.e., myoglobin or hemoglobin).

Patient Presentation

Oliguria or anuria is the most common presenting finding. However, in the postsurgical period, nonoliguric renal failure with azotemia is the most common presentation.

Histology

Light Microscopy

The glomeruli appear normal, for the most part, although they may occasionally contain fibrin thrombi that occlude vascular loops. More commonly, however, they appear bloodless and often collapsed, resulting in an enlargement of Bowman's space. In these cases, the parietal epithelial cells are cuboidal in shape.

Table 13–1. Causes of Acute Tubular Necrosis

Ischemia

Shock/sepsis/burns
Rhabdomyolysis
Incompatible transfusion
Hepatorenal syndrome

Toxins

Heavy metals: Mercury
              Bismuth
              Gold
Paraquat
Ethylene glycol
Phosphorus

Drugs

Lithium
Sulfonamides
Antibiotics (polymyxins, kanamycin, cephalosporins,
    gentamicin, tobramycin, rifampicin)
Chemotherapeutic agents (cisplatin, streptozotocin,
    bleomycin, vinblastine)
Anesthetics (Fluothane, halothane)
Mushroom poisoning
Contrast medium
Hypertonic solutions
Carbon tetrachloride
Chelating agents

The most characteristic histologic finding is that the intersitial region is widened by edema (Fig. 13–1). There are few interstitial inflammatory cells, although occasional lymphocytes or plasma cells may be seen. In fact, the paucity of interstitial inflammatory cells, and their absence between tubular epithelial cells (so-called tubulitis), are the most useful features in the differentiation of lesions that are primarily tubular in origin from those that originate in the interstitium. Thus, when acute tubular necrosis is accompanied by a dense interstitial inflammatory infiltrate, either the lesion must be considered to be both interstitial and tubular in origin, or it is assumed that the initial lesion originated in the interstitium.

The tubules frequently show mild and focal lesions. In these cases there is often a complete absence of tubular cell necrosis or sloughing of cells into the lumen. Rather, the tubular epithelial cells may show mild injury consisting of dilation of the tubular lumen and thinning of the epithelial cell cytoplasm, so-called tubular simplification (Fig. 13–1). In most cases there are few casts, but cytoplasmic fragments may be visible in the lumina. When present, casts are most often seen in distal tubular segments and contain either hyalin or granular material. Pigmented or hemoglobin casts,

which have a granular appearance and a brown-orange color, are conspicuous only in patients with hemolysis or rhabdomyolysis. In patients with polyethylene glycol toxicity, calcium oxalate crystals are found in the tubular lumina and in the tubular epithelial cells. The presence of large casts, multilaminated casts, or casts with a surrounding cellular reaction should signal the presence of a dysproteinemia, especially multiple myeloma (see Chapter 9).

The brush border of the proximal tubules is always altered, being either completely or partially absent. This is best appreciated in periodic acid–Schiff (PAS)-stained sections. Fine cytoplasmic vacuolations are most marked in patients who have received infusions of *hypertonic solutions* (low-molecular-weight dextrans or mannitol). This histologic lesion is called osmotic nephropathy. This lesion is also seen following *radiocontrast administration* (Fig. 13–2). Occasional tubular cells may be sufficiently damaged to lead to sloughing, but true necrosis is rarely observed.

The term *lower nephron nephrosis* was formerly used to describe the distal tubule lesion in ischemia. This finding is often a terminal event, and it is almost always associated with lesions in other tubular segments. The term is no longer used to describe a tubular injury because nephrosis now carries the connotation of a glomerular change leading to proteinuria.

Normally the tubular basement membranes are continuous when examined by PAS or silver stains. However, in areas of severe epithelial cell injury with necrosis and karyorrhexis, the basement membranes may be disrupted or fragmented, a finding which signals that the repair process will be accompanied by fibrosis. Calcifications are often found several weeks or months following the acute injury.

The accumulation of leukocytes in the vasa recta of the medulla is a very common lesion at autopsy in patients with acute tubular necrosis. Since leukocytes are often restricted to the medulla, they are not commonly found in renal biopsies.

Whatever segment is involved, regeneration can be recognized by the presence of cells with hyperchromatic nuclei and basophilic cytoplasm. This may be the only feature present in biopsies performed more than 1 week after the acute injury.

The blood vessels are not affected, and changes therein reflect pre-existing lesions.

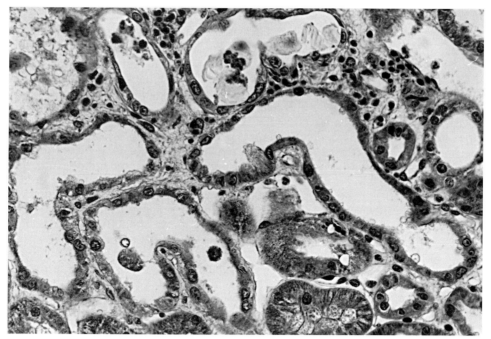

Figure 13–1. Acute tubular necrosis, ischemia. The tubular epithelium is "simplified," i.e., the lumina are dilated, the epithelium is low lying, and the brush borders of the proximal tubules are absent. A small number of casts and desquamated tubular epithelial cells are present. There is diffuse interstitial edema, containing a sparse mononuclear inflammatory cell infiltrate. Note the absence of inflammatory cell invasion of the tubular epithelium (so-called "tubulitis"). (Masson's trichrome, ×400.)

Immunofluorescence Microscopy

There are no deposits of immunoglobulins or complement. Fibrin-related antigens may be found in the peritubular regions, in the presence of capillary injury and/or passive congestion.

Electron Microscopy

The electron microscopic findings confirm the absence of glomerular lesions. Although the morphology of early tubular lesions could be of considerable interest, few detailed studies are available in humans.

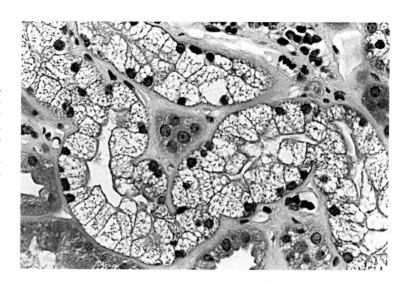

Figure 13–2. Acute tubular necrosis, radiocontrast media. The tubular epithelia are swollen, and the cytoplasm contains numerous fine, clear vacuoles. The brush borders of the proximal tubular cells are intact. There are very few inflammatory cells within the edematous interstitium. This is the so-called "osmotic nephrosis." (Hematoxylin and eosin [H&E], ×500.)

When present, the proximal and distal tubular changes consist of vacuolation and swelling of the cytoplasm and loss of the brush border microvilli. There is concomitant loss of the basal and lateral infoldings of the cell membranes. Myeloid bodies are occasionally present in the cytoplasm and probably represent modified lysosomes. They are most common in patients who have received aminoglycosides.

Regenerating tubular epithelial cells may also lack a brush border and the lateral interdigitations and may also have a small number of cytoplasmic organelles. The cytoplasm of regenerating cells is scanty, and the cell height is reduced, compared with normals.

Prognosis

The prognosis is nearly universally excellent if the condition(s) causing the renal injury is reversed within a short period of time. The acute renal changes almost always completely resolve without sequelae. The only exceptions appear to be those unusual instances in which the injury was of sufficient severity to result in dissolution of the tubular basement membranes and interstitial framework. These lesions heal with scarring and disruption of the architecture.

SELECTED READINGS

1. Olsen S, Solez K: Acute renal failure in man: Pathogenesis in light of new morphological data. Clin Nephrol 27:271, 1987.
2. Racusen LC, Fivush BA, Li YL, et al: Dissociation of tubular cell detachment and tubular cell death in clinical and experimental ''acute tubular necrosis.'' Lab Invest 64:546, 1991.
3. Solez K, Morel-Maroger L, Sraer JD: The morphology of ''acute tubular necrosis'' in man. Analysis of 57 renal biopsies and a comparison with animal models. Medicine (Baltimore) 58:362, 1979.
4. Wilson DM, Turner DR, Cameron JS, et al: Value of renal biopsy in acute intrinsic renal failure. Br Med J 2:459, 1976.

ACUTE INTERSTITIAL NEPHRITIS

Acute interstitial nephritis is a clinicopathologic entity defined by the presence of acute renal failure and infiltration of the cortical interstitium by inflammatory cells. The syndrome has multiple causes and diverse clinical manifestations (Table 13–2). The classic histologic finding, which differentiates this lesion from acute tubular necrosis, is the presence of a prominent inflammatory infiltrate and tubulitis in acute interstitial nephritis, and the absence of inflammatory cells in acute tubular necrosis.

The most common cause of the pathologic lesions was scarlet fever; thus, this nephritis virtually disappeared after the introduction of antibiotics. In fact, acute interstitial nephritis was considered to be a curiosity in 20th century medicine until the 1960s, when it emerged again as an important entity. The reasons for the reappearance of acute interstitial nephritis were fourfold.

First, several new classes of therapeutic agents with renal toxicity were introduced into general clinical use. The drugs that initially were most commonly associated with interstitial lesions were antibiotics of the penicillin group and nonsteroidal anti-inflammatory agents.

Second, the use of renal biopsy became widespread, revealing interstitial lesions that had previously been difficult to appreciate.

Third, a systemic syndrome consisting of uveitis and interstitial nephritis was recently recognized.

Finally, the group of hemorrhagic fevers initially called nephropathia endemica were discovered. The etiologic agent was quickly found to be the Hantaan virus, and, as evidenced by many subsequent cases documented in the current literature, this disease remains a significant cause of acute interstitial nephritis.

Table 13–2. Causes of Acute Interstitial Nephritis

Infections	Sepsis
	Streptococcal infections
	Leptospirosis
	Legionellosis
	Hantaan virus
	Other infections
Systemic Diseases	Sarcoidosis
	Sjögren syndrome
	Systemic lupus erythematosus
Drug Reactions	Antibiotics
	Nonsteroidal anti-inflammatory agents
	Others
Idiopathic	With immune deposits
	Without immune deposits
	With uveitis

Infectious Disease with Acute Interstitial Nephritis

Sepsis

Histology

LIGHT MICROSCOPY

It is not common to perform a renal biopsy in a patient suspected of having an acute infectious renal disease. The observation of a leukocytic interstitial infiltrate and leukocyte casts suggests the presence of an acute infectious interstitial nephritis.

IMMUNOFLUORESCENCE MICROSCOPY

Although few studies have been published, our experience and that of others is that immunoglobulins are not present in the kidneys. Small, scattered, granular deposits of C3 may be found in the mesangium and along the basement membranes of the tubules and Bowman's capsule.

Hantaan Virus or Hemorrhagic Fever or Muroid Virus Nephropathy

It is not clear whether this lesion should be considered to be an acute interstitial nephritis or acute tubular necrosis. Hemorrhagic fever with renal manifestations has been recognized in several countries. It was first described in Korea, but cases have been reported in North America, Belgium, France, Scotland, Scandinavia, and Eastern Europe. The disease consists of fever, loin pain, acute renal failure, and transient thrombocytopenia.

Pathogenesis

The infectious agents are RNA viruses, which have been grouped together under the heading of Hantaviruses. They belong to the Bunyaviridae family. Previously called muroid viruses, they are transmitted by exposure to rodent excreta.

Patient Presentation

The renal signs appear 4 to 10 days following the onset of fever and loin pain. The evidence of significant renal involvement is most often short lived. Few patients have other than a brief episode of oliguria, and few require hemodialysis. Proteinuria is seldom present in more than trace amounts; however, heavy transient proteinuria may be present.

Histology

LIGHT MICROSCOPY

The glomeruli and blood vessels are normal. There are interstitial edema and scattered inflammatory cells consisting of lymphocytes and plasmacytes. Neutrophils are uncommonly a part of this infiltrate. Foci of dilated tubules associated with flattened epithelial cells are present but are not a prominent feature.

Foci of medullary hemorrhage are the most conspicuous lesions. They are not associated with significant numbers of inflammatory cells.

Finally, we observed interstitial and glomerular deposits of Tamm-Horsfall protein in some cases in our series. This suggests that focal tubular disruption and obstruction, with reflux of tubular fluid, may be one of the mechanisms involved in the renal lesions.

Drug-Induced Acute Interstitial Nephritis

Drug-induced acute interstitial nephritis has become a common cause of acute renal failure. The mechanism is thought to be allergic, and the nephritis usually follows the use of the drug(s) in what is considered to be the usual therapeutic range. The categories of drugs that have most often been incriminated are beta-lactam antibiotics, antimicrobial agents, nonsteroidal anti-inflammatory agents, and diuretics (Table 13–3). Other drugs have also been postulated to be causal, although they represent a smaller number of cases.

Pathogenesis

The pathogenesis of acute lesions of the interstitium is complex, but many lesions are thought to be immunologically mediated. The frequency of lesions in this compartment has greatly increased with the introduction of a large number of new therapeutic agents, many of which have the potential for triggering an inflammatory reaction when concentrated by the renal tubules or are capable of inciting an allergic response. If the kidney is a major site of drug metabolism or excretion, the interstitium is often the site of the adverse reaction. Drugs in this category include antibiotics and

Table 13–3. Drug-Induced Acute Interstitial Nephritis

Antibiotics	Nonsteroidal Anti-inflammatory Agents	Other Drugs
Beta-lactam antibiotics	Fenprofen	Analgesics
Methicillin	Indomethacin	Paracetamol
Penicillin G	Diclofenac	Glafenin
Ampicillin	Piroxicam	Diuretics
Cephalothin	Phenylbutazone	Thiazides
Other antibiotics	Salicylazosulfapyridine	Triamterene
Rifampicin	5-Aminosalicylic acid	Furosemide
Ciprofloxacin		Anticonvulsive agents
Vancomycin		Diphenylhydantoin
Sulfonamides		Others
Co-trimoxazole		Phenindione
Acyclovir		Allopurinol
		Cimetidine
		Ranitidine
		Captopril
		Alpha-interferon

the nonsteroidal anti-inflammatory agents. A number of animal models support the concept of an immunologic cause. These include models in which antibodies to tubular basement membrane antigens induce an acute reaction, closely paralleling that in methicillin-induced acute interstitial nephritis. Cell-mediated immunity has also been considered to be a candidate mechanism, based on animal and human studies in which T-lymphocytes are part of the interstitial infiltrate. The concurrence of interstitial granulomas further strengthens the suspicion of a hypersensitivity reaction. Finally, some patients demonstrate a positive skin test to the antigen implicated in causing acute interstitial nephritis.

Patient Presentation

The presentation of drug-associated acute interstitial nephritis varies widely, depending on the underlying cause. The number and variety of drugs that have been implicated in acute interstitial nephritis are large. We have chosen to discuss and/or list only those that have been reported in a relatively large number of patients (Table 13–3). Some cases of drug-related acute interstitial nephritis are accompanied by fever, rash, and eosinophilia. These features suggest a drug hypersensitivity reaction. This symptomatic triad may be absent, particularly in hospitalized patients who may be receiving multiple therapeutic agents, some of which may mask the signs of hypersensitivity. Thus, the presence of acute interstitial

nephritis may be difficult to recognize, and even when suspected, the offending agent may be difficult to identify.

Regardless of the actual basis of the injury, many patients with acute interstitial nephritis present with nonoliguric renal failure. Macroscopic hematuria may precede the development of azotemia, but proteinuria is either very mild or absent. The presence of eosinophils in the urine, signaling a hypersensitivity reaction, is a helpful finding in making the diagnosis of drug-related acute interstitial nephritis.

General Histologic Features

In all drug-induced acute interstitial nephritis, the renal histology reveals edema of the interstitium, associated with infiltrates of mononuclear cells. Eosinophils may be seen in some cases, but they are far from constant and their number varies widely. Tubular lesions are patchy. In some instances there is only minimal tubular damage, with atrophy of the tubular epithelium within the regions where the cellular infiltrates are the most prominent. In others, the tubular lesions are more extensive, with marked tubular atrophy and dilation of the lumina, suggesting acute tubular necrosis. In the majority of the cases the glomeruli are unaffected. However, since many of these cases occur in older patients, there may be chronic vascular lesions and ischemic glomeruli, which are believed to antedate the AIN. Thus the diagnosis relies on a combination of histologic and clinical features. Finally, most patients receive a combination of drugs, which may render the identification of a single culprit more difficult.

Histology

Light Microscopy

As in other forms of acute interstitial nephritis, the glomeruli and blood vessels are normal, although they may be surrounded by an intense inflammatory infiltrate. The tubules may become atrophic.

The principal lesion in a toxic reaction to nonsteroidal anti-inflammatory drugs is an intense, often diffuse, inflammatory infiltrate. The nature of the infiltrate varies, but lymphocytes are always a major component. Several studies have shown that the lymphocytes are mainly T-cells. There is no general agreement about the frequency with which each subclass is represented. Neutrophils are uncommon components of the infiltrate. Eosinophils have been noted in a few cases. Therefore, the presence of eosinophils is indicative, but not diagnostic, of a hypersensitivity acute interstitial nephritis. Finally, the presence of granulomas is relatively rare except in penicillin-associated AIN, but it has been reported.

Antibiotic-Associated Acute Interstitial Nephritis

The beta-lactam antibiotics, penicillins, and cephalosporins are common causes of AIN.

Methicillin was the first antibiotic to be reported as a cause of acute interstitial nephritis. Since the first reports, this has been a well-documented and frequently reported association. White men appear to be more affected than women.

The dose of antibiotic is not excessive in most instances, but the duration of therapy is usually prolonged. General symptoms include rash, fever, and eosinophilia in approximately two thirds of the patients. Hematuria, macro- or microscopic, is constant and is often associated with eosinophiluria. Most patients exhibit nonoliguric renal failure.

Histology

Light Microscopy

The interstitial lesions following exposure to beta-lactam antibiotics sharply differ from those in nonsteroidal anti-inflammatory drug toxicity. The infiltrate is more diffuse and includes a larger proportion of plasma cells and lymphocytes; eosinophils are scattered throughout or are in large aggregates (Figs. 13–3, 13–4). Epithelioid cells and multinucleated cells are often present, and they may form granulomas (Fig. 13–5). Finally, there are often breaks in the tubular basement membranes, with infiltration of the tubular epithelial cell layer by inflammatory cells.

Immunofluorescence Microscopy

Few cases have immune reactants in renal tissue. Essentially the only findings are in those

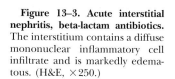

Figure 13–3. Acute interstitial nephritis, beta-lactam antibiotics. The interstitium contains a diffuse mononuclear inflammatory cell infiltrate and is markedly edematous. (H&E, ×250.)

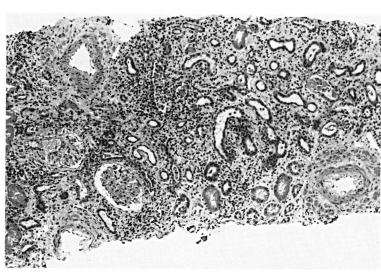

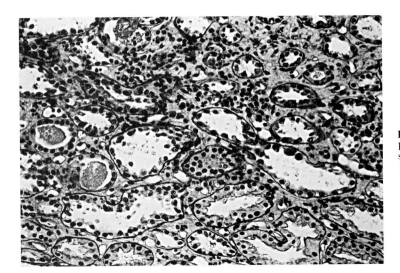

Figure 13–4. Acute interstitial nephritis, beta-lactam antibiotics. Lymphocytes are abundant in the interstitium. (Periodic acid–Schiff [PAS], ×400.)

patients with methicillin-induced acute interstitial nephritis in whom there may be antibodies against tubular basement membranes. In this instance there are linear, diffuse deposits of IgG along the tubular basement membranes (Fig. 13–6).

Electron Microscopy

There are seldom podocyte changes, but some reports mention the presence of elec-

tron-dense deposits along many tubular basement membranes.

Sulfonamide-Associated Acute Interstitial Nephritis

Sulfonamides may induce AIN. Combinations of drugs such as trimethoprim-sulfamethoxazole appear to favor the occurrence of AIN.

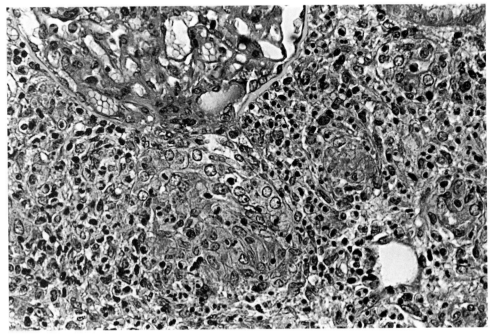

Figure 13–5. Acute interstitial nephritis, vancomycin. The interstitium contains numerous inflammatory cells, including eosinophils and granulomas. (H&E, ×400.)

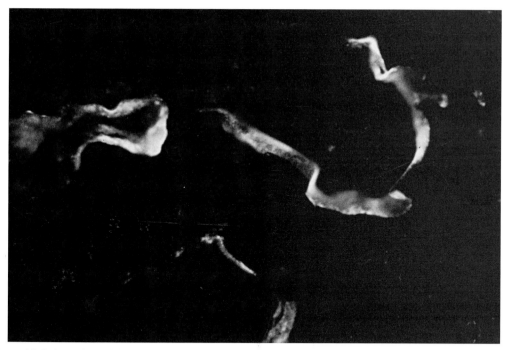

Figure 13–6. Acute interstitial nephritis, methicillin. Linear deposits of IgG are present along the tubular basement membranes. (Immunofluorescence micrograph, ×400.)

Another drug with renal toxicity is rifampicin. In most cases, the renal symptoms appear in patients having intermittent therapy; when therapy is resumed, these patients experience acute flank pain, hematuria, and acute renal failure, which may be oliguric.

Histologically, the infiltrate is often minimal, and many patients have a picture more suggestive of acute tubular necrosis than AIN. These cases emphasize that the histologic distinction is not always clear-cut.

Diuretics

Diuretics, including thiazides, chlorthalidone, furosemide, and ticrynafen, may all cause AIN, especially in patients with prior renal disease that may complicate the histologic analysis, since the underlying disease is associated with multiple acute interstitial infiltrates and acute tubular lesions.

Nonsteroidal Anti-Inflammatory Drugs

Nonsteroidal anti-inflammatory drugs (NSAIDs) have frequently been associated with acute interstitial nephritis. This complication is usually restricted to patients over the age of 50 years who are receiving the drug for prolonged periods (months or even years). Acute renal failure is progressive and usually is not accompanied by any symptom associated with hypersensitivity. It is to be remembered that the most common cause of renal failure due to NSAIDs is acute tubular necrosis. In some cases the acute interstitial nephritis is associated with a nephrotic syndrome. Hematuria is exceptional.

Histology

Light Microscopy

Some histologic features may help in differentiating lesions induced by nonsteroidal anti-inflammatory drugs from those caused by beta-lactam antibiotics. In the former, the interstitial inflammation is predominantly composed of small lymphocytes and occasional plasma cells, but eosinophils are absent or rare. Arteriolosclerosis and obsolescent glomeruli are commonly present in biopsy samples from these patients. In addition, the lesions by electron microscopy are quite different.

The principal lesion in a toxic reaction to nonsteroidal anti-inflammatory drugs is an in-

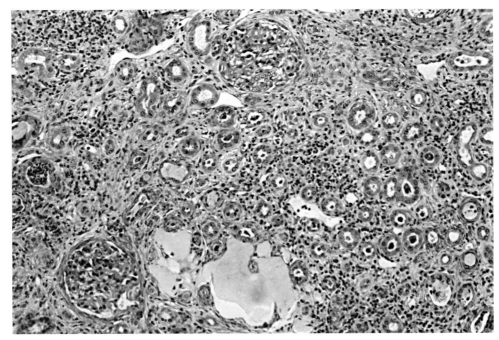

Figure 13–7. Acute interstitial nephritis, nonsteroidal anti-inflammatory drugs. There is massive interstitial cellular infiltration and edema, with tubular atrophy. Multiple tubules are destroyed. There are proteinaceous masses in the interstitium. (Masson's trichrome, ×100.)

tense, often diffuse, inflammatory infiltrate and tubulitis (i.e., infiltrating inflammatory cells in the epithelial cell layer) (Figs. 13–7, 13–8, 13–9). The nature of the infiltrate varies, but lymphocytes are always a major component. Several studies have shown that the lymphocytes are mainly T-cells. There is no general agreement about the frequency with which each subclass is represented. Neutrophils are uncommon components of the infiltrate. Eosinophils have been noted in a few cases. Therefore, the presence of eosinophils

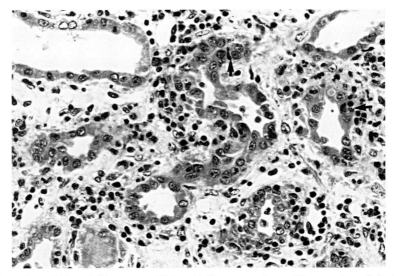

Figure 13–8. Acute interstitial nephritis, nonsteroidal anti-inflammatory drugs. Edema and a cellular infiltrate separate the tubules. There is also tubulitis *(arrow)*. (H&E, ×300.)

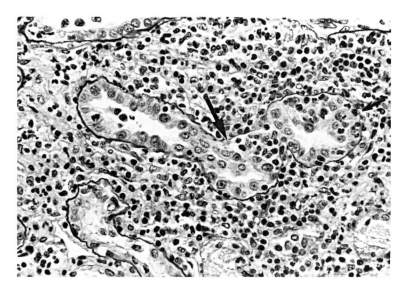

Figure 13–9. Acute interstitial nephritis, nonsteroidal anti-inflammatory drugs. The intense interstitial infiltrate and edema are associated with interrupted *(breaks)* tubular basement membranes *(arrows)*. There is also tubulitis. (PAS, ×400.)

is indicative, but not diagnostic, of a hypersensitivity acute interstitial nephritis. Occasional patients may have interstitial granulomas.

Electron Microscopy

The glomeruli in patients with lesions induced by nonsteroidal anti-inflammatory drugs often have spreading of the pedicels when they have proteinuria. They do not have deposits along the tubular basement membranes. These glomerular lesions stand in sharp contrast to those in patients with a hypersensitivity reaction to beta-lactam drugs.

Other Drugs

Many other drugs have been implicated as a cause of acute interstitial nephritis, including glafenin, an analgesic drug used in France, and the anticoagulant phenindione. It is to be expected that as the pharmacologic armamentarium expands, the list will change. Because renal lesions are one of the significant complications of drug therapy, it is important to be alert to the possibility of kidney involvement with the introduction of each new agent.

Granulomatous Interstitial Nephritis

We first described the occurrence of interstitial granulomas consisting of epithelioid cells and giant cells in two patients who had methicillin-induced acute interstitial nephritis (see

Fig. 13–5). Granulomatous lesions are also common in patients exposed to other beta-lactams. They have also been encountered in patients using sulfonamides, thiazides, phenindione, NSAIDs, and an analgesic widely used in France (glafenin). The granulomas may be small and sparsely distributed, but in some biopsy specimens they may occupy the major part of the renal interstitium. In the latter case, the granulomas may be confluent and resemble the histologic pattern seen in sarcoidosis.

Prognosis

If the cause of the renal lesion can be determined early in the course and removed from the patient's environment, the prognosis is generally excellent. If, however, the lesions at onset are severe or are not recognized, renal failure may ensue. In our experience, patients with a large number of interstitial granulomas seem to be particularly prone to develop progressive renal failure.

Interstitial Nephritis and Uveitis

Acute interstitial nephritis and uveitis was first described in 1975, and there are now many reported cases. Eighty-five per cent of the patients are young women. The presenting symptoms are an anterior uveitis, enlarged lymph nodes, and acute nonoliguric renal failure. The renal findings may precede the onset or discovery of the ocular abnormalities.

Histology

Light Microscopy

The interstitial lesions are diffuse and are characterized by a heterogeneous cellular infiltrate consisting of lymphocytes, plasma cells, and a large number of eosinophils (Fig. 13–10). Eosinophils, although considered to be characteristic of this syndrome, are present in only one half of the reported cases. When present, they are abundantly admixed with the mononuclear cells. Small foci of epithelioid cells with occasional multinucleated cells have also been described. They are restricted in size, and large granulomas have not been reported. The infiltrate is associated with prominent interstitial edema.

The tubular lesions (principally atrophy) parallel and appear to be secondary to the severity of the interstitial lesions (Fig. 13–10).

The glomeruli and blood vessels are unremarkable.

Immunofluorescence Microscopy

There are no deposits of immune reactants.

Interstitial Nephritis, Miscellaneous Causes

Sarcoidosis

The renal lesions in sarcoidosis are rarely of sufficient severity to cause acute renal failure.

Histology

LIGHT MICROSCOPY

The histologic lesions are characterized by interstitial infiltrates and the frequent presence of granulomas. The granulomas, surrounded by lymphocytes and plasma cells, are identical to those in patients with drug-induced acute interstitial nephritis (Figs. 13–11, 13–12). It has recently been shown by immunofluorescence microscopy that some cells of the granulomas possess angiotensin-converting enzyme. The significance of this observation is unknown.

Prognosis

The long-term prognosis appears to be excellent despite the residuum of interstitial fibrosis that persists after resolution of the interstitial infiltrate.

Interstitial Nephritis with Antineutrophilic Cytoplasmic Autoantibodies (Granulomatous Acute Interstitial Nephritis)

A new syndrome characterized by the presence of rapidly progressive renal failure associated with general symptoms of acute inflammation, acute interstitial nephritis, and antineutrophilic cytoplasmic autoantibodies (ANCA) has been recently identified. The fre-

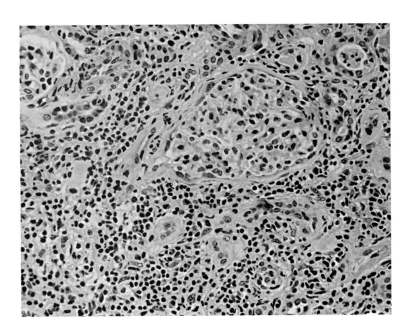

Figure 13–10. Acute interstitial nephritis and uveitis. There is a diffuse interstitial infiltrate, with considerable tubular atrophy. The glomeruli and blood vessels appear unaffected. (H&E, ×250.)

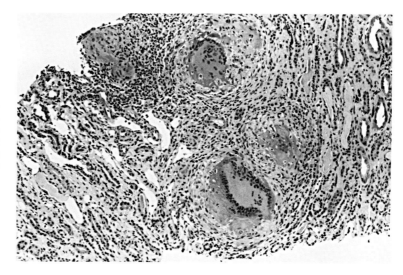

Figure 13–11. Interstitial nephritis, sarcoidosis. Multiple nodular granulomas, containing multinucleated giant cells, are present in the interstitium, which also has massive tubular atrophy and interstitial fibrosis. (H&E, ×125.)

quency of this syndrome is not known yet and awaits further studies.

In a few patients with rapidly progressive renal impairment associated with a clinical profile suggesting the presence of acute inflammation, including ANCA, we have found a renal biopsy picture of acute interstitial nephritis and no glomerular lesions. In three cases the lesions were characterized by extensive, intense inflammatory cell infiltrates in the interstitium, with sparing of the glomeruli. The inflammatory cells consisted of macrophages, epithelioid and multinucleated giant cells, and neutrophils. These often formed granulomas. It is important to recognize this syndrome, since it responds to specific immunosuppressive therapy.

Histology

Light Microscopy

In three of these cases, the lesions consisted of an extensive, intense inflammatory infiltrate consisting of macrophages, neutrophils, and multinucleated giant cells (Fig. 13–13). The latter were associated with the formation of numerous granulomatous nodules. It is interesting that there were no granulomas around the arteries or veins. The glomeruli did not show any lesions.

Prognosis

These patients respond dramatically to immunosuppressive therapy, similar to those with

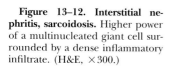

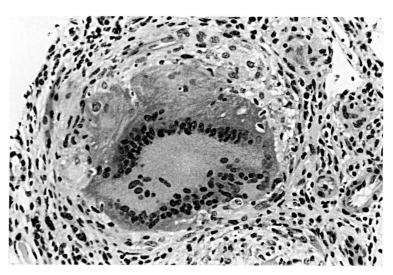

Figure 13–12. Interstitial nephritis, sarcoidosis. Higher power of a multinucleated giant cell surrounded by a dense inflammatory infiltrate. (H&E, ×300.)

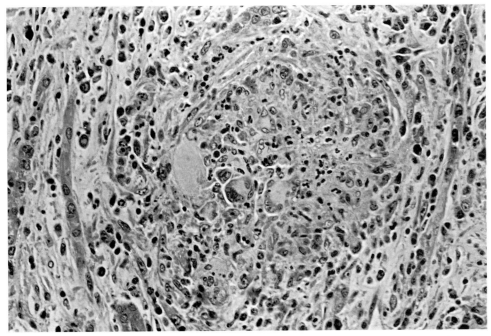

Figure 13–13. ANCA-positive granulomatous interstitial nephritis. There is a large interstitial granuloma containing neutrophils, monocytes, and giant cells. There is a surrounding, loose interstitial edema with inflammatory cells. (Masson's trichrome, ×300.)

ANCA-associated vasculitis and glomerular lesions. Therefore, it is important to recognize this histologic picture.

Megalocytic Interstitial Nephritis

Although megalocytic interstitial nephritis is a rare entity, the diagnosis is readily made by routine histologic techniques. Involved kidneys are seen to be enlarged, often irregularly, by imaging methods.

Histology

Light Microscopy

There are nodular or diffuse infiltrates consisting of large macrophages, which may contain cytoplasmic PAS-positive inclusions. The tubules are displaced by the interstitial infiltrates but do not appear to be a part of the primary process.

Electron Microscopy

The macrophage inclusions are seen to be lysosomes with crystalline electron-lucent structures.

Prognosis

It has been assumed that this disorder is a minor form of malakoplakia, differing only in the absence of Michaelis-Gutmann bodies. The prognosis is unknown, but in the few reported cases, it was found that if an underlying infectious process can be treated, the lesions may regress.

SELECTED READINGS

1. Andres GA, McCluskey RT: Tubular and interstitial renal disease due to immunologic mechanisms. Kidney Int 7:271, 1975.
2. Bender WL, Whelton A, Beschorner WE, et al: Interstitial nephritis, proteinuria, and renal failure caused by non-steroidal anti-inflammatory drugs. Immunologic characterization of the inflammatory infiltrate. Am J Med 76:1006, 1984.
3. Burnier M, Jaeger PM, Campiche M, et al: Idiopathic acute interstitial nephritis and uveitis in the adult. Report of one case and review of the literature. Am J Nephrol 6:312, 1986.
4. Buysen JG, Houthoff HJ, Krediet RT, Arisz L: Acute interstitial nephritis: A clinical and morphological study in 27 patients. Nephrol Dial Transplant 5:94, 1990.
5. Cameron S: Aspects immunologiques des nephrites tubulo-interstitielles primitives et secondaires. In Crosnier J, Funck-Brentano JL, Bach JF, Grunfeld JP (eds):

Acta Nephrol Hôpital Necker. Paris, Flammarion Medicine-Sciences, 1988, pp 223–261.

6. Cheng HF, Nolasco F, Cameron JS, et al: HLA-DR display by renal tubular epithelium and phenotype of infiltrate in interstitial nephritis. Nephrol Dial Transplant 4:205, 1989.

7. Colvin RB, Burton NE, Hyslop NE, et al: Penicillin-associated interstitial nephritis. Ann Intern Med 81:404, 1974.

8. Dobrin RS, Vernier RL, Fish AJ: Acute eosinophilic interstitial nephritis and renal failure with bone marrow–lymph node granulomas and anterior uveitis. A new syndrome. Am J Med 59:325, 1975.

9. Gerhardt RE, Loebl DH, Rao RN: Interstitial immunofluorescence in nephritis of Sjögren's syndrome. Clin Nephrol 10:201, 1978.

10. Kelly CJ, Roth D, Meyers CM: Immune recognition and response to the renal interstitium. Kidney Int 39:518, 1991.

11. Kikkawa Y, Sakurai M, Mano T, et al: Interstitial nephritis with concomitant uveitis. Report of two cases. Contrib Nephrol 4:1, 1977.

12. Kleinknecht D, Vanhille P, Morel-Maroger L, et al: Acute interstitial nephritis due to drug hypersensitivity: An up-to-date review with a report of 19 cases. Adv Nephrol 12:277, 1983.

13. Kourilsky O, Solez K, Morel-Maroger L, et al: The pathology of acute renal failure due to interstitial nephritis in man with comments on the role of interstitial inflammation and sex in gentamicin nephrotoxicity. Medicine (Baltimore) 61:258, 1982.

14. Kuncio GS, Neilson EG, Haverty T: Mechanisms of tubulointerstitial fibrosis. Kidney Int 39:550, 1991.

15. Lockwood CM: Antineutrophilic cytoplasmic autoantibodies: The nephrologist's perspective. Am J Kidney Dis 18:171, 1991.

16. Mignon F, Mery JP, Mougenot B, et al: Granulomatous interstitial nephritis. Adv Nephrol 13:219, 1984.

17. Neilson EG: Pathogenesis and therapy of interstitial nephritis. Kidney Int 35:1257, 1989.

18. Papadimitriou M: Hantavirus nephropathy. Kidney Int 48:887, 1995.

19. Ten RS, Torres VE, Milliner DS, et al: Acute interstitial nephritis: Immunologic and clinical aspects. Mayo Clin Proc 63:921, 1988.

20. Van Ypersele de Strihou C, van der Groen G, Desmyter J: Hantavirus nephropathy in Western Europe: Ubiquity of hemorrhagic fevers with renal syndrome. Adv Nephrol 15:143, 1986.

21. Wilson CB: Nephritogenic tubulointerstitial antigens. Kidney Int 39:550, 1991.

CHRONIC INTERSTITIAL NEPHRITIS

As described in earlier sections, chronic lesions affecting the tubulointerstitial compartment occur as a common consequence of many glomerular, tubular, and vascular diseases. The name *chronic interstitial diseases* should be reserved for those cases in which the lesions can be assumed to be primary in the interstitial compartment. The etiologic agents are multiple, and although some are historic curiosities, many new lesions have appeared during the past few decades as a result of the myriad new drugs and environmental toxins to which patients are exposed.

The most common cause of interstitial nephritis is the use of a therapeutic agent that has renal damage as an important side effect.

A less common cause, but nonetheless important, is the presence of a systemic disease that is immune mediated. We will describe the general characteristics of these diseases and try to identify the histologic features that are helpful in differentiating the various types of chronic interstitial nephritis.

Chronic interstitial nephritis can be classified according to the etiologic causes as follows:

1. Infection
2. Therapeutic agents and toxins
3. Metabolic
4. Systemic diseases (sarcoidosis and Sjögren's syndrome)
5. Unknown

This categorization encompasses most varieties of chronic interstitial nephritis encountered in a renal biopsy practice. We have deliberately excluded conditions that have only historic interest or are rarely subjected to renal biopsy (e.g., Balkan nephritis, tuberculosis, and syphilis).

The following descriptions consider only those findings that have general applicability to chronic interstitial nephritis. The specific etiologies will be considered after the general description, and features unique to a particular disease will be considered in the appropriate sections.

Histology

Light Microscopy

The glomeruli are usually unaffected in the early stages of this process, even in patients with severe interstitial fibrosis. The earliest glomerular lesion is thickening and multilamination of Bowman's capsule, detectable by PAS or silver stains. As the interstitial disease progresses, the glomeruli become progressively ischemic, as manifested by increasing wrinkling and thickening of the glomerular basement membranes. The glomerular vascular spaces shrink, and the glomerulus slowly becomes sclerotic. Bowman's space is initially enlarged because of the shrunken glomerular tuft, and it later fills with connective tissue. The resultant obsolescent glomerulus is small and shrunken but remains recognizable by PAS or silver stains, as an ischemic glomerulus. The mesangial spaces are not enlarged in these diseases, and cellularity is normal in the early stages, becoming progressively more hypocellular as the sclerosis proceeds. The glomeruli may appear much closer together than normal as the interstitium shrinks and tubules disappear.

The tubulointerstitial lesions are often patchy and irregular in distribution. For this reason, the renal biopsy material may not give an accurate assessment of the distribution of this lesion. The lesion is characterized by a combination of cell infiltrates and areas of fibrosis (Fig. 13–14). The nature of the infiltrate may provide insight into the pathogenesis of the disease. In the case of granulomatous infiltrates or eosinophils, for instance, a drug sensitivity reaction might be suspected.

Periglomerular fibrosis and Bowman's capsule thickening may be the earliest signs of interstitial damage. The accumulation of interstitial extracellular matrix (fibrous connective tissue) along the tubular basement membranes is a conspicuous finding in all these diseases, regardless of the underlying etiology. It is accompanied by atrophy of the adjacent tubular epithelium.

Casts are often present in the neighboring tubules and should be carefully examined, as their appearance and composition may be of use in determining the etiology of the lesions.

For instance, plasma cell dyscrasias are associated with characteristic Bence Jones casts (see Chapter 9).

Tubular atrophy accompanies the zones of interstitial fibrosis. The tubules entrapped within these areas are small in diameter and casts fill their lumina, resulting in the histologic appearance reminiscent of the thyroid—thus the use of the descriptor "thyroidization."

The areas of interstitial fibrosis and tubular atrophy often alternate with zones where there is compensatory hypertrophy of both the tubules and glomeruli. The tubular cells are hypertrophied, and the overall tubule diameter is increased. Similarly, the individual glomerular cells are hypertrophied. These tubular and glomerular changes are the histologic markers of compensatory hypertrophy due to partial nephron loss. They are much more frequently seen in biopsies of children and young adults than in patients older then 50 years.

The blood vessels may show chronic changes consisting of medial hypertrophy, duplication of the elastic laminae, and arteriolar sclerosis. These changes parallel those of the interstitium.

Immunofluorescence Microscopy

For the most part, there are no immune reactants in biopsy specimens of the chronic tubulointerstitial diseases, except for those associated with some of the systemic immune-mediated diseases. Immunoglobulins or complement components are restricted to the scle-

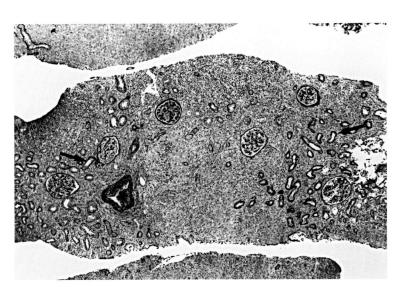

Figure 13–14. Chronic interstitial nephritis. Large areas of the interstitium are densely but irregularly fibrotic. The tubules are quite atrophic in the fibrotic areas. Some are dilated and contain casts, others are very small with thickened basement membranes *(arrows)*. The glomeruli appear normal. (Periodic acid–silver methenamine [PASM], ×50.)

rotic zones and are in the amounts typical of this phenomenon in other conditions. Namely, there are small amounts of IgM and C3 within the sclerotic areas, particularly within glomeruli. Such deposits are considered to represent nonspecific trapping.

Electron Microscopy

The nature of the cellular infiltrate may be best appreciated by electron microscopy, but otherwise there is nothing further to be learned by this technique over light microscopy.

Specific Conditions

Bacterial Infections

Chronic bacterial infections are often associated with urinary tract obstruction and infection. A chronic inflammatory reaction is almost always present, and the infiltrate is composed of lymphocytes and plasma cells. Lymphoid follicles may occasionally be seen in the cortex.

Miscellaneous

Other forms of chronic interstitial nephritis are rare in practice and therefore they are uncommonly a renal biopsy diagnostic entity. They include the following:

Malakoplakia. This condition, most frequently observed in patients with long-lasting urinary tract infections, is characterized by the presence of an intense interstitial infiltrate principally consisting of large macrophages. Occasionally there is giant cell formation. The cytoplasm of the macrophages is expanded by large lysosomes, some of which contain PAS-positive crystalline inclusions that are also silver positive. They have been given the name Michaelis-Gutmann bodies and are found in no other renal condition. The particles have a unique ultrastructure consisting of lysosomes that contain structures composed of a crystalline core surrounded by a multilaminated structure.

Tuberculosis and Histoplasmosis. These infections are very rare in the Western world and are not usually the subject of a biopsy. However, they should be considered in patients with granulomatous cortical lesions, especially if they are immunocompromised (Fig. 13–15).

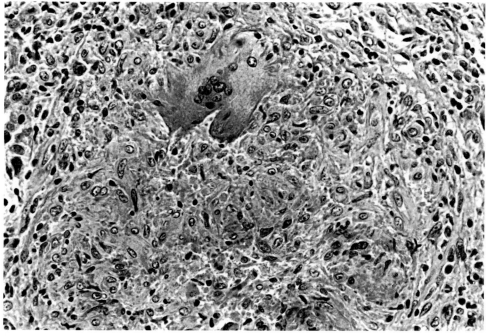

Figure 13–15. Chronic interstitial nephritis, tuberculosis. A well-formed interstitial granuloma is present, containing a multinucleated giant cell. The tubules and interstitium are severely disrupted. (Masson's trichrome, ×300.)

Drugs and Toxins

Analgesics

The prolonged, heavy use of analgesic compounds, especially if they contain phenacetin, results in chronic tubulointerstitial nephritis. It has been estimated that the patient must ingest more than 5 kg of these compounds before the lesions become manifest. Such consumption obviously requires several years to realize, and the lesions are thus chronic, cumulative, and difficult to detect because of the insidious nature of the process. One of the consequences of this abuse is the occurrence of papillary necrosis, a diagnosis that is rarely achieved by renal biopsy. However, the cortex develops irregular areas of interstitial lesions. There is prominent tubular atrophy and interstitial fibrosis (Figs. 13–16, 13–17). The atrophied tubules are filled with hyaline casts, and the epithelial cells contain lipofuscin pigment in their lysosomes. There is often a modest mononuclear interstitial infiltrate.

A recent report has linked the chronic abuse of acetaminophen to chronic renal disease, but the histologic lesions have not been described. This association awaits independent confirmation.

Lithium

The existence of a renal lesion following chronic lithium ingestion is not established beyond doubt. However, some patients who have no other obvious cause of chronic interstitial disease have a history of chronic lithium ingestion. The fact that acute tubular injury may follow acute lithium toxicity lends credence to the supposition that chronic ingestion of lithium in low doses might be a cause of chronic interstitial disease. The lesions consist of patchy zones of fibrosis and tubular atrophy. The occurrence of multiple cortical microcysts has been described in as many as 40% of the cases.

Heavy Metals

Lead. Chronic exposure to heavy metals usually occurs at the workplace; this is especially true for lead. The only histologic marker of chronic lead intoxication is sparsely scattered nuclear inclusions in tubules. The inclusions may mimic viral inclusions and are best seen in hematoxylin and eosin (H&E) sections. By electron microscopy, the inclusions appear as dense, often multiple, intranuclear masses.

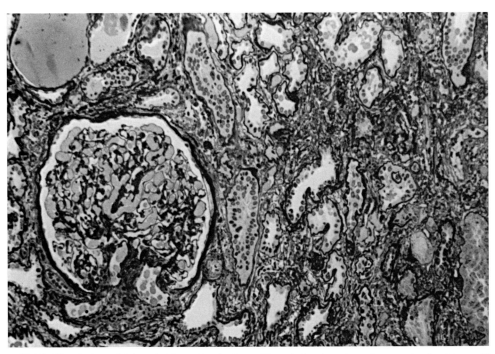

Figure 13–16. Chronic interstitial nephritis, analgesic abuse. The tubules show irregular atrophy, low-lying epithelium, and thickened basement membranes. The interstitium is increased in amount, in an irregular fashion. The glomerulus is relatively normal. (PASM, ×250.)

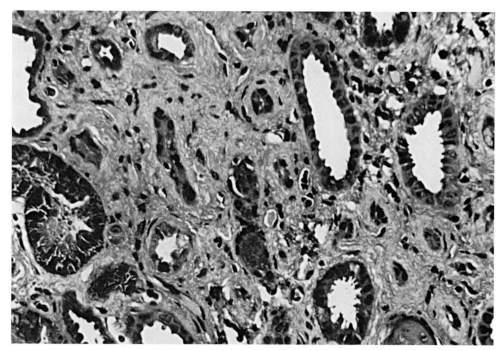

Figure 13–17. Chronic interstitial nephritis, analgesic abuse, late lesion. The interstitium is diffusely fibrotic, and the surrounding tubules are atrophic. (H&E, ×300.)

They may appear to be bounded by a single layered membrane.

Cadmium. Cadmium is a known nephrotoxin, and a tubular lesion has been produced in experimental animals. Little information is available about renal effects in humans.

Cyclosporine

Renal lesions due to cyclosporine are reviewed in Chapter 11. The use of cyclosporine in conditions other than renal transplantation has led to the clear demonstration that it can cause chronic tubulointerstitial and vascular disease.

Antineoplastic Agents

Many antineoplastic agents are thought to cause tubular and interstitial toxicity. The lesions are often acute, but they may also be chronic. The list of offending agents includes *cis*-platinum, nitrosoureas (methyl CCNU, streptozotocin), and mithramycin. The renal lesions have most frequently been observed as postmortem findings, and the diagnosis has therefore been retrospective. In general, these agents cause acute, severe tubular injury, followed by progressive interstitial fibrosis. Be-

cause most patients receive a combination of chemotherapeutic agents and are often infected with unusual organisms, it may be difficult to determine the exact agent that caused the chronic renal lesion.

Balkan Nephropathy

This is a chronic interstitial nephropathy that is endemic in certain valleys in the Balkan states. Both kidneys have diffuse cortical interstitial fibrosis. The lesions progress to end-stage renal failure within a few years. The etiology is unknown, although toxins are suspected since family members who locate in other geographic regions do not have this lesion.

Chinese Herbs

The presence of a rapidly progressive interstitial nephritis following the use of a Chinese herb was first reported in Belgium. This lesion affected young women taking medications thought to promote weight loss. The toxin is not identified, but it could be aristocholic acid, an agent also incriminated in Balkan nephropathy.

Patient Presentation

Four to eighteen months following treatment, these young women presented with rapidly progressive renal failure, bilateral cortical atrophy, and no hypertension. The course to end-stage renal disease is 1 to 2 years.

Histology

LIGHT MICROSCOPY

The lesions predominantly affect the cortex. There is severe interstitial fibrosis, containing a small number of inflammatory cells. Diffuse tubular atrophy with thickened tubular basement membranes is associated with relatively spared glomeruli. Bowman's capsular basement membrane is multilaminated. The blood vessels show lesions characteristic of cortical atrophy, i.e., increased extracellular matrix and reduced diameters.

IMMUNOFLUORESCENCE MICROSCOPY

No deposits are present.

Metabolic Disturbances

Several types of metabolic disturbances are associated with chronic tubulointerstitial damage. Although they are seldom the subject of renal biopsy, they are mentioned here because they may be missed unless special stains are used in their detection.

Hypercalcemia

Calcium deposits may be found along the tubular basement membranes, the basement membrane of Bowman's capsule, and the basement membranes of the arteriolar wall smooth muscle cells. They also occur in the tubular epithelial cell cytoplasm and in the lumina of the tubules. When present in the interstitium, they are surrounded by an inflammatory cell reaction that may include macrophages. Calcium deposits are recognized by von Kossa's stain and by polarizing microscopy.

Urates

Urates are highly soluble in water, so the tissue must be processed in absolute alcohol, including the fixation steps. The crystals have a characteristic elongated, rectangular shape and are present in the interstitium. They are often surrounded by inflammatory cells and macrophages, forming small granulomas known as tophi. Many of these inflammatory foci are found in the medulla.

Oxalosis

These deposits are found either in patients with a hereditary primary enzyme deficiency or in those who have been exposed to certain toxins, such as polyethylene glycol. Oxalates are also soluble, and special care must be taken in the fixation and processing of tissues to ensure their preservation. The crystals have a characteristic rhomboid shape, often arranged in rosettes, and may be admixed with calcium precipitates.

Cystinosis

See Chapter 8.

Hypokalemia

Prolonged, severe hypokalemia results in proximal tubular cytoplasmic lesions consisting of vacuolation and swelling of tubular epithelial cells and interstitial fibrosis. The vacuoles are larger than those present after exposure to hyperosmotic solutions. The interstitial fibrosis is not associated with an interstitial infiltrate and is often of modest degree.

Granulomas, Including Sarcoidosis

Granulomatous lesions in the interstitium may be observed in patients with chronic tubulointerstitial disease. Although they are uncommon, their discovery may provide important diagnostic information. We reported on 13 patients with this finding in 1983. At that time, we noted that the granulomas contained macrophages and occasional multinucleated giant cells. They were surrounded by large infiltrates of lymphocytes. Several categories of diseases were found in association with the interstitial granulomas.

Sarcoidosis

The granulomas in patients with sarcoidosis may sometimes be differentiated from those due to other causes if the multinucleated giant cells contain asteroid bodies as cytoplasmic inclusions. It has recently been reported that cells in the infiltrate stain positively when tested with an antibody to angiotensin-converting enzyme. Finally, the patients are often hypercalcemic, and calcium deposits may accumulate in the interstitium.

Granulomatous Interstitial Disease

Granulomatous interstitial disease is an idiopathic entity, but before the diagnosis can be made, other causes of interstitial granulomas must be thoroughly investigated. These include tuberculosis, drug hypersensitivity, and vasculitis.

Systemic Diseases, Including Sjögren's Disease

The interstitium is affected in many of the systemic diseases. However, only in Sjögren's disease do the interstitial lesions constitute the principal renal manifestation. Approximately 20% of patients with this syndrome develop chronic tubulointerstitial disease. It is often recognized because of the appearance of acidosis.

Histology

LIGHT MICROSCOPY

The glomeruli are normal in most instances. There have been some reports of mild mesangial hypercellularity, but this is by no means a common finding.

The interstitium contains a homogeneous, monotonous infiltrate and may be mistaken for a lymphoid malignancy (Fig. 13–18). The composition of the infiltrate is almost solely small lymphocytes, with occasional plasma cells and a rare neutrophil. There is seldom significant interstitial fibrosis. The infiltrate may displace the tubules, and those present in the areas of dense infiltrate have flattened epithelium and thickened basement membranes. There are few casts within the tubules.

IMMUNOFLUORESCENCE MICROSCOPY

The glomeruli are usually negative. It is common to find granular deposits of IgG and complement components in a coarse pattern along the tubular basement membranes and occasionally along the intertubular capillary basement membranes (Fig. 13–19). IgG may be present in the nuclei in a lightly speckled pattern. This finding of uncertain significance is shared by some of these patients and some of those with systemic lupus erythematosus.

Idiopathic

A group of patients with chronic interstitial nephritis have no recognizable etiology or associated disease. These are exasperating cases not only because one is unable to establish an etiology, but also because one is obligated to consider the multiple known causes of chronic tubulointerstitial disease.

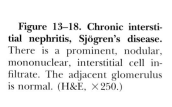
Figure 13–18. Chronic interstitial nephritis, Sjögren's disease. There is a prominent, nodular, mononuclear, interstitial cell infiltrate. The adjacent glomerulus is normal. (H&E, ×250.)

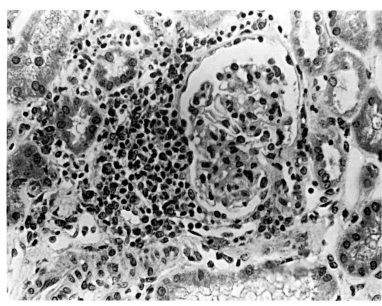

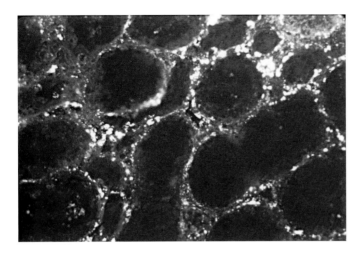

Figure 13–19. Chronic interstitial nephritis. Sjögren's disease. There are granular IgG deposits along the tubular basement membranes. (Immunofluorescence micrograph, ×400.)

It must be emphasized that any advanced renal disease may be associated with interstitial scarring. In these instances, there is often a sparsely scattered infiltrate of lymphocytes. This histologic picture is not the consequence of a primary interstitial disease process, and it is therefore not accurate to label it as chronic interstitial nephritis.

Histology

LIGHT MICROSCOPY

The lesions consist of a chronic interstitial nephritis without distinguishing features.

IMMUNOFLUORESCENCE MICROSCOPY

Linear or granular deposits of immune reactants may provide an indication of an immune pathogenesis, but for the most part these studies are negative.

Prognosis

The clinical course of chronic interstitial nephritis is characterized by the slow deterioration of renal function, which parallels the amount of tubular loss. Histologically, the increase in interstitial connective tissue is associated with a thickening of the tubular basement membranes and atrophy of epithelium. The accentuation of the multilamination of the Bowman's capsule, which is characteristic of the disease, also progresses. Chronic vascular lesions lead to ischemic obsolescence of glomerular tufts and tubular atrophy. In late lesions, the remaining glomeruli are closely approximated due to the advanced tubular atrophy.

The rate of progression varies with the extension of the lesions and with the nature of the etiologic factors. The progression may be considerably delayed or prevented if the cause of the disease can be identified and removed. The best examples are analgesic agents and infectious diseases. It is currently thought that these disorders progress at a slower rate than glomerular diseases.

SELECTED READINGS

1. Depierreux M, Van Damme B, Vanden Houte K, Vanherweghem JL: Pathologic aspects of a newly described nephropathy related to the prolonged use of chinese herbs. Am J Kidney Dis 24:172, 1994.
2. Dobynan DC, Truong LD, Eknoyan G: Renal malacoplakia reappraised. Am J Kidney Dis 22:243, 1993.
3. Hannedouche T, Grateau G, Noel LH, et al: Renal granulomatous sarcoidosis. Report of six cases. Nephrol Dial Transplant 5:18, 1990.
4. Marcussen N: Atubular glomeruli in cisplatin-induced nephropathy. An experimental stereological investigation. APMIS 98:1087, 1990.
5. Mignon F, Mery JP, Mougenot B, et al: Granulomatous interstitial nephritis. Adv Nephrol 13:219, 1984.
6. Pirani C, Valeri A, D'Agati V, et al: Renal toxicity of nonsteroidal anti-inflammatory drugs. Contrib Nephrol 55:159, 1987.
7. Spondlin M, Moch H, Brunner F, et al: Karyomegalic interstitial nephritis: Further support for a distinct entity and evidence for a genetic defect. Am J Kidney Dis 25:242, 1995.
8. Szabolcs MJ, Seigle R, Shanske S, et al: Mitochondrial DNA deletion: A cause of chronic tubulointerstitial nephropathy. Kidney Int 45:1388, 1994.
9. Vanherweghem JL, Depierreux M, Tielemans C, et al: Rapidly progressive interstitial renal fibrosis in young women: Association with a slimming regimen including Chinese herbs. Lancet 341:387, 1993.

Index

Note: Page numbers in *italics* refer to illustrations; page numbers followed by t refer to tables.

ISBN 0-7216-6412-1